When Your Child Is Ill

SAMUEL KARELITZ, M.D.

When
Your Child Is Ill

A Guide to Infectious Diseases

in Childhood

COMPLETELY REVISED

WITH THE LATEST MEDICAL DEVELOPMENTS

Random House · *New York*

I acknowledge with gratitude the great
help of Mrs. Bess Brand and Mrs. Bess Schaul
in the preparation of the manuscript.
Mrs. Nan Talese, my editor, was most helpful
in the preparation of this book.

To my wife, Ethel, my most ardent supporter

Preface

The many difficulties encountered in writing a manual on children are well known to me, as I have written a book on child care with Dr. William Rosenson. There already exist several very popular books on this subject. If, therefore, a very well-known pediatrician has an urge to write a volume on childhood diseases, he must have a particularly deep interest in the subject and a feeling that he can approach it from an original point of view. And this has been accomplished in this outstanding book by Dr. Samuel Karelitz.

In his very large pediatric practice, Dr. Karelitz has had daily opportunity to learn of the many problems that worry mothers in the care of their sick children. His thought was not to tell mothers how to treat their children but rather to tell them what symptoms to look for and what signs constitute danger signals so that nothing of importance is missed. When a mother understands these things, she will consult the pediatrician at the earliest possible moment.

Furthermore, Dr. Karelitz feels that the mother can derive a general understanding of childhood diseases by reading the book and become conversant with the daily problems of caring for her children. The result will be that she will ask the pediatrician more pertinent questions and will better comprehend his answers. There is always the difficulty of knowing how far to go in giving mothers instructions, lest they believe they can replace the family doctor. Dr. Karelitz has solved this difficulty extremely well.

If you will read, for example, the chapter on poliomyelitis or the one on colds, you will understand what I mean. Parents want to know the essential facts, the important symptoms, the methods of treatment and prevention of diseases. Having this knowledge and the realization of the dangers, they will more eagerly and more intelligently carry out the orders of the family physician, who will also benefit when attempting to answer satisfactorily points puzzling the mother.

In a similar way this book will be helpful to nurses in their discussions with parents concerning the phases and symptoms during the course of a particular disease, both before the family physician arrives and particularly after he has left the home. In her excitement, the mother often forgets many of the questions she wanted to ask her physician. We doctors know how important it is to treat not only the child but also the parents.

I enjoyed very much reading many chapters of this book. Therefore, I know how much satisfaction parents, nurses, interns, resident and family physicians will derive from a study of it.

I wish to congratulate Dr. Karelitz on his having written so intelligently a book for intelligent readers.

BELA SCHICK, M.D.

Contents

Part Two: Common Childhood Diseases

Introduction

More than twelve years ago I wrote a book, *When Your Child Is Ill,* which described most of the common and some of the less frequent infections of childhood and indicated how to recognize them and what to do about them until the doctor comes.

My friends thought that the book would be current for a few decades on the knowledge of infectious diseases. Neither they nor I anticipated the tremendous progress in identification, treatment and, most important, the prevention of many of our most common serious infections.

I had anticipated the discovery of vaccine against polio and measles since Professor John Enders had already successfully isolated the viruses and learned how to culture them. Today, polio is a very rare disease in the United States. From an average annual thirty-six-thousand-plus cases with some five per cent deaths and many more severely handicapped by paralyses of various degrees, we now have less than a hundred cases annually in an ever-increasing population, and relatively few cases with severe paralyses.

Measles is now destined to share the same fate. Physicians who used to see five to fifty cases a month during epidemic periods, which occurred every two to three years, may see only one or two a year.

Mumps vaccine is now available, and German measles vaccine will probably be available for general use by the time this book is published.

The need for help in identifying the cause of fevers, pink spots and red rashes and for suggestions on what to do about them is ever increasing since house calls are now reduced to a minimum and are destined to become an anachronistic way of treating sick patients.

This manual will not convert the average parent, nurse, camp director or school teacher into a diagnostician, a therapist, or a public health officer who works in preventive medicine. It may, however, serve as a guide in alerting the layman to conditions which necessitate prompt medical attention.

Hopefully the questions and answers will be helpful. I have tried to include most questions asked of me by parents of my patients, by nurses working in schools, camps and in public health, by physicians who are usually less concerned with the subject of infectious diseases and by innumerable others.

I have canvassed groups and suggested that they ask me any question which came to mind when the children had measles, whooping cough and so on.

How many times have you taken your child to his doctor, was told what Johnny had and what to do about it, left the office, and then thought of a dozen questions you forgot to ask or did ask and did not understand, or forgot the answer?

Perhaps you will find some of the answers to such questions in this book.

                                                       −S. K.

About Causes, Symptoms & Prevention

1: Allergy

The word *allergy* means altered reactivity. If a person is allergic to a substance, he reacts to it differently from the way a person does who is not. There are many kinds of allergic reactions. The most common ones are:

Hives: A skin condition in which there appear intensely itchy red blotches with white raised centers either in a few places or distributed widely over the body. They appear and disappear in crops.

Eczema: A condition in which the skin is rough, reddened, swollen and finely blistered in patches. The blisters are very small, hardly visible and easily become infected. They ooze serum which dries and crusts. A dry form of eczema appears scaly.

Asthma: A lung condition characterized by spasms of the bronchial tubes, swelling of their linings and excessive secretion of mucus, all of which cause coughing, wheezing, breathing difficulty and a feeling of constriction of the chest.

Hay Fever: An acute condition involving the nose, eyes and sinuses in which there is sneezing, running nose, intense itching of the eyes and inside of the nose and often headache.

Vasomotor Rhinitis: Stuffiness and running of the nose caused by expansion of the blood vessels of the nasal-lining membrane and increased secretion of mucus.

Intestinal Allergy: A reaction to food which causes spitting up, vomiting, colic, diarrhea and, rarely, blood in the stools.

Allergic Headache: The kind commonly called "sick head-ache," the same as migraine headache, involving intense pain in the head, nausea and sometimes visual disturbances.

Serum Sickness: A hypersensitivity which is not strictly an allergy. A reaction to animal serum (frequently horse serum), characterized by hives, joint swelling pain, fever and some-times swollen lymph glands, frequently follows the use of diphtheria or tetanus antitoxin, which is made from horse serum. Similar reaction sometimes follows the use of antibiotics and other drugs.

If an infant who is fed nothing but cow's milk develops eczema, he is probably allergic to the milk. A child whose eyes and nose itch or who sneezes when he is in a dusty room is probably allergic to the dust in that room and maybe to dust in general. A child who repeatedly develops asthma when he is near a horse, a dog or a cat is probably allergic to either the hair or the scurf of the animal. If he often gets croup or asthma with colds he is probably allergic to the infection.

DIFFERENT KINDS OF ALLERGIES

Allergies are divided into several groups: (a) food allergy, caused by eating a food to which the child is sensitive; (b) in-halant allergy, which is caused by breathing the provocative substance, such as dust, fungus, feathers, or the pollens of weeds, grasses and trees; (c) contact allergies, which are caused by having the allergenic substance in contact with the skin, as in poison ivy, poison oak, poison sumac, wool, silk, some drugs and chemicals, such as mercury, glue, lacquer, and many other substances; (d) bacterial allergy, the kind caused by infection, as in the child who gets asthma because of an infection of the nose and throat. Reactions differ according to the manner in which the child comes in contact with the al-lergenic substance. Also, different children react differently to the same substance. A child might be sensitive to a sulfa drug and develop a rash over his entire body if he swallows some of the drug or takes it in the form of nose drops. If the drug is applied to his skin in the form of an ointment, he may have a skin irritation only where the ointment was applied, he may break out in a local eruption followed by a general rash, or both. A child who is sensitive to wool may develop eczema from a woolen blanket, or an itchy nose or asthma from breathing the wool particles.

ALLERGIES AND HEREDITY

Allergic conditions occur universally in all people. The allergic tendency is inherited and may show up anytime from infancy to old age. However, it may be acquired. If one parent has a major allergy (hay fever, asthma, etc.) his child may or may not be allergic. The chances of his being allergic are about one in four. If both parents are allergic, most of their children will probably be and their allergies may appear at an earlier age than they would otherwise. Approximately 10 per cent of the population at large is afflicted with one allergy or another. While the tendency to be allergic is inherited, the individual allergy to a certain substance may not be. A parent may have asthma due to ragweed, and the child eczema due to milk.

ACQUIRED ALLERGIES

Allergy may be acquired. For example, a child who is not born allergic to a sulfa drug may become so if the drug is applied to his skin or given to him internally over and over again. He may develop an allergy to penicillin or another antibiotic in the same way. He may acquire an allergy or hypersensitivity to chemical substances, to blood serums of other animal species (such as the horse serum used for tetanus antitoxin) and to bacteria and fungi.

CONTAGION

Allergies are neither contagious nor infectious. A child cannot become allergic or catch an allergy by being with someone who has asthma, hay fever or hives.

ALLERGY AND AGE

From infancy until two years of age, reactions to food are
most common. Spitting, vomiting and/or diarrhea—rarely with
blood—running nose, skin rashes, eczema and sometimes hives
occur. After age two, food reactions are less common, and the
region involved is more often the respiratory tract, the nose,
the sinuses, the throat, the bronchial tubes and the lungs. Hay
fever starts most often at four to eight years of age, and at
the same time other allergic reactions like hives and allergic
headaches become more prominent. Asthma may occur in the
first month of life and increase in frequency until puberty, but
may begin at all ages. I would like to emphasize that while
the reactions I have mentioned are more common at these
ages, there is no special age for the development of any of
them, particularly asthma. Any one may occur at any time.

DURATION

Allergic sensitivity and the resulting reaction may be permanent, but they are not necessarily so. The sensitivity may persist, but the reaction may change or disappear. An infant who
develops eczema because he is allergic to cow's milk is very
likely to continue to have this reaction to cow's milk until he
is one year to eighteen months old. After that, some continue
to have eczema for a long time, in some the eczema clears up
temporarily, but returns from time to time, and some children
outgrow the eczema, but are still allergic and later develop
other symptoms such as hay fever, vasomotor rhinitis or
asthma due to the same or other allergen. A child who has
attacks of asthma with nose and throat infections (bacterial
allergy) sometimes stops having this type of asthma when the
infections become less frequent. However, occasionally after
puberty such a child may have asthma again, though it is not
necessarily associated with infection. It may recur for many
other reasons. In some instances, it follows emotional upsets.

RESISTANCE AND DESENSITIZATION

It is also possible to overcome or to develop resistance to some allergenic substances. For example, a young child may become allergic to penicillin and then, after weeks or months of not having it, he may be able to take penicillin again without noticeable reaction. His penicillin allergy has become weakened with the passing of time. In other allergies like allergy to horse serum, time alone may not alter the sensitivity enough and a second injection of horse serum might cause alarming symptoms and serious harm. If a child who is sensitive to horse serum should be in need of treatment with a horse serum preparation such as diphtheria or tetanus antitoxin, he must be helped to become less sensitive to it by a process called desensitization. This is done by giving a very minute dose of the horse serum at first, and by increasing the dose every twenty to thirty minutes until the child is able to tolerate larger amounts without ill effects, usually within three or four hours. Another type of desensitization is the type usually done in the case of hay faver, in which the patient is given injections of the pollens he is sensitive to in gradually increasing doses over a period of months, starting long before the pollination season starts and continuing until it is over. This type of treatment is often successful in hay fever and in other forms of allergy, e.g., food, fungus. Some physicians prefer to give these injections at less frequent intervals throughout the year. Another method is to give only four to eight injections of longer-acting material. This method is growing in disfavor because reactions are more likely to occur and are more difficult to treat. This form of desensitization is commonly used in hay fever and other inhalant and food allergies.

WHAT INFLUENCES ALLERGIES?

One important factor in allergic reaction seems to be the level of tolerance for the substances to which the child is allergic.

If this tolerance is exceeded, symptoms occur. A child might be able to eat an egg once a week with no difficulty, but has a reaction if he eats one a day. A child who has hay fever due to weed pollen might be quite comfortable when exposed to small amounts of pollen, but is sick when the pollen is abundant. An injection of a small amount of horse serum might or might not cause ill effects, but a very small amount may be dangerous if injected in the person who has had horse serum before.

This tolerance can be influenced temporarily by many other things besides the amount of the allergen. For example, physical illness, infection, emotional strain, fatigue—any of these may lower the tolerance. If a child has a tendency to develop colic as an allergic reaction to eating chocolate, but does not develop symptoms unless he eats three chocolate bars at a time, he may develop colic after half a bar under any of the above conditions. The child's tolerance for chocolate has been temporarily reduced and the threshold above which he develops symptoms of allergy has been temporarily lowered.

Emotional strain is one of the most important causes of recurrent asthma. Unhappiness, an unhappy home, problems in school can and may increase the frequency, intensity and duration of the attack. In dealing with such a child, his whole environment must be carefully evaluated and suitable treatment instituted. This may require separation of the patient from his family for an extended period of time, during which the child and family are helped to learn to live together. While emotional upsets and the other factors I have mentioned influence allergies only temporarily, or periodically, conditions such as puberty, menstruation, pregnancy and severe illness sometimes result in long-lasting as well as temporary changes in the allergic pattern. Some allergic sensitivities disappear altogether, and new ones may develop.

INFECTION AND ALLERGY

Since this book deals primarily with infection, it is important to comment further on allergy associated with infection. The rashes which occur with some infections and hives, purpura (skin bleeding), erythema nodosum (a purplish-red, firm, painful and tender, bumpy eruption) may be the result of allergic reaction. Bacterial allergy, or sensitivity to infectious agents, is also of considerable importance in causing such symptoms as frequent running nose, repeated colds, sneezing, coughing, croup and asthma.

TREATMENT AND PREVENTION

If you know your child is allergic to a food—egg, for example—the most successful treatment is, of course, to eliminate eggs and all foods containing eggs from his diet. If the reaction is traceable to something he touches, it is important to avoid it. A child who develops a rash from glue or lacquer should not handle glue and lacquer.

The problem is more serious and more difficult to solve in the case of allergy to infection. If a child gets asthma with a cold, it is important that his colds be kept down to a minimum by scrupulously avoiding people who have them, by being careful about exposure to severe weather, and by eliminating, if possible, the source of infection.

Antibiotics may be valuable in avoiding some allergic reactions to bacteria because they prevent infection with them. In rare instances, a child is better off being in a warm, dry climate during the season when respiratory infections are most abundant at home.

If your child is allergic to a food or a drug, such as penicillin, be sure to tell this to his doctor, the schoolteacher and the camp director. Give your child a card which indicates his allergies.

ANTIHISTAMINIC DRUGS

Antihistamines are helpful for minimizing and, in some instances, for preventing allergic reactions. They are particularly helpful in hay fever and allergic rashes, such as hives. In treating a cold or the grippe, these drugs make the child more comfortable because they eliminate some reactions like excessive running nose, stuffiness and irritated eyes, but they do not cure the cold and occasionally they may be harmful. If these drugs are given, the child should be kept under close observation for a day or two after they are stopped since he may still be sick and the antihistamine may have only served to obscure the symptoms.

Adrenalin, cortisone and A.C.T.H. are the most powerful antiallergic drugs known. An injection of adrenalin may stop an attack of asthma or make hives disappear within a few minutes, and its effect may last up to several hours, but it rarely is a cure. It is not used for eczema, colic, migraine, hay fever, etc. Cortisone, given by mouth or injection, and A.C.T.H., given by injection, are far more potent, and the effect may last for a much longer period—even days or weeks. They do not cure the allergic condition either, but they relieve the child for a longer time and are useful in almost all allergies. They even cause temporary improvement in rheumatic fever and the rarer collagen diseases, and in hypersensitivity conditions like lupus, dermatomyositis and nephrosis. Cortisone ointment is also very effective when applied to skin affected by eczema or other allergic eruptions. Cortisone is often used to relieve asthma. It or similar drugs may be continued for months, even for a year or two. When these drugs are taken for a long time, a month or more, the child eats more, gets heavier and may develop side effects, such as skin ridges on the thighs and, less frequently, other complications.

ALLERGY TESTS

There are several kinds of tests for discovering what is responsible for allergic reactions. Most of them are skin tests, but frequently the elimination diet is used when a child has eczema and food seems to be responsible.

ELIMINATION DIET

The child is given a very limited variety of the foods he is used to, for example, milk, one cereal, one fruit, one vegetable and vitamins, for a week or two. If the eczema clears up or improves, it indicates that the child tolerates these few foods well and that one or more of the eliminated foods was responsible. Then other foods are introduced, one at a time, at intervals of one or two weeks. As soon as allergic symptoms show up again, it is possible to tell which food is responsible since it is the only one which has been added recently.

SKIN TESTS

If a child gets a running or itchy nose and repeated colds during any time of year, if he develops hives or asthma with or without an infection, it is often difficult to decide whether the child is suffering from an infection, an allergy or a combination of both. By means of skin tests, it is often possible to determine just what the child is allergic to. Skin tests are made in several ways.

Scratch Test: The material to be tested is placed on a scratch made on the skin, and if the child is allergic, a raised welt surrounded by redness appears in five to fifteen minutes. These are the easiest skin tests to make, and many substances can be tested at one time, a dozen or two on the skin of the back, for instance.

Intradermal Test: *Intradermal* means within the skin, and as the name implies, the solution to be tested is injected into the skin. A raised welt appears in five to fifteen minutes if the child is allergic to that substance. These tests are more sensitive and more reliable than scratch tests, but fewer can be done at a time and naturally they are less popular with children.

Patch Test: A piece of gauze impregnated with the material to be tested is placed on the skin and kept in place with tape for one or two days. A positive reaction is shown by the skin becoming irritated where the allergenic substance was applied. These tests are usually made in diagnosing contact allergies.

Passive Transfer: Passive transfer tests are done when the patient's skin is so extremely involved with eczema that there is not enough clear skin for testing or when the allergy is so severe that direct testing might result in a severe reaction. Small amounts of blood serum made from the blood taken from the allergic child are injected into the skin of a person who is known to be free of allergies. These prepared sites are tested by the intradermal technique. The results are similar to those noted in the direct testing of the patient's skin, but since this is an indirect form of testing, it is not considered as reliable as testing on the patient himself.

Skin tests often reveal allergies that could not be discovered otherwise, but in all instances the history of the child and his reaction to the allergen must be considered as well as the results of the skin tests, because the tests do not always show a positive result even though the child is allergic to the substance tested. If a child has a positive skin test for chocolate, but has no ill effects from eating it in moderation, he might continue to eat small quantities of chocolate. If a child develops asthma or eczema or a stuffy nose after eating chocolate and the skin test is nevertheless negative, the test should be ignored and chocolate should be withheld. If a child develops an itchy nose and eyes, if he sneezes a good deal and his nose becomes stuffy during the hay fever season, he should be treated for hay fever even if his skin test is negative for the pollens which usually cause it. If he has asthma repeatedly with infection of the upper respiratory tract, he has bacterial allergy even though skin tests for bacteria are negative. The technique of doing proper skin testing is simple, but the interpretation of the reactions is often difficult and must be done by an experienced doctor or a person trained in this field.

The control of the symptoms of hay fever will also reduce infection of the nose and sinuses (which is more likely to result when the nasal membranes are inflamed) and sometimes lessen the possibility of developing the asthma due to hay fever, pollen asthma. Desensitization, antihistaminic drugs to some degree, and in some instances cortisone are very helpful for this purpose. Having a child immunized against diphtheria and tetanus with injections of toxoid will make it unnecessary to treat him later in an emergency with horse serum antitoxins and will thereby avoid the possibility of serum sickness or shocklike reactions.

As already indicated, a change in the child's environment may result in dramatic improvement. This is often true of a stay in a hospital for as short as a week or two.

EYE TEST

This is particularly useful when one wants to determine whether the patient is allergic or sensitive to horse serum, which is commonly part of tetanus or diphtheria antitoxin. A drop of horse serum is dropped into the eye. If the eye gets very red in five to fifteen minutes, the patient is sensitive to horse serum. This reaction passes quickly and will not injure the eye.

QUESTIONS & ANSWERS

Q. *Is there any geographic influence on allergies?*

A. Yes. Hay fever depends on specific pollens of weeds, grasses, flowers or trees. If a person is allergic only to ragweed pollen and there is no ragweed in the area, he will not have symptoms of hay fever.

Q. *Are all racial and national groups similarly allergic?*

A. I am not certain that the answer is well established. I would think that there are probably many variations, possibly due to different living habits and environment, and possibly due also to variations of racial and national origin.

Q. *Does cold or bad weather influence allergies?*

A. Yes. There are people who break out in hives when exposed to cold weather, to sunlight, to close contact with ice. Also temperature and humidity may influence the absorption of allergens through the skin or otherwise alter the skin's reaction to them.

Q. *Is there an incubation period to allergic conditions?*

A. Yes, especially to the hypersensitivity type. For example, a child gets an injection of horse serum and in seven to fourteen days he develops serum sickness. If he gets a second injection of it within two weeks, he may have an accelerated reaction—one that comes within two to five days instead of seven to fourteen. If the second injection is three or four months after the first, the reaction may come within a few minutes to one day. This latter reaction is sometimes very severe and very dangerous, even fatal.

In the case of reactions like hives, asthma and hay fever, the incubation period may be so short as to be almost nonexistent, and in migraine headaches, eczema and intestinal allergies it is longer.

Q. *What is the difference between an allergy and an infection?*

A. Allergy can be caused by an animate or inanimate object. Infection is produced only by living bacteria, viruses, fungi, protozoans, etc. The symptoms of both allergy and infection are manifestations of the body's reaction to the causative substance, but they are caused by different kinds of bodily reactions.

Q. *Are allergies ever purely psychological or emotional?*

A. No, but allergic people become more so under emotional stress, and some symptoms of allergy may be produced by emotional disturbance or even by hypnosis. This reaction to emotion is similar to blushing or the red blotches on the neck and chest that some people get when they are embarrassed or frightened. Chronic hives are frequently caused by emotional upset. Asthma is often made more severe and more frequent.

Q. *Is there any way by which allergy can pass from one person to another?*

A. Yes. If blood from an allergic person is injected into a person who is not allergic, the second person may temporarily develop an allergy to the substance to which the first person was allergic. But allergy cannot be transmitted by personal contact as infection can. Of course, mother's allergic tendencies can be transmitted to the unborn infant.

Q. *Are breast-fed children more or less likely to have food allergies?*

A. Less likely when they are fed only breast milk, but there is no difference after they begin to eat food like cow's milk and wheat.

Q. *Can children who are breast-fed develop long-lasting allergies to foods the mothers eat?*

A. Yes, it is possible.

Q. *Do mosquito bites or bee stings cause allergic reactions?*

A. Yes. People have very different reactions to mosquito bites. The itchy welt around the bite is similar to an itchy hive, and some people never develop it at all. A bee sting is the same, only more severe. Some hypersensitive people even develop shock from a bee or wasp sting.

Q. *Do you become more sensitive to bee and wasp stings if you are stung several times?*

A. Not usually, but reactions are not always identical.

Q. *Are antihistamines taken internally or applied locally good for stings and mosquito bites?*

A. Yes, either way. If the reaction is a very severe one, antihistamines taken internally are more effective. But in the case of local itching or stinging, locally applied antihistamines are usually enough.

Q. *Do snake bites produce allergic reactions?*

A. No. They produce poisonous or toxic effects.

Q. *Is psoriasis an allergic disease?*

A. No.

Q. *You said that cortisone and A.C.T.H. are useful for rheumatic fever. Does that mean that rheumatic fever is an allergy?*

A. No, not exactly. It is the result of the body becoming hypersensitive to some part or parts of the Beta Hemolytic streptococcus of group A. Only a small percentage of streptococcus infections results in rheumatic fever. Cortisone and A.C.T.H. are very effective in the treatment of hypersensitivity diseases, no matter what the agent is to which the body is hypersensitive.

Q. *What is "physical allergy"?*

A. Allergic reactions, such as hives and other skin rashes, which are produced by heat, cold and sun are called physical allergies.

Q. *Is motion sickness related to allergy?*

A. No.

Q. *Are cold sores ever caused by allergy?*

A. No, they are caused by the herpes simplex virus.

Q. *Are canker sores in the mouth an allergic reaction?*

A. Yes, sometimes.

Q. *If a child has a severe reaction to, say, whooping cough vaccine, is it because he is allergic to it?*

A. Sometimes it is. Do not repeat the vaccine injection in full dose; let your doctor advise you.

Q. *Do children ever outgrow their allergic tendencies, or do they always crop up later in the same or a different form?*

A. Some outgrow them, but the majority do not.

Q. *My son can take penicillin by mouth, but he gets hives when it is injected. Why is that?*

A. This does not usually happen. It may be because the dosage is greater when it is injected or more of it is absorbed by his body, or he may be allergic to the substance the penicillin is mixed with for injection. In any event, avoid giving it by mouth as well as by injection.

Q. *Are allergic headaches the same as migraine headaches, and do children ever have them?*

A. Yes, they are, and children do have them.

Q. *Is "bacterial allergy" really only an allergy to bacteria, or does it also include allergy to viruses, fungi, etc.?*

A. Bacterial allergy only applies to bacteria, but one may be allergic to viruses and fungi, too.

Q. *If a child is allergic to wool when he swallows particles of*

Q. *Is that how you know that there are fifteen different viruses that produce influenza?*

A. Yes. There are probably more.

Q. *Can you prevent virus infections?*

A. Some of them. For example, measles and hepatitis (liver infection) can be temporarily prevented by gamma globulin. Influenza and yellow fever can be prevented for a longer time by vaccine. We are now able to prevent polio and measles by vaccine, probably for life. Vaccines against mumps are now available and one for German measles will soon be available, hopefully.

Q. *Are the antibiotics or sulfa drugs helpful in treating virus infections?*

A. Most virus infections do not respond to them. Some of the exceptions are diseases caused by a few of the larger viruses like the one causing psittacosis (parrot fever). Recently a drug effective in smallpox has been developed; another is being recommended for influenza, but this one requires further evaluation. The Eaton Agent, causing atypical pneumonia, etc., was considered to be a virus but is now known not to be.

Q. *Then why is penicillin or other antibiotics often given in case of a virus infection?*

A. If the infection is definitely known to be caused by a virus, most antibiotics will not be helpful. Often it is not possible to eliminate bacteria as the cause. Antibiotics are therefore given as a precaution. Should the disease (even a very serious disease like meningitis) be caused by a bacterium, drugs in common use now will destroy most of the usual bacteria known to cause it.

Some people who have influenza become infected with bacteria after the virus infection has started. This may cause even more trouble than the virus infection, and most of these bacteria do react to treatment with antibiotics or sulfa drugs. Many physicians feel that antibiotics should not be used when an infection is known to be caused or is strongly suspected of being caused by a virus, except as already indicated.

Q. *Are cold sores caused by a virus?*

A. Yes. While this virus causes cold sores, it may also produce other conditions, even encephalitis, and other infections such as ulcers in the mouth and, rarely, a general infection or an infection of the central nervous system. In the newborn infant this virus can produce serious disease.

Q. *You indicate that some warts are caused by viruses. I thought warts were growths, like tumors.*

A. They are growths, but viruses are known to stimulate the development of some warts.

Q. *Are vaccines made of dead virus effective?*

A. Yes, they are, but the immunity or protection produced is temporary. Those made from attenuated live viruses are more effective, result in long-lasting immunity and are therefore preferable.

Q. *Then why is there so much discussion about the lasting quality of the immunity produced by the Salk vaccine or the killed measles vaccine?*

A. It is known that immunity from killed virus vaccine, such as the Salk or killed measles vaccines, are temporary. It is therefore preferable to give the live vaccines which result in long-lasting, probably permanent, immunity.

Q. *If it is true that the killed virus vaccines produce immunity for even a few months or a year, are they not still worthwhile?*

A. Some doctors use only killed vaccine, especially since immunity can be maintained by frequent booster injections. However, since the immunity is not permanent, there is always danger that the temporary immunity produced by killed vaccine will disappear and the child will again be susceptible to the disease. Recently reactions to live-measles-virus vaccine and to measles itself have been described in children who were previously injected with killed measles vaccine. Killed measles vaccine is therefore being discouraged.

Q. *Are there any other killed virus vaccines?*

A. Yes, but not commonly used at present.

Q. *If a vaccine is made from a live virus which has been*

made harmless, could the virus regain its ability to produce disease?

A. If it occurs at all it does so rarely. It is therefore not a significant hindrance to the use of live vaccine.

Q. *You mentioned a hundred and thirty APC viruses. Are they all different?*

A. Yes. A vaccine has been made from some strains of APC viruses. These have been protective in a high percentage of those vaccinated.

Q. *You indicated there are three types of polio viruses. Are there many types of viruses producing measles, etc.?*

A. This varies with the disease. Only one virus is known to produce measles. Some fifteen types of influenza viruses are known to produce influenza; more than one may produce hepatitis. Many can cause croup, bronchitis, and a large number may produce encephalitis—thirty-five or more.

Q. *Why do doctors assume that any disease for which they cannot find the cause is a virus disease?*

A. Most doctors do not, and if any does, he probably implies that the infection behaves like one caused by a virus rather than bacteria. Occasionally the term is used loosely for a disease which cannot be identified. There are some diseases like roseola and infectious mononucleosis which are presumed to be caused by viruses because no bacteria have been found to cause them, and experiments have suggested that they are caused by a virus.

3: Fever

If your child's temperature is 100° F. (37.5° C.) or over, he has fever. This is equally true whether the temperature is taken by mouth, by rectum or by armpit. Probably it means that your child is sick, but it may not be very significant since the normally active child may have a daily range of temperature from 98° to 99.5° F., and sometimes slightly higher. If the child has been very active, running about or playing hard, his temperature may rise to 100° or even to 101° and return to normal after he has rested for about half an hour. This tendency for body temperature to rise after exercise is also true of adults, but the fluctuations are not as great except after severe and continuous exertion. (Temperatures of 103° and 104° have been recorded after a four-mile crew race.) It is important for a child to rest for at least twenty minutes to get a true temperature measurement.

The temperature may be different at different times of the day, lower when fasting, higher after eating, lower when the child is asleep than when he is awake. If the child's temperature is 99.5° when he is asleep, it is more likely to signify fever than the same temperature would at other times.

In the newborn and very young infant, a few days old, and even more so in the case of the prematurely born infant, the temperature control center in the brain functions inefficiently as compared with that of the older child and adult. For example, if a newborn infant is too heavily clothed, or if the temperature of the nursery is kept very high, 90° to 100°, the baby's temperature may rise to 101° or 103°, and even more. On the other hand, if he is inadequately covered, or if the room temperature is too low, below 68°, his temperature may drop to 95°, 94° or even lower. Older children and adults exposed to 90° to 100° heat may also have a rise in temperature of one degree or a little more, but rarely to any level as high as an infant reaches. The infant's body may not be able to adjust its temperature until he is one or two weeks old, or older, but after the first week or two of his life, his temperature will become more or less stable.

Premature infants have such poor temperature control mechanisms that they are routinely placed in incubators immediately after birth. The temperature in the incubator may have to be kept between 80° and 90° and higher to keep the infant's temperature close to normal. As the infant's temperature becomes stabilized, the temperature in the incubator is reduced, and finally when the infant is able to maintain a temperature approaching normal, he is moved to an open crib. This transition period may last as little as two or three days, or as long as two months, depending, to some extent, on the size of the infant. In general, the smaller and more premature the infant, the longer it takes for the development of normal temperature control.

TAKING THE TEMPERATURE

If you call your doctor because your child is ill, you should know what his temperature is before you call. The doctor will want to know it, and whether you are giving him a rectal or an oral reading. All thermometers used to measure body temperature are carefully calibrated. They differ only in the bulb. An oral (mouth) thermometer has a long, thin bulb which is constructed to measure temperature quickly. A rectal thermometer has a rounded, heavier bulb which is considered less likely to cause rectal injury. You can use an oral thermometer to measure rectal temperature and a rectal thermometer in the mouth. Either one can be used in the armpit.

Before and after using a thermometer, you should clean it with soap and *cool* water. Before starting to take your child's temperature, shake the thermometer down until it registers below 97°. To do this, take hold of the end opposite the bulb and shake the bulb end downward with a snapping motion. Then, if you are taking a temperature by rectum, coat the bulb well with Vaseline or cold cream. Turn the child on his side or on his stomach on the bed, or if he is a baby, hold him on his stomach across your knees. Spread his buttocks with the thumb and forefinger of your left hand and insert the greased thermometer gently into his rectum with your right hand for about an inch. Let the thermometer find its own course. Don't push hard. Never leave the thermometer unguarded in an infant or a child who is not cooperative. You must have constant control of it. Gently resting a finger on the thermometer, or holding it between two fingers with the palm of your hand across his buttocks is enough to keep it in and you will be able to withdraw it quickly if necessary. The thermometer is usually left in about three minutes, but you will notice that the mercury reaches close to its maximum rise in less than a minute. If the child is restless and there is danger of breaking the thermometer, pull it out. The actual height of the temperature may not yet have been recorded, but you can get a fair idea of it from the mercury level at 45 to 60 seconds. Usually you take temperatures by rectum or by armpit until a child is five or six years old because before that time he can't keep the thermometer under his tongue.

When you take a mouth temperature, the child must be able to support the thermometer with his tongue and lips and be sitting up or lying on his side or back. You should place the bulb under his tongue and his lips should be closed over the thermometer for about three minutes. When temperature is taken in the armpit, you place the thermometer across the armpit with the bulb in the hollow of it. Then the child holds his arm close against his side for three minutes. All newborn infants and infants who have diarrhea should have their temperatures taken in the armpit.

TEMPERATURE AND PULSE

Ordinarily the temperature and pulse go up together and down together. In most infections the temperature and pulse both rise. In fact, doctors estimate a rise of ten pulse beats per minute for each degree of fever above 100°. In some infections, though, the temperature and pulse do not rise and fall together. For example, in typhoid fever the temperature may be high and the pulse relatively normal. In the newborn infant, the temperature is often subnormal while the pulse is very fast.

In other circumstances both the temperature and the pulse are low. After a child has recovered from an illness like pneumonia or typhoid fever, it is not unusual for the temperature to drop to 96° or 97° and stay at this level for a week or two until convalescence is well along. During this time the pulse may drop to 60 in a child who normally has a pulse of 80 or 90. When the child becomes active again, the pulse returns to normal.

Pattern of Temperature: If a child is sick, his temperature is usually lower in the morning and higher in the late afternoon and evening, but in some diseases the temperature is higher in the morning. Although a sick child's temperature usually goes up once a day, it may go up and down more than once. In fact, two peaks of temperature a day is characteristic of some diseases.

When a temperature rises to 104° or 105° and in the same day drops to 99° or 100°, and this pattern is repeated for several days, it is called a septic temperature and the doctor may suspect an infection in the blood. But this pattern also occurs sometimes in pneumonia and other diseases. A child may have a chill as his temperature begins to rise, after which the temperature climbs to a high level. On the other hand, as the temperature begins to drop, he may have a sweat.

CONVULSIONS WITH FEVER

Young children under five years of age (rarely older) are sometimes delirious or have a convulsion when the fever reaches 104° or more. This is because the high temperature disrupts the normal functions of the body, especially the brain. Such a convulsion in a young child is similar in some ways to a chill in an adult. It is as if the child is having a chill, but lacks the ability to control the rapid contractions of the muscles so that the muscles become so tense as to produce a convulsion. Although convulsions occur in some children when the temperature reaches 104° or 105°, in others they may not occur until 106° or more. On the other hand, I have seen children who become disoriented and have muscular twitching with as little as 102° or 103°. Often more than one child in a family has a tendency to have convulsions with fever, but it does not necessarily follow that because one child has them his brothers and sisters will, also.

Children who have convulsions with fever are more likely to have epileptic attacks later than are children who never had convulsions with high fever. Children with a tendency to have febrile convulsions upon getting sick should be treated promptly with drugs to lower the temperature and to reduce his irritability.

A fever which reaches 107° or 108° or higher and stays there for some time may cause permanent injury to the brain. However, children's temperatures have been known to reach 110° and the children have survived without any apparent injury.

REDUCING TEMPERATURE

If you suddenly notice that your child's eyes look dull, small and tired, and that his skin is warmer than usual, and you find that he has a fever of more than 101°, it is wise to try to reduce it, especially if the child tends to react badly to high temperature. Sponging his body with lukewarm water followed by rubbing his skin with alcohol is usually effective. You sponge only one part of the body at a time while you keep the rest covered. Keep this up until the entire body has been sponged. Occasionally an enema with tepid water (95° to 100°) is helpful in reducing temperature. When the fever is 104° or more, it may be necessary to use a wet pack if these other measures fail. You undress the child and wrap around his naked body a thin blanket or a sheet which has been soaked in lukewarm water (100°) and wrung out. You then put the wrapped child on a rubber sheet or some other waterproof material and cover him with a dry blanket. If he is kept in such a pack for about an hour, his temperature usually drops several degrees. These measures—sponges, enemas and wet packs—are extremely important and sometimes most urgent for children who are prone to have convulsions with fever. Except for emergencies, you should consult your doctor before proceeding with them.

In many instances, fever may be a natural defense of the body against infection. In such cases, the doctor may not want to reduce the temperature unless it reaches 105° or more. But that decision can only be made by a doctor who knows your child well.

Aspirin is an excellent drug to reduce temperature. Of course, there are many other drugs also, and your doctor may prefer one of the others. These others are especially helpful if a child cannot tolerate aspirin.

ASPIRIN POISONING

At this point I would like to stress a very important subject— aspirin poisoning. You should be warned against the indiscriminate use of aspirin, especially for little children. More infants and children are brought to the hospital with poisoning due to aspirin than to any other drug. Aspirin is harmful if you give too much of it. It must be used correctly and according to the doctor's orders, otherwise it is just as dangerous as some of the more toxic and less commonly used drugs. The taste of aspirin seems to please little children. Some children two and three years old will, if given the chance, chew and swallow most of the contents of the aspirin bottle. This is more true now than ever before, since so many brands of aspirin have been flavored to make them quite attractive to children. Be sure to keep aspirin and other drugs from the reach of your children.

Another source of danger is misunderstanding the doctor's orders. I have seen several cases admitted to the hospital in whom the aspirin poisoning was due to the fact that the mothers had given ten grains of aspirin every three hours to children of eighteen months. The doctor had ordered two grains, and the mother thought that a grain meant an ordinary aspirin tablet which actually has five grains of aspirin. The doctor's orders should be precise and, if possible, in writing. And whether in writing or by telephone, both the doctor and the parents should be sure that the directions are exactly understood.

Too much aspirin stimulates the breathing center in the brain. Breathing becomes very rapid, the child later develops fever, acidosis (an overproduction of acid by the body) and may become drowsy, stuporous or even unconscious. I have seen permanent brain damage and even deaths from aspirin poisoning. Aspirin, nevertheless, is an extraordinarily good drug with which to bring down temperature and is perfectly safe, if used correctly. It is almost indispensible in the practice of medicine.

Dosage of Aspirin: A dose of one grain per year of age given about every four hours is enough for infants and children. You should not give this much or more than this without a doctor's specific directions. Thus, a child of three years of age could have three grains of aspirin every four hours, or a five-year-old five grains every four hours, if he needed it. If the child is asleep, do not awake him for aspirin, unless asked to do so by the doctor. Some doctors mean only four times a day when aspirin is ordered every four hours. The night is excluded. Be sure you know exactly what the doctor prescribed. A ten-year-old may not require ten grains every four hours (five grains is often a large-enough dose), but most children of that age will tolerate ten grains, or more if needed, without difficulty. Adults can take ten to fifteen grains and more every four hours without trouble, but individual tolerance for drugs must be taken into account. One person may do well with ten grains while another of the same age may be made uncomfortable by the same dose. The four-hour interval between doses applies if the drug is to be continued for a whole twenty-four-hour period or longer, but need not be adhered to if, for example, the first dose has not been successful or its effect has lasted only two hours. A second dose might be ordered in two or three hours, but intervals of two hours should not be continued if the drug has to be given much longer.

Aspirin Sensitivity: There are people who are sensitive to aspirin as to every other drug. These people should let the doctor know about themselves or their children when drugs are ordered. Unless you know that your child can tolerate aspirin, a small dose should be given at first, perhaps a half or a third of what you would ordinarily give, and if there are no bad effects within an hour, the full dose may be given.

In general, it is wiser and safer to give the aspirin under the doctor's direction than to give it by yourself without knowing exactly what is the cause of the temperature, and whether aspirin is the best medicine to give. For example, if your child has 102° or 103° fever and you call the doctor, he may tell you to give a definite, usually small, dose of aspirin before he sees the child, or he may prefer to see the child before you give him anything.

Reducing a child's temperature by drugs gives you a false sense of security for a period of three to six hours, sometimes as much as twelve hours. It is rare for the drugs which reduce the temperature also to cure the disease, although there are exceptions like quinine, which both lowers the temperature of malaria and cures it. On frequent occasions when someone has telephoned me to see a sick child with a high temperature, I have recommended that a small amount of aspirin be given before I arrive. The aspirin usually lowers the temperature in an hour or two and the child looks and feels better. Then I may receive a second telephone call saying that I need not come because the child is well, then a third, frantic call several hours later, often late at night, when the fever has risen again. The child looks sicker and the parents are afraid to go through the night without knowing what is wrong and how to treat him. You must not be deceived as to the severity of an illness because the temperature has been reduced by aspirin. I want to emphasize that while aspirin will lower the temperature of pneumonia, tonsillitis and many other diseases, it will not cure them. To assume that a child is getting well because his fever drops after a dose of aspirin may delay more specific treatment of a serious illness which should be treated quickly.

Aspirin is quickly absorbed from the stomach. It is therefore imperative that a doctor see the child promptly after he has taken an excessive dose. If the doctor cannot be reached, the child should be taken to the emergency room of a nearby hospital. Time is important. Try to make a child vomit by giving him a teaspoonful of syrup of ipecac, or by tickling his throat with your finger. If you put your finger in his mouth, be sure you put something like a tongue depressor or the handle of a teaspoon in one corner of the child's mouth so that he does not bite your finger.

QUESTIONS & ANSWERS

Q. *What is the normal temperature of the human body?*

A. It is 98.6° Fahrenheit or 37.5° Centigrade, but it fluctuates about one degree (F.) in twenty-four hours.

Q. *Is it the same whether you take it by rectum or mouth?*

A. Yes, but mouth temperatures are usually lower because they are not easily recorded unless the person is cooperative and holds his mouth completely closed with the thermometer bulb under his tongue.

Q. *Is it correct that the true temperature of the body is the rectal temperature and that that is one degree higher than the oral?*

A. Essentially, except that the difference is nearer half a degree.

Q. *Can you take a rectal temperature with a mouth thermometer?*

A. Yes.

Q. *Why are the thermometers we buy in drugstores marked in Fahrenheit, when in hospitals they use Centigrade thermometers?*

A. The Centigrade scale is used by everyone in all countries except England and the United States, and hospitals prefer to use the universal methods for the sake of uniformity.

Q. *Do people who live in warm climates have higher temperatures than people in cold ones?*

A. No, the temperature stays about the same in either climate. It the weather is very hot, the body loses heat trying to keep the temperature down. If it is very cold, the body tries to manufacture heat faster to keep the temperature normal, and these processes keep the temperature constant.

Q. *Is it true that the bodies of infants are not able to regulate temperature as adult bodies do?*

A. Yes. As a result, infants' temperatures fluctuate with external heat and cold much more than adults' temperatures.

Q. *What should the temperature of a newborn infant's room be?*

A. For a full-term infant, it should be between 72° and 76°. Many nurseries are kept much warmer, but when they are, the babies are not as heavily clothed. If an infant is prematurely born, his body is even less able to regulate temperature, so he has to be put in an incubator where the temperature is kept at a higher level, usually 90° to 93° at first, lower later.

Q. *When an incubator or a room is kept very warm for an infant, doesn't the air become too dry?*

A. It would if no moisture was added. Humidity is very important in the environment of newborn infants. It should be about 55 to 65 per cent for very small and premature infants, 85 to 95 per cent until the infant's temperature is 96° or 97°.

Q. *When my child is ill and has a fever, how often should I take his temperature?*

A. Two or three times a day—morning, noon and late afternoon—unless the temperature stays high, in which case you may have to take it every four hours or more often, especially when you are trying to lower it by artificial means.

Q. *When my child is sick, should I wake him to take his temperature?*

A. No. Sleep is very valuable for a sick child. He should not be disturbed except when special treatment is necessary. Taking his temperature is usually not as important; feeling the skin may be sufficiently informative.

Q. *Is it safe to reduce a child's temperature very sharply in a short time?*

A. Yes, except when a high temperature is reduced to a subnormal level very quickly.

Q. *What might happen if you did that?*

A. If a child had 105° fever and you dropped it to below 99° in an hour, for instance, usually nothing would happen except that the child would sweat, but an occasional child might become limp and exhausted.

Q. *I have been told that fever is one of the body's ways to fight disease. Why, then, should you make an effort to reduce it?*

A. With infants and children who are prone to have convulsions with very high temperatures, it seems wiser to reduce the fever to below the level which stimulates the convulsions. This level varies with individual children—104° in some, 102° in others. Sometimes a child's temperature is raised artificially and kept high as a form of treatment for a disease.

Q. *How is that done?*

A. Sometimes by wrapping him in blankets and keeping him warm, sometimes by keeping him in a very hot room, and sometimes by exposing his body to radio short waves which raise his temperature, or by the injection of bacterial vaccine.

Q. *Do children stop having convulsions with fever at any particular age?*

A. Yes, usually at about five years of age. If the convulsions continue for a long time after that, especially if they come with relatively low temperatures, or if they start after five years, you should suspect something more than just a convulsion with fever—possibly epilepsy. I have occasionally seen convulsions in children six, eight and ten years old as a result of high fever, but these children usually had had convulsions when they were younger, too, and are more likely to have epilepsy.

Q. *How can you tell a convulsion caused by fever from one due to a condition like epilepsy?*

A. The convulsions may be identical, but if it is true epilepsy, they will also occur without fever. The majority of children who have convulsions with fever do not have epilepsy, but epilepsy is much more common among those who do have febrile convulsions than among those who do not. The presence of epilepsy can be determined with some degree of accuracy by a test known as an electroencephalogram, which usually, but not always, shows it. Some doctors believe that a child who has had more than one febrile convulsion lasting half an hour or more is an epileptic. I have not found this always to be the case—unless a single convulsion is regarded as evidence of epilepsy.

Q. *If a child with a high fever wants food, is it safe to give it to him?*

A. Yes, if he is able to take it and keep it down. Some children with high fevers lose their appetites completely and they vomit if the food is forced. If the child has a fever for many days, he may lose a great deal of weight unless he is fed. It is now customary to give such patients high-calorie diets (rich in milk, sugar, cream, cereals, breads, etc.) so that they will not lose weight during the illness.

Q. *What about the idea of starving a fever?*

A. It is old and out of place in many conditions. It may be correct if the child is unable to take food for a day or so. Personally, I feel encouraged if a child who is ill keeps his appetite and takes enough food and fluid. I feel that he is improving and will undoubtedly recover.

Q. *Can you have an infection without fever?*

A. Yes. Mild infections often occur without fever. If an infant or child is very weak, he may even have a severe infection with no fever. Usually, though, if the infection is general, there is some fever. Small premature infants have such poor temperature control mechanisms that they may not respond to infection with elevated temperature. It is therefore very important to promptly investigate the reason why such an infant stops eating, becomes drowsy, dull and so on.

Q. *How high should the temperature be before you call the doctor?*

A. I think you should call the doctor when your child gets sick whether his temperature is high or not. Of course, if it is high, the doctor will feel that the call is more urgent, but even 100° or 100.5° in a child who was normal before, indicates that he is sick, and you ought to talk the matter over with your doctor.

Q. *Can you get a fever with an allergic reaction?*

A. Yes, with some kinds, especially a reaction to a drug, such as an antibiotic, or to a serum (serum sickness). Serum sickness often causes very high temperatures.

Q. *If a child has had an infection and afterward keeps on having a temperature of 99° and 100°, does it indicate that he still has the disease?*

A. That is difficult to answer. In general, my feeling is this: When a child first becomes ill and has a temperature near 100°, I think the temperature is abnormal and represents a fever. But if a child has that kind of temperature after an illness of four or five days during which he had 102° or 103° fever, and if he is feeling fine, I think of that as a low-grade fever without very much significance, although it may mean there is still some low-grade infection.

Q. *Would you let a child with a low-grade temperature like that be up and around?*

A. Yes, I would, if I feel that he may be better off out of bed.

Q. *Could I send my child to school if his temperature stays around 100°?*

A. Usually not, but if the 100° has persisted over a period of several days to weeks, and I am absolutely sure the child has no illness which he can spread or complication of an illness for which he must remain at home, I suggest he return to school.

Q. *But if the child continues to have a temperature of about 100°, doesn't it mean that there is a hidden infection somewhere?*

A. Perhaps it does, but when it is impossible to find it we have to rely on our own judgment, which is based on experience, on how the patient feels, looks and acts. One way of finding out whether this 100° temperature means anything is to take it after the child has been resting for about half an hour. Usually, it will go below 100° after the rest period. If that happens often enough, I usually feel that the child is ready to go back to school, but is not ready for a great deal of hard physical activity.

Q. *You suggested giving an enema for bringing down temperature. What temperature should the water be—cold or warm?*

A. It should be tepid, about 95° to 100°.

Q. *Should the enema be plain water?*

A. Water with bicarbonate of soda or ordinary table salt in the proportion of one teaspoonful of soda or salt to a quart of water.

Q. *How much of that solution should I inject?*

A. It depends on the size of the child. A newborn infant gets two ounces, a child ten or fifteen years old, a quart.

4: The Wonder Drugs

ANTIBIOTICS

The word *antibiotic* means, literally, "against life," or "tending to destroy life." An antibiotic is a drug, a chemical substance which is made from living objects such as bacteria, fungi or molds and which is capable of destroying or stopping the growth and multiplication of other bacteria, viruses, molds or protozoa. Antibiotics combine in the body with substances which bacteria require for growth and multiplication. In some cases, this completely destroys the bacteria. The antibiotic is then "bacteriocidal." In others, when the antibiotic merely stops the growth and multiplication of the bacteria, the body is able to get rid of the infection by natural processes because it is no longer overwhelmed by the numbers of infecting agents. This type of antibiotic is "bacteriostatic."

CHEMOTHERAPEUTIC AGENTS

After the chemical make-up of an antibiotic becomes known, it may be produced synthetically from basic chemical substances in the laboratory. It is then known as a chemotherapeutic agent (an agent which acts by chemical treatment). These, like antibiotics, are capable of destroying bacteria, molds and some viruses, or of arresting their growth and multiplication, but they are not made from living objects. Chloromycetin, first made from a soil mold, is an antibiotic which has since been synthesized. All of the sulfonamides (sulfa drugs), the antisyphilis arsenic-containing drugs, quinacrine (the antimalarial drug) and innumerable other such substances are chemotherapeutic agents rather than antibiotics in that they are made from chemical substances, not from living objects.

Today the tendency is to call chemotherapeutic agents antibiotics, too, as a matter of simplicity, since they perform the same functions and since some of them can be made either way.

MOLDS AND SOIL BACTERIA

The influence of molds on infection has been known for a long time. Farmers used to put moldy bread on infected fingers or hands because they knew it would stop the infection. Men working in the Roquefort cheese caves in France knew that their cuts and other skin injuries were not likely to become infected. Bacteriologists working in laboratories had noticed that when a mold contaminated a bacterial culture, the area surrounding the mold was free of bacteria. These molds are considered a nuisance by most of us, but Sir Alexander Fleming made use of this nuisance and realized that the mold actually prevented the growth of the bacteria. From the mold that Dr. Fleming observed, Abraham, Chain and Florey later produced penicillin, to date the most useful antibiotic yet discovered.

It was also known that many ordinary disease-producing bacteria are destroyed in the soil. One of the reasons is that the soil contains some bacteria which have the ability to destroy others. As a result of these and other similar observations, samples of molds and soil have been gathered from all over the world, and thousands of them have been studied in an effort to obtain disease-destroying antibiotics. Millions of dollars have been spent by research laboratories in universities and by pharmaceutical manufacturers in the quest for new antibiotics. Many have been isolated which were found effective against bacteria, but unfortunately they are too toxic for man or higher animals.

Of the thousands studied, an ever-increasing number have

fulfilled the requirements that they be safe for man and be capable of destroying bacteria. Some of the commonly used and generally safe ones are penicillin compounds, semisynthetic penicillin-like drugs (e.g., Staphcillin, Oxycillin, Penicillin V, Ampicillin, Keflin, Loridin, Cephaloglycin), the tetracycline drugs (Aureomycin, Achromycin, Terramycin and Tetracyn), Chloromycetin, Erythromycin, Furadantin, isoniazid and streptomycin. Neomycin, polymycin and bacitracin are excellent drugs, but they are more toxic than the others and are reserved for infections resistant to other antibiotics when they may be effective in smaller, less toxic doses. They and tyrothrycin are widely used externally for skin and eye infections. Mycostatin and Griseofulvin have been found to control the growth of some molds. New antibiotics are being developed, and we hope that soon there will be some which will be effective against virus infections. One said to be effective against the influenza viruses and another against the smallpox virus are available. More and more effective agents are urgently needed.

THE SULFONAMIDES

The sulfa drugs came into use in 1936. Only those of us who practiced pediatrics before the discovery of sulfanilamide, sulfathiazole, sulfapyridine and sulfadiazine can realize how close to the truth was the name given to them and to the antibiotics—"the wonder drugs."

We now have a large series of sulfa drugs. The first three are not in common use, but sulfadiazine is still very widely used and effective. Others like Azosulfadine are widely used for intestinal infections, but because some types of bacteria have become resistant to them, their range of usefulness has become limited. Antibiotics have replaced a good many of them.

INFECTION SINCE DISCOVERY
OF ANTIBIOTICS

Sulfonamides and antibiotics have changed the effects of infection. The physician who entered the practice of medicine since the discovery of sulfanilamide, which was very useful against the streptococcus, and sulfapyridine to combat the pneumococcus, and penicillin to fight both of these and many other bacteria can hardly appreciate how vast those changes are.

Before sulfapyridine was available, 40 per cent of infants who contracted pneumonia in the first year died. In the year following its discovery, how dramatic was the announcement by a group of my pediatric friends that out of three hundred infants with pneumonia who were treated with sulfapyridine, only one died!

Mastoiditis has become rare because the ear infections which precede it are readily cured. Erysipelas has become infrequent, and neither one of them is any longer a particular threat.

Meningitis now responds to antibiotics and sulfa drugs, and the recovery rate is 80 per cent to almost 100 per cent, depending on the type. Even tuberculous meningitis which was formerly always fatal is cured in 50 to 80 per cent of cases since the introduction of isoniazid.

The antibiotics and sulfa drugs are extremely useful in the treatment of diphtheria, scarlet fever, strep throat, whooping cough, sinusitis, cervical adenitis, croup, the rickettsial diseases, gonorrhea and syphilis, dysentery and innumerable others. They are also effective in atypical pneumonia caused by the Eaton Agent. In these and in others, such as influenza and other viral disease, where they have no effect on the original infection, they may, if used correctly, cut down the number and severity of the complications.

In streptococcal infections, the antibiotics not only cure them, but have vastly reduced the number of cases of rheumatic fever and nephritis which may follow them. In children who have had rheumatic fever, antibiotics given as preventives have for years cut down the incidence of relapses by 60 per cent.

Antibiotics are also useful in the prevention of scarlet fever, diphtheria and meningitis in children who have been exposed to them, and they are used extensively before and after many surgical procedures to guard against postoperative infection.

There is no doubt that antibiotics have brought longer and healthier life to man and domestic animals. They have increased the rate of growth of chickens, turkeys and pigs, bringing them to market at lower cost and in shorter time.

CORRECT USE OF THE WONDER DRUGS

In spite of their great value, antibiotics and sulfa drugs can be dangerous, as all drugs can be. Aspirin, for instance, is a wonderful drug. It is used in almost every home; but some people are allergic to it and too much aspirin is one of the most common causes of poisoning in little children. Antibiotics, like other drugs, must be used correctly to be useful. If they are not, they can definitely be harmful.

Each antibiotic has a certain sphere of activity. Some are effective against one type of bacteria and others against another group. For their best effect, each must be given in a certain dosage and continued for the proper period of time, depending on the type of infection, its severity, its location, its accessibility to the antibiotic and on the patient's past experience with the drug and his ability to tolerate it.

Some antibiotics have to be injected because they are not absorbed into the blood stream from the stomach or intestines. Some may be taken by mouth because they are absorbed. Some are also taken by mouth because they are meant to act on the intestines locally as an ointment acts on the skin. These would not be effective in an infection of the lungs or kidneys, even though the bacteria causing it were easily destroyed by them, because the drugs, not being absorbed into the blood stream, would not act on the lungs or the kidneys.

DISADVANTAGES OF ANTIBIOTICS

Unfortunately, most viruses and some bacteria are not disturbed by antibiotics. The viruses which cause the common cold, influenza, polio and the various forms of encephalitis are in this group. Unfortunate, too, is the fact that some bacteria which are easily destroyed by an antibiotic may, if they are not completely eradicated, undergo changes (mutations) and become resistant to the antibiotic. The staphylococcus is the prime example of this. It causes boils and impetigo, and in infants it is a common cause of pneumonia. At first, penicillin was the choice drug against the staphylococcus, but gradually, over the years, the staphylococci which were resistant enough not to be destroyed by penicillin in moderate doses, and were not attacked by penicillin in lethal doses, have multiplied until in some hospital wards the incidence of penicillin-resistant staphylococci has risen as high as 60 to 85 per cent. In the case of mutations, the succeeding generations of bacteria which survive the attack of the antibiotics do not necessarily become more resistant; their structures change, so that while they may cause the same disease, they are not harmed by the same antibiotic. The process is very much the same as the evolutionary development of man or animals, in which, because of outside influences, only those flexible enough to change were able to survive. Fortunately, other antibiotics can be given in place of penicillin, just as there are substitutes for most of the antibiotics to which resistance appears, but there are more and more cases of treatment which must be changed because of resistant bacteria.

The body, when its functions are not interfered with by antibiotics, appears to have a fine balance between its various bacteria and molds so that they keep each other under control. Another handicap resulting from the widespread and excessive use of antibiotics is that some of these bacteria and molds which seemed harmless before the bacteria which controlled them were eliminated by antibiotics, have now become a threat. For instance, the mold which is the cause of thrush, and which is often present in the mouths of perfectly healthy children and adults, overgrows when its enemy bacteria are eliminated and produces changes on the tongue, the pharynx, the bronchial tubes (but rarely the lungs) and in the intestines. The staphylococcus, which ordinarily does not produce disease in the intestines, may overgrow and cause diarrhea if an antibiotic which does not disturb the staphylococcus eliminates bacteria harmful to it in the intestines.

Because of this upset in balance, bacteria which were previously not important in producing disease now sometimes cause very stubborn infections in wounds, in the kidneys and elsewhere. These bacteria, known as Pyocyaneus, Proteus, etc., do not respond readily to antibiotics, so they are particularly troublesome. Since the discovery of antibiotics, there has been a tremendous increase in diseases caused by viruses and more in diseases caused by molds. We may well wonder whether this is because we are now able to identify them more easily, or whether by eliminating many of the bacteria in the body, we have removed the barriers against invasion by viruses.

Allergy: Some people who are allergic to or become allergic to antibiotics react with rashes, swollen glands, painful joints and fever. This occurs in about 1 to 2 per cent of children and 10 to 15 per cent of adults who get penicillin. Allergies to other antibiotics are less frequent, but they do occur.

Toxicity: Some antibiotics which are toxic or injurious to specific parts of the body may cause disturbances of balance, kidney damage, irritation and itching around the anus and vulva and irritation of the stomach and intestines resulting in loss of appetite, nausea, vomiting and diarrhea. Dihydro-streptomycin, one of the antibiotics used in treating tuberculous meningitis, may cause temporary or permanent deafness in some patients, but it is one of the few drugs available for treatment of this otherwise always fatal disease. It is no longer recommended.

The antibiotics which cause toxic symptoms are sometimes effective and less toxic in smaller amounts, but usually others have to be substituted.

THE CHOICE OF AN ANTIBIOTIC

The doctor's choice of an antibiotic for any given infection depends on very special knowledge. He must know what bacteria are causing the infection and what antibiotic is most effective against those bacteria. If more than one would be effective, he must know which is most suitable for the particular child. He must know the amount to give, by what method to give it, in what doses and how long to keep up the treatment. Now, this is more than any parent could possibly be expected to know and yet many parents insist on giving advice to the doctor on antibiotics. Parents should neither insist on nor resist the use of antibiotics for a given infection, nor should they try to influence the choice, the dosage or the manner of giving an antibiotic.

If the doctor feels that penicillin is not necessary for a cold or the grippe, parents should not press him to give it. If he wants to give penicillin by injection instead of by mouth, the parents should not try to prevent it because a child dislikes having a "shot." Sometimes parents use antibiotics to treat a child's illness without consulting the doctor, because they feel that the illness is the same as the one for which the medicine was originally prescribed. Since they actually have no way of knowing this, and since, even if it is the same disease, the doctor may want to prescribe different medication or different dosages, he should be asked about it before any medicine is given.

More Than One Antibiotic: There has been a great deal of discussion in medical literature about using more than one antibiotic at the same time. Many doctors question this practice because in some cases one antibiotic interferes with the action of another so that the combination is less effective than one alone would be.

It is generally agreed that it is best to choose a single antibiotic whenever possible, but there are conditions which justify the use of more than one at a time. These are:

1. When there is a mixed infection and no one antibiotic is effective against all of the bacteria involved. For instance, in peritonitis caused by a ruptured appendix or a ruptured ulcer, all of the different bacteria in the intestines may enter the peritoneal cavity.

2. When the antibiotic most suitable for the infection cannot reach it as quickly as other, less effective, drugs, as in some forms of meningitis. Although sulfadiazine is less effective then either Chloromycetin or streptomycin against the influenza bacillus which causes one type of meningitis, sulfadiazine penetrates into the brain and spinal canal more quickly and helps to some extent until the more potent drugs gain entrance. Newer drugs, such as Ampicillin, may replace these.

3. When bacteria quickly develop a resistance to one antibiotic, as the tubercle bacillus does to streptomycin. In treating tuberculosis, para-aminosalicylic acid is used with streptomycin to hasten the destruction of the tubercle bacillus and to avoid or delay its development of resistance to the streptomycin.

4. When the best antibiotic for a certain infection, e.g., streptomycin, is known to be relatively ineffective against another germ, such as the staphylococcus, and the staphylococcus is given free rein after the first infection has been eliminated, an additional antibiotic, such as penicillin or one of the tetracyclines, may prevent the staphylococcus from producing a second disease on top of the first one.

5. When large amounts of one antibiotic cause toxic or allergic reactions, sometimes smaller doses of two antibiotics will be effective and they are less likely to cause the reactions.

Incomplete Treatment: Many children with recurrent fevers due to upper respiratory infections, ear, lymph gland and kidney infections are examples of incomplete treatment. Occasionally a change of antibiotic or the addition of a second is needed. More often, larger doses continued for a longer time are effective.

Cost: Some antibiotics are expensive, others less so. Doctors take this into consideration and choose the less costly one when there are two which are equally effective. There are some diseases, however, which can only be treated with expensive antibiotics, often in large doses or over a long period of time. Children who have such a disease and whose parents cannot afford the proper medication are much better off in hospitals where they can get the most effective treatment.

QUESTIONS & ANSWERS

Q. *Are antibiotics available in every drugstore?*

A. Most of them are. Some of the less frequently used ones may not be stocked in every one. When traveling away from the United States, there may be some difficulty in getting the less common ones, but effective agents are found almost everywhere, especially in hospitals.

Q. *If I find that my druggist does not have the antibiotic my doctor prescribed, is it all right to take the substitute he offers?*

A. Only if the pharmacist first discusses it with your doctor. The doctor may have good reason for wanting a particular preparation. For instance, there are several liquid penicillin preparations. They come in several flavors; some lose their potency in a week, others retain their strength for a year or two. Some can be taken at any time, others may not be taken when there is food in the stomach. Your doctor selects a preparation which suits your child's needs, and a substitute may or may not fulfill all the requirements.

Q. *Why does my doctor sometimes give penicillin by injection instead of by mouth?*

A. There are several reasons. He may feel that the illness requires more rapid and more certain concentration of penicillin in whatever part of the child's body is involved. He is sure that the child will not spit out part of it, that he will not lose any by vomiting, and that the penicillin will not be destroyed by digestion in the stomach. He can inject a kind of penicillin which is slowly absorbed and which produces higher levels in the blood for longer periods which he may not be able to accomplish with penicillin given by mouth. If a child resists taking medicine, a single daily injection is much less trying for him and the family and more certain to help him than a struggle every four hours around the clock.

Q. *My child vomits most medicines. Is there any way of masking them?*

A. Yes. They may go down and stay down better with some milk, or a favorite soft drink, or mixed in some strong-flavored food like chocolate syrup or jam.

Q. *Is it all right to take antibiotics with food?*

A. Yes, in fact with some it is preferable. Some penicillin preparations are destroyed in the stomach when the digestive juices are abundant. Other antibiotics and the sulfa drugs are less likely to have any nauseating effects if they are taken with food, particularly milk.

Q. *Isn't it just as effective to give a large dose of an antibiotic once or twice a day as to give it in smaller amounts every three or four hours?*

A. Yes, with some of them. To be effective against bacteria certain concentrations of antibiotics are needed in the blood of the patient. They are eliminated from the body in certain periods of time. Aqueous (water solution) penicillin, for instance, given by mouth, produces effective levels in the blood for three or four hours. After this time, the penicillin concentration which remains in the body is not enough, so another dose is needed. Giving a larger dose does not always lengthen the time it takes the body to eliminate the penicillin. However, we have longer-acting penicillin, which may be effective for twelve hours or longer, and one type supplies an adequate concentration for some streptococci for two to three weeks. Some antibiotics are effective for six to eight hours. In these cases, the drugs may be given less frequently. Your doctor has this in mind when he gives you directions for the use of all medicines.

Q. *If the antibiotic concentration in the body must be kept at a certain level by giving regular doses, why does my doctor tell me to give my child penicillin at four-hour intervals during the day, but to let him sleep at night?*

Won't the penicillin be eliminated during the twelve hours of the night while he sleeps?

A. Yes, it will, but experience has shown that a high concentration several times a day, or for part of the day, is better than a low one day and night. In a relatively mild infection, such as a sore throat, twelve hours are not enough time for the bacteria to damage the body. In a serious and virulent infection like meningitis, however, your child would be given large doses of antibiotics day and night, so the concentration would be constantly high. In an infection of this kind, the bacteria might do great damage in less than twelve hours.

Q. *Can antibiotics be given by rectum?*

A. Yes, but they are not as effective because we cannot rely on them to be absorbed from the rectum.

Q. *Are antibiotics useful when they are given as a very fine spray into the mouth and nose?*

A. Yes. They are given this way for certain bronchial and lung conditions, and for sinusitis.

Q. *Are they effective in nose drops?*

A. They are often helpful for local infection. Of course, their effect is almost entirely in the surface bacteria with which they come in contact.

Q. *If I let my child get penicillin for a mild infection, will he become immune to it and not be able to take it later for a more serious infection?*

A. This question shows that you need more information about the body's reaction to penicillin. Children do not become immune to drugs. Some bacteria become resistant to the action of penicillin. If the resistance is not too great, larger doses may be used. If it is, a different antibiotic may become necessary. If your child's second infection is due to some other germ which also responds readily to penicillin, then penicillin should be given and it will be effective. About 2 per cent of children develop allergic reactions, rashes, swollen glands, fever, etc. Most are not serious or dangerous and the tendency to react to penicillin is not necessarily permanent. Often these children are able to take it again after an interval of not having had it.

Q. *My child developed diarrhea the last time he took an antibiotic. Does this mean I should not give him the same one again?*

A. No, not if the diarrhea was mild. In any event, remind the doctor of this next time he prescribes it. He may order a substitute unless he feels that the same one is best. Many antibiotics cause mild side reactions, but a single experience with a drug need not determine its future use. Smaller amounts or less frequent doses, or mixing the drug with other substances may avoid the unpleasant reaction.

Q. *My child developed a rash after taking an antibiotic. Must he have a different one the next time?*

A. If another antibiotic would be equally effective, it should be substituted for the one that caused the rash, but if it is necessary to use the same one because it will work better than another, the child should be watched and the antibiotic stopped if there is any unusual reaction. Sometimes allergic reactions are prevented by giving antihistaminic drugs along with the antibiotic. Only your physician can decide what to do.

Q. *My child had an inflamed ear and a swollen lymph gland. Now his temperature is normal and he feels fine. Must he continue taking antibiotics?*

A. It is quite common for an ear or gland infection to flare up again unless treatment is continued for several days after all signs and symptoms have disappeared. Other diseases, too, have to be treated long after the temperature is normal and the child seems well. Bone infection, peritonitis, meningitis and others may have to be treated for as much as three or four weeks after the child appears to be cured. Your doctor is the best judge of when to start an antibiotic, which one and how much.

Q. *Are any of the antibiotics effective against viruses?*

A. Very few are. There is one against influenza, another against smallpox, and some are effective against parrot fever and a venereal disease called lymphogranuloma venereum and against atypical pneumonia caused by the Eaton Agent. (The Eaton Agent is no longer included among the viruses.)

Q. *If antibiotics are not effective against the measles virus, why are they recommended in measles by some doctors?*

A. Some doctors recommend antibiotics in measles because the danger of infection is greater for some individuals— especially infants in the first year or two of life, or others who have tuberculosis or some other active infection. They fear possible complications in general. Antibiotics are not useful in an uncomplicated case of measles. Instead, the patient should be watched carefully and complications which are amenable to treatment should be given appropriate protection. This is equally true for influenza, mumps, chicken pox and other viral diseases. In some parts of the world, bacterial complications of measles are so destructive that early treatment with suitable antibiotics is justified.

Q. *Are antibiotics used very often as preventives rather than cures for disease?*

A. Yes, children who have had rheumatic fever are given penicillin for long periods of time to prevent infection with a streptococcus which may cause a recurrence of rheumatic fever. Streptococcus infections such as scarlet fever, even if they are mild, are treated to avoid rheumatic fever and kidney infections. Children who have almost constant nose and throat infections may avoid them if they are given small doses of antibiotics during the winter and spring. Children who suffer from many other diseases are given antibiotics to prevent the complications which often follow them. Antibiotics are often given to prevent the spread in a household of such diseases as scarlet fever and epidemic meningitis to members of the family who have been exposed to them. It is almost routine to give antibiotics before and after such operations as a tonsillectomy, tooth extractions, operations on the intestines and operations to prevent other infections or the spread of infection in children with heart or chronic lung disease.

Q. *Antibiotics are very expensive. Can one use less expensive drugs?*

A. Many conditions can be treated with the less expensive sulfonamides, but not all of them. Some diseases do not need either the sulfa drugs or antibiotics. Other drugs may serve. In each case where cost of medicine is a factor, your doctor has probably thought of the expense when he ordered the antibiotic. If you think he does not know of the need for economy, you might mention it to him. There are some diseases which can be helped only by certain antibiotics, and only if given in certain doses. Children with such diseases are probably best treated in hospitals if you cannot afford this kind of care at home.

5: Immunization

Children are immune to disease when they have antibodies (protective substances) in their body fluids which effectively overcome the germs which cause the infections. For example, if a child comes in contact with someone who has measles but does not catch it, he is probably immune to measles, and probably has antibodies against the measles virus. This is so in about 83 to 85 per cent of children who do not catch measles on exposure. In the remaining 15 to 17 per cent, the child may be thoroughly exposed to measles and yet not develop it even though he has never had measles and does not have these antibodies to protect him against the measles virus. Later, this same child might catch measles, even though he is only casually exposed. It is not easy to determine why a particular child reacts this way, because there are so many possible explanations for it and so many speculations on why it happens.

A child who is poorly nourished, sickly or tired contracts infections more easily than one who is well nourished, strong and rested.

The amount of infection the child is exposed to may also decide whether or not he comes down with the disease. If a child with measles coughs into the face of a susceptible child, it is likely that the susceptible child has received a large amount of measles virus. If the well child is sitting ten or twelve feet away, he will receive a smaller amount of infection, possibly not enough to produce the disease.

The length of time a child is exposed to infection may also influence his chances of getting the disease. For example, if a child lives in the same room with a measles patient, the chances of his getting measles increase the longer he stays there.

In general, however, a child is immune to a disease either because he possesses antibodies to the germ which causes it or because he has the ability to produce these antibodies quickly when he is exposed to it.

Antibodies against infection can be acquired in four ways. Two of them are called *active immunity,* and two are called *passive immunity:*

A. THE FIRST KIND OF ACTIVE IMMUNITY RESULTS FROM THE CHILD'S ACTUALLY GETTING THE DISEASE. His body reacts to the infection by producing enough antibodies to overcome it and end the disease. In addition, his body produces more antibodies than it needs, and these last in the body fluids for weeks or months, possibly indefinitely. While this process is going on, the child's body acquires the ability to make antibodies to this disease in larger amounts and with greater speed when it is infected again later.

B. THE SECOND KIND OF ACTIVE IMMUNITY IS THE SAME TYPE OF IMMUNITY AS IS PRODUCED BY NATURAL INFECTION, BUT IT IS PRODUCED DELIBERATELY. It is developed when the child's body reacts to injected vaccine made from dead, weakened or live bacteria or viruses, from toxins and from toxoids (toxins which have been made less irritating). Immunization with vaccines and toxoids also makes the body able to produce antibodies rapidly and in large amounts when it is injected again within a limited period of time. This is known as the booster or recall reaction.

C. THE FIRST TYPE OF PASSIVE IMMUNITY IS THE IMMUNITY OF THE NEWBORN INFANT. He has antibodies which he has obtained from the blood of his mother before birth when they had a common bloodstream. Only some kinds of maternal antibodies are able to cross over the placenta to the infant, for antibodies to some diseases may be too large. Of course, only antibodies for infections which the mother has had or has been vaccinated against are available to the infant. This immunity is temporary, lasting from three to six months and less frequently to nine months. It becomes progressively weaker after birth.

D. THE SECOND KIND OF PASSIVE IMMUNITY IS AN IMMUNITY BORROWED FROM THE BLOOD OF PEOPLE OR ANIMALS WHO HAVE HAD THE DISEASES OR HAVE BEEN VACCINATED AGAINST THEM. If a child is given an injection of blood serum or gamma globulin (a protein fraction of blood which includes most antibodies) made from the sera obtained from these people or animals, he gets enough antibodies to protect him for two to five weeks against the disease in question. These antibody preparations are used for both the prevention and the treatment of disease, but they are not effective against all of them. In general, gamma globulin is preventive and sometimes curative, and antiserum is frequently both preventive and curative.

In this chapter I shall take up mostly the types of immunity described in B and D.

ACTIVE IMMUNIZATION

As I have said, it is possible to stimulate the development of immunity to an infection in a child without his actually having the disease. After being injected with a small amount of vaccine or toxoid, the human or animal body reacts by producing antibodies. For example, when diphtheria toxoid is injected into a child (or an adult), his body reacts by producing antibodies to diphtheria toxin. These antibodies enable the child to combat diphtheria. In addition, because his body has once produced these antibodies, it has learned to produce them with great speed and in greater quantities. Once the child has been inoculated with diphtheria toxoid and an immunity has been established, the immunity lasts for a considerable length of time, possibly several years. But it becomes much weaker at the end of one or two years because the antibodies become less abundant or disappear, and are perhaps not sufficient to protect the child against diphtheria. If, at the time when the antibody concentration is dropping, another injection of toxoid is given—even a very small amount of it—the toxoid stimulates the production of antibodies far more than the original injection did. This is known as a booster or recall injection and it serves to maintain immunity at a high level. Probably we maintain some immunities for life by being stimulated often through repeated exposure or by carrying the germ in our bodies indefinitely.

In the last forty years the practice of immunizing infants and young children by injections of toxoids, toxins and vaccines has become very widespread all over the world, perhaps most extensively in the United States. In the following section I shall describe the immunizations against some of the more common or more feared diseases: smallpox, diphtheria, whooping cough, tetanus, typhoid, influenza, tuberculosis, poliomyelitis, measles, mumps, etc.

DIPHTHERIA

Begun on a large scale in 1925–27, immunization against diphtheria caused a sharp drop in the frequency of the disease. A survey of the U.S. Public Health Service reports shows how extraordinarily valuable these immunizations have been. Soon after they were begun, some cities of 100,000 to 150,000 population reported having no cases of diphtheria in a whole year, whereas before immunization was introduced, diphtheria was always present. Today in the United States it is quite difficult to show medical students a case of diphtheria. Some doctors go for many years without seeing one. Although I have seen several hundred cases, I have had only two in my own practice since 1927. All of my patients have been immunized against diphtheria.

In New York City, diphtheria cases have dropped from several thousand to less than one hundred a year. No cases were reported in the past few years. Some of this drop occurred spontaneously, but most of it seems to have followed the beginning of immunization.

All children should be immunized against diphtheria between two and six months of age. Three injections of toxoid given at monthly intervals result in immunity in almost everyone. This immunity does not develop immediately, but some antibodies begin to appear about a week after the first injection. It may take six to twelve weeks, however, to develop enough immunity to be able to withstand a diphtheria infection. This immunity stays at a high level for six months to a year, after which time it slowly diminishes. In some instances it has dropped to an unsafe level by the end of a year. So it is necessary to give another injection, the first booster dose, one year after the last injection. After this, it is customary to give booster doses every two years until school age, and some doctors continue them every three or four years until puberty. Others do a Schick test (which tells whether or not the child is still immune) every two or three years, and if it is positive they give a booster injection. A booster is also given if the immunized child is exposed to diphtheria. There are several different preparations of diphtheria toxoid in use, all of which are effective. The doctor will decide which one to use. When the child has been exposed to a person with diphtheria and is being given a booster because of that, doctors prefer to use a kind of toxoid which builds the immunity much more quickly. This is called fluid or clear toxoid. The routine injections are usually made with alum-precipitated toxoids which take a longer time to become effective, but last longer.

Diphtheria injections in infants and young children usually cause no ill effects, but if the same dose of toxoid is given to a child over six or an adult, it is much more likely to produce reactions, and they are likely to be more severe. There may be local pain, redness, swelling at the injected site, or a general reaction with fever and a grippe-like feeling, or both. Therefore we only give injections to older children and adults after making a skin test with a small dose of diluted toxoid (the Moloney test). If the Moloney test is negative, the toxoid injections may be given as they are for young children except in smaller amounts. If it is positive, it indicates that the person has had previous experience with the toxoid and probably can do without it, or with only a small booster dose of toxoid. A toxoid preparation especially produced for children who are six years or older and adults is now available.

About 65 per cent of infants are born with immunity to diphtheria which has been transmitted to them from their mothers. This passive immunity lasts from three to nine months, but weakens progressively. Since it may have dropped to a level which leaves the infant susceptible at three months, it is not safe to rely on it beyond this time. That is why I usually begin diphtheria toxoid injections at three months. About 35 per cent of infants have no immunity because their mothers are not immune, and for this reason some doctors like to start the injections at one or two months. We can tell by a Schick test whether the infant is immune at birth, and the test can be done either on the mother or the infant, for if the mother is immune, the infant will be also. It is easier to give the toxoid than to test for the presence of immunity.

WHOOPING COUGH

Three doses of whooping cough vaccine injected at monthly intervals stimulate immunity in most infants and children. The immunity is not as reliable as the one produced by diphtheria toxoid, but there is enough favorable evidence to make whooping cough immunization worthwhile. In a test done in a town in England, half of the children received whooping cough vaccine and half did not. Afterward the disease was much more common and more severe in the unvaccinated group. Although I have seen a number of cases of whooping cough in children who had had the vaccine six months to three years before, I have seen much more whooping cough in children who had never had the injections.

Usually whooping cough vaccine is mixed with diphtheria and tetanus toxoids and the three are injected together, but it may be, and often is, given separately. Since the immunity resulting from whooping cough injections does not last as long as the immunity from diphtheria and tetanus toxoid, booster injections should be given more often, every two years, or annually if there is danger of infection, and again if the child is exposed.

Whooping cough is most dangerous in the first year of life, so it is important that infants get this vaccine very early, especially if they live in congested communities.

Whooping cough vaccine produces many more reactions than diphtheria and tetanus toxoids do. Some doctors prefer to give the whooping cough vaccine separately and the two toxoids together for this reason. On rare occasions, after an injection of whooping cough vaccine, an infant develops a very severe reaction, high fever (104° or 105°) and, rarely, a convulsion. In such cases the doctor may decide to give it in small doses of only the aqueous type or he may discontinue the whooping cough vaccine. If the infant is later exposed to whooping cough, he can be helped by an injection of hyperimmune serum or gamma globulin made from the blood of a person who has high immunity to whooping cough. The pertussis vaccines now available are being reevaluated. It is possible that they will be modified so that they cause less reaction and actually induce greater immunity.

TETANUS (LOCKJAW)

Tetanus immunization is probably the most successful of all. The immunity develops quickly after the injections of toxoid and lasts a long time. In World War II there was almost no tetanus among soldiers who had been immunized, while in World War I, when there was no immunization, the cases were numerous.

Tetanus toxoid is usually given in three doses. In the case of infants and young children, it is given as part of a triple vaccine mixed with diphtheria toxoid and whooping cough vaccine, but it may be given separately at any time. It is made as a clear fluid or as a milky alum-treated toxoid. The immunity to tetanus, once established, lasts longer than the whooping cough and diphtheria immunities do. Boosters given periodically after the first one are not required more often than every five years, except when the child is injured in a way that breaks the skin. Then it is wise to give a booster injection if the last dose of toxoid was given more than a year before. This does not, of course, mean that a booster should be given for every scratch or small cut. When the doctor wants to stimulate immunity quickly in case of injury, he uses the *fluid toxoid* rather than the slower *alum-precipitated toxoid*.

If a person has not been immunized with tetanus toxoid and sustains an injury involving a laceration or a puncture wound, he is usually injected with tetanus antitoxin so that he will not develop lockjaw. Antitoxin is generally made from horse serum which may produce a reaction called serum sickness. This can be mild and insignificant or severe and most annoying. If it is repeated or if the child has previously had another horse serum, such as diphtheria antitoxin, it may even be dangerous to life. If everyone were immunized with toxoid, the need for antitoxin would be eliminated, and in my opinion everyone—child and adult—should be. In many clinics when tetanus antitoxin must be given because the patient has not been previously immunized with toxoid, the first dose of toxoid is included in the antitoxin injection, especially if the patient has had antitoxin before.

Antitoxin made from the blood of persons recently immunized with tetanus toxoid is now available in limited amounts. It is choice but quite expensive. It is a great comfort both to the patient and the doctor to know that treatment with antitoxin will not be necessary because the patient is already immune to lockjaw from the injections of toxoid.

COMBINED OR TRIPLE VACCINE

Combinations of diphtheria toxoid, tetanus toxoid and whooping cough vaccine are available and are used extensively. There are several different types of this triple vaccine. They differ mainly in that they are prepared with or without alum. The difference in their effect is primarily the speed with which they are absorbed after being injected into a muscle or under the skin. The ones which are absorbed more slowly last longer and usually stimulate a higher level of immunity. The quickly absorbed ones are more quickly dissipated, though they stimulate antibody production more rapidly. The slow ones are alum-precipitated and the fast ones are called fluid or clear vaccines. Three injections at monthly intervals are usually started at three months of age, often earlier. A booster dose is given one year after the last initial injection, another two years after the first booster, and then boosters every two or three years until school age. Some doctors keep up the regular boosters until puberty.

While most children do not have severe reactions to these injections, occasionally one does. If this happens, it is wiser to give only the diphtheria and tetanus toxoids in the next injections and to eliminate the whooping cough vaccine, which usually accounts for the severe reactions.

Vaccination against smallpox, introduced by Edward Jenner in England in the eighteenth century, was the first kind of immunization practiced. Jenner found that if a person was infected with cowpox (*vaccinia*), he became immune to both cowpox and smallpox. Most vaccinations against smallpox are still done with vaccine made from the cowpox virus.

Vaccination is usually done in the first year of life. Some doctors vaccinate infants during the first few days after birth, others wait two or three months, still others vaccinate between six, nine or twelve months. If there is smallpox in the community, an infant should be vaccinated no matter what his age is. *An infant should not be vaccinated if he or a member of his family has eczema or some other open skin disease,* since a person with eczema easily becomes infected with the cowpox virus and may develop a generalized eruption which resembles smallpox. He should not be vaccinated while being treated with cortisone or A.C.T.H.

Ordinarily, the immunity lasts for several years, but it does drop progressively and the vaccination should be repeated at the end of five to seven years. If you live in an area where smallpox occurs from time to time, it is wiser to be vaccinated every three years, and if the disease is prevalent, as often as every year. No matter when a person has been vaccinated before, if he is actually exposed to smallpox he should be revaccinated immediately. If a person travels outside the United States, he must have proof that he has been vaccinated within three years before he may reenter the country.

Vaccination is done differently in different parts of the world. Some of us, including myself, use the puncture technique. We put a drop of vaccine on the skin of the arm in the case of a boy, or the outer surface of the thigh in a girl, and with a sharp, pointed needle puncture the superficial layers of skin through the drop of vaccine ten to twenty

times. Some doctors make one to four scratches of about a
quarter to half an inch long and supply the vaccine to the
scratched area, or apply the vaccine to the skin first and
scratch through it. Those who use multiple scratches believe
that the immunity which results is greater than the immunity
which follows the use of the puncture technique. The vaccination is not covered until the blister stage when a loose
bandage is put over it so that it will not stick to clothing.

A vaccination shows signs of taking in four or five days
when a small red spot appears. This gets larger and the
center becomes blistered. A red swelling about an inch and a
quarter wide or more develops around the blister. In more
than a third of the children vaccinated, fever between 100°
and 104° develops on the seventh to ninth day and lasts for
one to three days. The glands in the armpit or groin, depending on whether the vaccination is on the arm or leg, usually
become swollen and tender. The blister shrinks, dries and a
scab forms, as the swelling and redness disappear. The entire
course is about two weeks, and the scab falls off in the third
week. This is called a "typical reaction."

If the child has fever from the vaccination which lasts
longer than three days, or returns a day or two later, some
complication may have set in and you should call the doctor.

A person who has been vaccinated before often gets what is
known as an "accelerated reaction." The red spot may develop
in two or three days, and this usually blisters, but the whole
process develops quickly and is over quickly, leaving little
or no scar and usually causing no severe reaction.

An "immune reaction" usually occurs in a person who is
still immune to smallpox from a previous vaccination. The red
spot may come in only a few hours and then disappear rapidly.
There is no scar and often no blister. Sometimes it all comes
and goes so quickly that the person is not aware of it.

If a vaccination does not take at all, it is usually due to
poor vaccine and it should be repeated with fresh vaccine. If
repeated vaccination is done with fresh vaccine known to take
in other children, the child is probably immune and vaccination may be deferred for six to twelve months.

Vaccinia, a complication of vaccination, is more common in
infancy. In countries like the United States where smallpox is
rare, vaccination after one year of age is recommended since

complications are less frequent after that age. Some physicians recommend that vaccination be used only for persons with a higher risk of getting the disease, persons living in areas where the disease is still prevalent or persons traveling to such areas. This recommendation is made only because drugs are now becoming available to combat smallpox. Personally, I am loath to recommend abandoning a procedure which has been successful in such large numbers of people over the entire world. New vaccines which are milder and cause less reaction are being investigated. They are available in limited quantities at present.

POLIOMYELITIS

Professor J. F. Enders was given a Nobel prize for discovering the method for culturing viruses. The production of virus vaccine is directly due to the discovery of polio vaccine, measles vaccine and mumps vaccine.

Vaccines against poliomyelitis have been available since 1955. For several years the vaccine prepared by Jonas E. Salk was recommended generally. It was made from the killed polio virus. It contained some of each of the three strains known to produce the disease. Three injections of this vaccine given at four- to eight-week intervals stimulate the development of immunity. To maintain the immunity with this killed vaccine, it is necessary to give repeated injections at least every two years, preferably every twelve or eighteen months.

The live-virus vaccine, known as the Sabin type, is made from attenuated live viruses and is fed by mouth in contrast to the killed vaccine which has to be injected. The vaccines are prepared separately for each type, I, II or III, or in combination of the three types, known as triple, or combined vaccine. It is recommended that they be given in the following order:

Type I: at two to three months of age, or anytime thereafter, up to eighteen years of age.

Type III: at four to eight weeks after Type 1.

Type II: at four to six weeks after Type 3.

If the triple vaccine is preferred, it is given in the same way as the individual types.

A year after these oral feedings of vaccine, a dose of combined vaccines, including types I, II and III, is fed the patient. It is given again before entering school, at about five or six years of age. If the child is in an area of a polio epidemic, a booster dose should be given immediately if he has had killed vaccine. In the case of live vaccine, a dose of the triple vaccine should be given if the last dose was received a year or longer before.

Salk vaccine, I.P.V., is made of all three types of the polio virus, and the viruses are *inactivated*. This is injected. Although very effective and quite free of reactions, it is not as effective as O.P.V., the live vaccine, or oral polio vaccine. The main differences are the following:

I.P.V.	O.P.V.
Killed-virus vaccine	Live-attenuated-virus vaccine
Less effective than O.P.V.	More effective than I.P.V.
Immunity—transient	Immunity—long-lasting, maybe permanent
Boosters required indefinitely	Boosters given, but may not be required after grade school
Polio possible if booster is omitted	Can be used for exposed children
	Can be used to stop epidemics

Poliomyelitis vaccine, the Salk and the Sabin, both have served to practically eliminate the disease from the United States. The past few years have seen a drop from an average of thirty-five thousand cases to less than two hundred annually, some of which have occurred in children who have received the killed vaccine. In most instances the booster doses were forgotten. Few cases of polio have been associated with the injection of the live vaccine. However, this has happened so infrequently that the danger is considered quite small, as compared with the beneficial effects.

Poliomyelitis vaccine should be given to all infants and young children. In this way the disease can be eliminated from our society.

It may be given to all under eighteen years of age who have not had it before, to persons of any age in, or traveling to or going through high-risk areas.

MEASLES

As a result of the work of Professor J. F. Enders and his associates, the measles virus was cultivated and a vaccine produced. As in the case of poliomyelitis a killed vaccine and a live vaccine were made available. The killed vaccine produces practically no ill effect. Three doses given at monthly intervals immunizes practically 100 per cent of susceptible individuals. This immunity lasts for a year or longer. It was my practice to give live attenuated measles vaccine one month after the second or third dose of killed vaccine. Reactions to the live vaccine were insignificant and practically 100 per cent became immune.

Recently observations have suggested that a year or more after a child has had two to three doses of killed measles vaccine, followed by live measles vaccine, a second dose of live vaccine causes a rise in immunity to measles, but may cause a reaction at the injected site. The reaction is usually an area of swelling, redness, fever and swollen lymph glands in the vicinity of the injection site. I have seen this type of reaction in five patients out of fifty who received the first injection of live vaccine about a year after being given three doses of killed vaccine.

Other observations indicate that infants who received killed vaccine and were exposed to measles after losing the temporary immunity developed a peculiar ailment, a rash starting on the legs, fever and in many instances pneumonia. This has *not* happened to children who were immune either because of having had measles or live virus vaccine. Killed vaccine is therefore no longer recommended and will not be manufactured in the United States.

Live-virus vaccine produces immunity which in almost all instances is long-lasting, possibly lifelong. It should be given to all persons who are not immune, beginning at ten or twelve months and at any other age.

There are many brands of live vaccine which differ in the method of preparation; yet all are effective. They vary in the illness they produce. Some produce fever, most commonly between six to nine days, less frequently on the tenth to fourteenth day after the injection, in about 50 per cent to 75 per cent of the children. A temperature of 103° or more occurs in 15 per cent, 25 per cent or 30 per cent, depending on the vaccine used.

Unlike the polio vaccine, the measles virus is not spread from one child to another, or to other members of the family. Complications resulting from measles vaccine are mild and infrequent. Ear infections, bronchitis, pneumonia and encephalitis, or dysentery are complications of regular measles. Only fever and rash occur after the vaccine. Other complications, especially pneumonia, are very rare and encephalitis hardly ever occurs.

A small amount of gamma globulin given at the time of the administration of the live measles vaccine results in reduction of the fever, rash, etc., and permits the child to be immunized. If, however, too much gamma globulin is given, the immunization effect of the live vaccine may be blocked. I personally reserve the use of gamma globulin for those patients for whom live measles-virus vaccine may involve some risk, such as children with leukemia, Hodgkin's disease or malignant tumors and children with a tendency to convulsions.

INFLUENZA

Virus vaccines against influenza are available and are quite effective. However, this vaccine is not recommended routinely for children. The influenza vaccine is recommended for children with chronic lung disease or with others debilitated by chronic ailments. It is recommended for aged and infirm adults and for those working in hospitals, since they are more likely to be exposed to the disease, and for all others who are at greater risk.

The vaccine is recommended during an epidemic, or where an epidemic seems imminent, and if the particular type of the influenza virus causing the epidemic is known, and if the vaccine available contains that particular strain of virus.

The vaccine available at present is made from several strains of the influenza virus, and is therefore likely to be helpful. A single injection may render immunity, but a second, given two to four weeks after the first, results in greater and longer-lasting immunity.

Influenza vaccine does not prevent the common cold or infections caused by viruses other than the influenza viruses.

ADENOVIRUS (APC OR ADENOIDAL-PHARYNGEAL-CONJUNCTIVAL) INFECTIONS

Some of these viruses, of which there are many, cause inflammation of the lymph glands in the neck, scratchy throat and redness of the eyes, occasionally pneumonia and, less often, encephalitis. Vaccines against some of these viruses are becoming available. These vaccines are not recommended routinely but may be useful in children's homes, institutions, camps and wherever children live in groups. They have been used primarily in military establishments with considerable success.

TUBERCULOSIS

B.C.G. is the name of the tuberculosis vaccine. The initials stand for the Bacillus of Calmette and Guérin, two French scientists. The vaccine is made from tubercle bacilli which have been weakened by being transferred from one culture medium to another repeatedly over a long time. The tubercle bacilli retain most of their usual characteristics, except the ability to produce generalized tuberculosis. When injected into nontuberculous children, instead of spreading through the body and producing widespread tuberculosis, the vaccine produces a small nodule in the arm or leg where it is injected. This infection is mild and remains localized, yet it causes the child to develop a reaction to the germ which can be established by a positive tuberculin test and which, we believe, protects him if he is later infected with disease-producing tubercle bacilli. Usually, a second injection of B.C.G. is given after two years, and where tuberculosis is prevalent, it is again given before entering school, and in some countries in the late teens or early in adult life. The incidence of serious tuberculosis has been reduced in the very groups among which a high rate of tuberculosis might have been expected.*

In the United States, B.C.G. is used for groups with a very high incidence of tuberculosis, like the American Indian. It may be given to individuals not previously infected who are likely to be exposed, such as nurses, medical students, and others working with patients with tuberculosis.

BUBONIC PLAGUE, CHOLERA, RICKETTSIAL DISEASES, YELLOW FEVER

Vaccines are available which stimulate the production of immunity to bubonic plague, cholera, the rickettsial diseases (Rocky Mountain spotted fever, Q fever, typhus, rickettsial pox, etc.), yellow fever and others. These are used almost entirely by people who live in or plan to travel to places where these diseases are prevalent. Yellow fever vaccine can be obtained through the United States Public Health Service, or through the Armed Forces clinics. Your local health department will tell you where you can get the other vaccines.

RABIES

While the Pasteur treatment for rabies gives long-lasting immunity and, therefore, comes under the heading of active immunization, it is never given except when the patient has been infected with or is suspected of having been infected

---

* B.C.G. is used routinely in countries where tuberculosis is prevalent, particularly the Eastern and Near Eastern countries, and some European countries, in the first week of life. When feasible, the newborn infant of a mother with active tuberculosis is removed immediately from the home and returned only when the mother is better and the infant's tuberculin test has become positive.

with rabies, in which case it is given along with antiserum. Rabies is transmitted by rabid dogs and carnivorous wild animals and, in the West Indies and South America, vampire bats. If a child is bitten by an animal, the animal should be captured alive whenever possible and kept under observation for ten days.

In 1960 a special committee of experts on rabies recommended to the World Health Organization the following procedure for immunization against rabies:

CONDITIONS FOR IMMUNIZATION AGAINST RABIES

Kind of Exposure	At Time of Exposure	During 10 Days Following	Treatment
No wound, indirect contact only	Rabid	———	Usually none, but start vaccine immediately if the child is too young to give a reliable account.
Licks: On unbroken skin	Rabid	———	Same as above.
On broken skin and broken or unbroken mucous membrane	(a) Healthy	(a) Healthy	(a) None.
	(b) Healthy	(b) Signs of rabies or proven rabid	(b) Start vaccine at first signs of rabies in animal.
	(c) Signs suggestive of rabies	(c) Healthy	(c) Start vaccine immediately. Stop treatment if animal is normal on fifth day after exposure. *or* (c) Give antiserum and withhold vaccine as long as animal remains normal.
	(d) Rabid, escaped, killed or unknown	(d) ———	(d) Start vaccine immediately.

Kind of Exposure	At Time of Exposure	During 10 Days Following	Treatment
Bites: Few on body	(a) Healthy	(a) Healthy	(a) None.
	(b) Healthy	(b) Signs of rabies or proven rabid	(b) Start vaccine at first signs of rabies in animal.
	(c) Signs suggestive of rabies	(c) Healthy	(c) Start vaccine immediately. Stop treatment if animal is normal on fifth day after exposure. *or* (c) Give antiserum and withhold vaccine as long as animal is normal.
	(d) Rabid, escaped, killed or unknown, or any bite by a wild animal	(d) ———	(d) Start vaccine immediately.
Multiple bites or bites on face, head or neck	(a) Healthy	(a) Healthy	(a) Antiserum immediately. No vaccine as long as animal remains normal.
	(b) Healthy	(b) Signs of rabies or proven rabid	(b) As above, but start vaccine at first sign of rabies.
	(c) Signs suggestive of rabies	(c) Healthy	(c) Antiserum immediately, followed by vaccine. Stop vaccine if animal is normal on fifth day after exposure.
	(d) Rabid, escaped, killed or unknown, or any bite by a wild animal	(d) ———	(d) Antiserum immediately, followed by vaccine.

IMMUNIZATION BY INJECTIONS
OF VACCINE OR TOXOID

Disease	Age for First Injection	Are Boosters Necessary?
Cholera*	Any age if needed.	Yes, if reexposure is possible.
Diphtheria	2–6 months and at any age thereafter.	Yes, first booster in 1 year. Subsequent boosters every 2 years.
Influenza	Any age, if needed.	Yes, if reexposure is likely.
Measles	After 10 months if mother had measles; 3 months if not. At 9 months, or earlier, in areas where measles is severe and dangerous.	Probably not needed after vaccination with live vaccine.
Mumps	Any age, if needed; preschool age, otherwise.	Not yet known. In prepuberty period?
Paratyphoid	Any age, if needed.	Yes, if reexposure is possible.
Plague*	Any age, if needed.	Yes, if reexposure is possible.
Poliomyelitis	2–3 months.	Repeat twice at 6–8 week intervals. Again a year later and at 5 years.
Q fever*	Any age, if needed.	Yes, if reexposure is possible.
Rabies	Any age, if needed.	Yes, if bitten again.
Rickettsial pox*	Any age, if needed.	Yes, if reexposure is possible.
Rocky Mountain spotted fever*	Any age, if needed.	Yes, if reexposure is possible.
Smallpox	First year and at any age thereafter.	Yes, every 5 to 7 years. More often if exposure is possible.
Tetanus (Lockjaw)	2–6 months and at any age thereafter.	Yes, every 3 to 5 years.
Tuberculosis	Any age, if needed.	Yes, after tuberculin test has become negative, about 2 years.
Typhoid	Any age, if needed.	Yes, if reexposure is possible.
Typhus*	Any age, if needed.	Yes, if reexposure is possible.
Whooping cough	2–6 months and at any age thereafter.	Yes, every 2 years.
Yellow fever*	Any age, if needed.	Yes, if reexposure is possible.
Rubella	1 yr. through adolescence	None indicated.

* Not common except in the few areas where the disease occurs.

RECOMMENDED SCHEDULE FOR ACTIVE
IMMUNIZATION AND TUBERCULIN
TESTING

Age

2–3	months	D.T.P.	O.P.V.*	Type I or trivalent
3–4	"	D.T.P.	"	Type III or "
4–6	"	D.T.P.	"	Type II or "
10–11	"	Tuberculin test		
11–12	"	Measles—live-virus vaccine; Rubella vaccine		
12–18	"	Smallpox		
18	"	D.T.P.	O.P.V. trivalent	
2 years		Tuberculin test		
3	"	"	"	D.T.P.
4	"	"	"	

Preschool
  5–6 years   Mumps vaccine—O.P.V. trivalent†
Preschool
  5–6 years   D.T.-Smallpox-tuberculin‡
  10–12 "   "   "   "
  10–12 "   Mumps vaccine, § if indicated by knowledge of
        status of immunity.

   * Oral Poliomyelitis Vaccine.
   † If immunization against polio is started later than 2 to 3 months,
the schedule for primary immunization should be followed.
   ‡ D.T. adult type.
   § Mumps vaccine is new. Exact procedure is not yet settled, but
should precede pubescence. If given at 5 to 6 years it may not be
needed at 10 to 12.

The recommendations of the World Health Organization committee apply even if the biting animal has been previously vaccinated against rabies.

Antiserum is usually prepared in horses. It is given in a
single injection twenty-four hours after the bite. If it is given
between twenty-four and seventy-two hours after exposure,
the quantity must be doubled or tripled. After seventy-two
hours the antiserum is not effective. Hyperimmune serum is
given for all severe exposures such as bites around the head
and neck.

The Pasteur treatment consists of fourteen daily injections
of vaccine. The injections are made into the muscle of the
abdomen. If the bitten child has already had rabies immunization on another occasion, the procedure may be modified

by giving fewer injections according to how long it has been since he received the first course and what his reaction is to the second one.

PASSIVE IMMUNITY

So far, I have discussed immunization by injections of toxoid or vaccine. This active immunity, produced through the production of antibodies, endures for a long time. There are, however, many situations in which it is not safe to wait until the child produces his own antibodies. If he has already been exposed to an infection, he must be protected immediately or within the next few days to keep him from developing the disease. This can be done by injecting him with antibodies to the specific disease which have already been produced by another person or an animal (*see* D on page 55).

Diphtheria antitoxin, tetanus antitoxin, scarlet fever antitoxin, distemper antiserum (for puppies), measles convalescent serum and human gamma globulin are examples of substances which contain antibodies against the respective diseases. The antibody-containing animal serums are prepared by injecting toxoid or vaccine into horses, rabbits, chickens, sheep, dogs, etc. The animals react to the various vaccines by producing antibodies to the diseases. These antibodies are in the animals' blood, and it is this blood from which the antitoxin or antiserums are prepared. Human hyperimmune serums are prepared from the blood of people who have had the disease in question, and are later given booster doses of vaccine to stimulate the production of more antibodies, as for whooping cough. This blood has a high antibody content which makes it especially useful.

While antibodies to some diseases can be produced in animals, some diseases, especially some caused by viruses, are quite limited to people, and attempts to infect animals with the germs are not very successful. To obtain antibodies to these diseases, for instance, measles and infectious hepatitis, it is necessary to use the blood of people who have recovered from the diseases.

MEASLES

If a child who has not had measles is exposed to it, and it is considered necessary to protect him, he must be supplied with antibodies to measles. This is done with an injection of human convalescent serum (blood serum taken from people who have recently recovered from measles) or gamma globulin, which is a substance extracted from the blood of people who have had measles. Convalescent serum and gamma globulin act in exactly the same way. If you know your child has been exposed to measles, you should tell his doctor promptly, since he may wish to inoculate the child with gamma globulin, either to prevent the measles entirely or to give the child just enough antibodies to make the disease milder. In most cases, it is more desirable to modify the measles because the mild form of measles is quite harmless and the immunity from it lasts many years, maybe for life. Only 1 to 2 per cent of children with modified measles develop complications as compared with 25 per cent of those with ordinary measles not treated with antibiotics.

The injection of gamma globulin or convalescent serum should be made between the first and sixth day, preferably on the third, fourth or fifth day, after exposure. If it is given on the seventh or eighth day, a larger amount of gamma globulin is needed and it may not modify the measles. When the injection is given very soon after exposure and in a large enough quantity to avoid the disease altogether, it is successful in about 80 to 85 per cent, causes modification in 10 to 15 per cent and has no effect in 2 to 5 per cent of all cases. Gamma globulin given to modify measles probably avoids the worst complication—encephalitis.

INFECTIOUS HEPATITIS

Infectious hepatitis (inflammation of the liver caused by a special virus) is influenced by the use of gamma globulin. If, therefore, a child is exposed, it is wise to try to avoid it entirely by giving him an injection of gamma globulin as soon as possible. The injection is not effective once the disease has begun. As in the case of measles, if infectious hepatitis breaks out in a school or an institution, it is often necessary to inject everyone who is liable to be exposed to it in order to stop the epidemic.

DIPHTHERIA

Susceptible children exposed to diphtheria used to be given antitoxin made from horse serum, but now they are given antibiotics, usually penicillin, instead. They are much safer, since there is no danger of serum reactions. They should be given immediately after exposure. Toxoid should be given promptly.

SCARLET FEVER

Convalescent serum or antitoxin is unnecessary since penicillin or other antibiotics rapidly destroy the streptococcus which causes the scarlet fever.

TETANUS

Children who sustain puncture wounds or other wounds in which there may be tetanus germs and have not been actively immunized with tetanus toxoid should be given tetanus antitoxin. First a test for serum sensitivity is made because the antitoxin is made from horse serum. Then the antitoxin is given in one injection. The injection should be given within twenty-four hours after the accident. If the period is longer, the dose must be larger. If the wound is not clean and healing after a week, the injection is repeated. When human hyperimmune serum is available it is preferred to horse serum antitoxin.

Disease	Substance Used	Effectiveness in Preventing or Modifying the Disease	Effectiveness in Treatment of Disease	Comment
Chicken pox	Convalescent serum or gamma globulin	Questionable Large doses suggested	Not known	Not recommended generally.
Diphtheria	Antitoxin	Very good	Excellent	Absolutely a must. Lifesaving as treatment.
Erysipelas	Penicillin	Good	Good	Penicillin is best.
German measles	Gamma globulin	Doubtful	None	Recommended only for pregnant women in early months of pregnancy, who are exposed.
Measles	Gamma globulin or convalescent serum	Very good	Fair	Slightly beneficial as treatment if given before rash appears.
Mumps	Convalescent serum or gamma globulin made from mumps convalescent serum	Fair	Not good, but doubtful results may be obtained when very large dose is injected early in disease	More valuable in prevention. Not recommended for treatment.
Poliomyelitis	Gamma globulin before exposure	Said to be good	Not good	Less effective after exposure.
Scarlet fever	Penicillin	Good	Good	Serums are rarely used. Sulfa drugs and antibiotics are preferable.
Tetanus	Antitoxin	Good	Fair to good	Human antitoxin is preferable.
Whooping cough	Hyperimmune serum or gamma globulin made from it	Fair to good	Fair to good	Used with antibiotics.

WHOOPING COUGH

When a susceptible child is exposed to whooping cough, he should be given immune serum or hyperimmune gamma globulin as soon as possible. These are usually given along with antibiotics.

CHICKEN POX, MUMPS

Gamma globulin and convalescent serum have been used in cases of mumps and chicken pox with doubtful results. They are not recommended for general use, but may be tried under special circumstances and may be more effective if given in large doses.

GERMAN MEASLES

It is considered unnecessary to immunize children against German measles (rubella); in fact, it is believed that girls are better off if they have had German measles before they are married. In the event of exposure to it, nothing should be done except in the case of a woman who has not had it and has been pregnant for less than 3 months. She should be given inoculations of large amounts of gamma globulin, 20 to 40 cc.'s might be given to try to prevent or modify the disease. This is especially important if the pregnancy is in the first three months, and is less significant later. There is some question as to how much good gamma globulin will do, but since it is the only substance which might possibly help, it is often recommended under these circumstances.

Vaccines against rubella are in the experimental stage and are very promising.

IMMUNITY TRANSMITTED FROM MOTHER
TO NEWBORN (PASSIVE IMMUNITY)
AND HOW LONG IT LASTS

Disease	Passive Immunity in Infant	Duration
Boils	No	———
Chicken pox	No	———
Common cold	No	———
Diphtheria	Yes	Up to 6 months, possibly 9 months.
Dysentery	No	———
Ear infection	No	———
German measles	Yes	3–6 months.
Impetigo	No	———
Influenza	Some in some infants, but not enough to ward off a heavy dose of infection.	———
Measles	Yes	6 weeks to 6–9 months.
Mumps	Yes	2–6 months.
Poliomyelitis	Yes	Exact period not known. Probably several months.
Roseola	No	———
Scarlet fever	Yes	Up to 6 months, but not to be relied on when treatment is considered.
Smallpox	Yes	Variable. Infants should be vaccinated.
Syphilis	No	———
Tetanus	Yes	Inadequate for protection. Toxoid should be given.

IMMUNITY TRANSMITTED FROM MOTHER
TO NEWBORN (PASSIVE IMMUNITY)
AND HOW LONG IT LASTS (*Continued*)

Disease	Passive Immunity in Infant	Duration
Tuberculosis	No	———
Typhoid	Probably yes	Not known.
Typhus fever	No	———
Whooping cough	No, although antibodies have been found in the newborn, especially when the mother had had whooping cough or injections of vaccine during pregnancy.	———

The chart above indicates the many diseases to which newborn babies may be immune. They can be immune only if their mothers are immune to the disease in question, and mothers can be immune only if they have had the disease or have been actively immunized. The immunity of the infant lasts varying lengths of time and becomes weaker and weaker as the infant grows older. Even when infants have some immunity to a disease, it is not wise or safe to expose them unnecessarily unless you plan to take advantage of the existing partial immunity to develop a mild infection and thereby give them lasting, possibly permanent immunity. This should never be done without a doctor's direction.

If an infant does not possess immunity to a disease, exposure to infection is particularly unwise, since infection in the newborn period and infancy is usually worse and more dangerous than after the first year.

RABIES

Rabies antiserum is discussed under active immunization because it is so often used along with rabies vaccine.

SKIN TESTS

Skin tests are made for three reasons. Some reveal whether or not a child is immune to the disease. Others indicate only whether the child has ever been infected with the disease. The third type of test is used to find out whether a child is sensitive to a certain substance. For example, a child who has hay fever may be sensitive to the pollen of ragweed, June grass or some other plant.

Skin tests are made in various ways: by injecting the testing material into the skin as in the Schick, Dick, tuberculin and allergy tests; by scratching the skin and applying the testing material to the scratch as in the Von Pirquet tuberculin test and allergy tests; or by impregnating gauze or blotting paper with the substance to be tested and keeping it in contact with the skin for one to two days. This is known as the patch test and is done for tuberculosis and for certain allergies. The choice of the type of test, when to do it, how often to repeat it, how to interpret it and what to do about it after the results are known are decisions which must be left to the doctor.

The tests most often used are the Schick test for immunity to diphtheria and the tuberculin test which tells whether a person has been infected with tuberculosis.

SCHICK TEST

A small but measured amount of diphtheria toxin is injected into the skin. If it is positive, an inflamed area about one centimeter in diameter will appear and persist for at least four to five days. If the test is negative, the skin will not be discolored after forty-eight hours. A positive Schick test means that the child's immunity to diphtheria is entirely absent, or that his level of immunity is too low to give a negative Schick test (too low to neutralize the small amount of diphtheria toxin injected into the skin), or that although he is immune, his skin has temporarily lost its ability to react to the injected diph-

SKIN TESTS

Test	Positive	Negative	Comment
Schick	Not immune to diphtheria.	Immune to diphtheria.	If positive, needs diphtheria toxoid.
Dick	Not immune to scarlet fever.	Immune to scarlet fever.	Needs medical attention if test is positive and child is exposed to scarlet fever.
Tuberculin	Infected with tuberculosis (infection may be healed or active).	Does not have tuberculosis or has old, healed infection.	If positive, a careful examination is necessary to find out where it is, and whether active or healed.
Mumps	Immune to mumps.	Not immune to mumps.	Test about 90% reliable.
Brucellosis	Infected at time of test or before.	Not infected.	————
Allergy	Sensitive to the testing substance.	Not sensitive to the testing substance.	Significance must be evaluated by a doctor.
Toxo-plasmosis	Infected.		A positive Sabin-Feldman test indicates infection sometime in the past.

theria toxin because of some acute febrile illness. If a child is given a Schick test during some acute illness, especially pneumonia, there may be a positive reaction even though the child is immune to diphtheria toxin. Within two weeks after his recovery from the acute infection, the same child will have a negative Schick test just as he did before his illness.

If a young child has never been injected with diphtheria toxoid, the Schick test should be, and usually is, positive. An infant, however, may have a negative Schick test up to six to nine months and occasionally longer because of the immunity transmitted to him from his mother. This immunity is gradually lost so that the results of the Schick test vary from month to month. It is negative in about 65 to 85 per cent of newborn babies, and by nine months of age only about 10 per cent of babies have negative Schick tests. Those whose tests have become positive after having been negative earlier have lost the passive immunity transmitted to them from their mothers.

TUBERCULIN TEST

The tuberculin test is usually done by the injection of a measured amount of tuberculin into the child's skin. This is done in various ways, by applying several small pinpricks with points covered with the tuberculin, or by injecting a measured amount of tuberculin or an extract of the tuberculin (P.P.D.). The test is positive if the injected area becomes red and elevated, and is about a half inch in diameter, and remains discolored for at least three to four days. A positive test indicates that the child has been infected with TB a minimum of six weeks before, or even many years before. The test must be done and interpreted by a person well acquainted with the reaction.

In a child who has been recently infected with tuberculosis, it takes five or six weeks for the skin test to become positive. If there is good reason to believe that a child has recently been infected and a test is made and found negative, another test with a larger amount of tuberculin should be made later to make sure. After a case of measles, after an injection of live measles vaccine and less frequently during or after other illnesses, the tuberculin test may be negative even though the child is known to have tuberculosis. These severe forms of illness cause what is known as tuberculin anergy, an inability to react to the tuberculin used for the test. This anergy lasts for about two weeks, occasionally up to four, after measles, but may last for months in very severe tuberculosis. Measles vaccine may also interfere with the reaction to the tuberculin test.

A positive tuberculin test is not necessarily a bad sign since a person can have a positive test for five, ten, fifteen years or even longer after the tuberculosis is healed. Some doctors feel that having a healed tuberculosis condition helps the person to combat later infection with tuberculosis. Since it takes twelve to eighteen months for tuberculosis to heal, a positive test in an infant is more significant. In the first year it would indicate an active tuberculous infection somewhere in the body, or one which has not yet healed completely. A positive test six months after a child has had a negative one means that he has been infected with tuberculosis during that six-month period and that his is an active case.

Every child should have a tuberculin test made before entering school. Some doctors make this test as a routine thing every year or two during their general examination of the child. This makes it possible to recognize an infection early and to start the necessary treatment.

IMMUNIZATIONS FOR FOREIGN TRAVEL

If you are planning to travel in foreign countries you will find that immunization against the diseases prevalent in those countries is either required or advised, and that to return to the United States you must have proof of immunization against smallpox. Be sure to ask your doctor when you should start having the injections. Some take a longer time to stimulate immunity than others, and some require more doses than others.

Smallpox: If you are traveling to an area where smallpox is prevalent, vaccination should be repeated even if the child was vaccinated a year before. To reenter the United States, you must be able to show evidence that you have been vaccinated within the past three years.

Typhoid, Paratyphoid: Vaccine is recommended for travel into any area with primitive sanitation or a poorly controlled water and milk supply. In these areas, do not eat raw shellfish or drink raw milk or ordinary tap or well water even if you have been immunized.

Tetanus: It is safer for everyone to be immunized. Get a booster if you have not had one within three years.

Diphtheria: Toxoid is recommended for children going to countries where diphtheria is prevalent or likely to occur.

Boosters are suggested for a young child who has not had toxoid for 2 years.

Plague: Plague vaccine* is not required by any country, but it is recommended by some for people entering endemic areas such as certain parts of India, Burma, Java, China, Madagascar and south, central and east Africa. Booster injections are needed every four to six months if you stay in an area where plague is a hazard.

Poliomyelitis: Poliomyelitis is still a common disease in some parts of the world. Be sure you have been immunized with live-virus vaccine within a year or with killed vaccine in the past six months before visiting these countries. The U.S. Public Health Service will tell you whether polio is a danger in the country you expect to visit.

Epidemic Typhus: Vaccination is recommended for those traveling to many parts of the world—Africa, the East and Near East, the Balkans, Poland, Russia. Boosters are needed annually where typhus is prevalent.

Cholera: Vaccination against cholera* is mandatory for travel to India and other parts of southeast Asia. Cholera is absent from the western hemisphere. A booster injection should be given every six months if you stay where danger of infection exists.

Yellow Fever: Vaccination* may be indicated where the disease is endemic to human beings and jungle primates in central and western Africa, the interior or jungles of Brazil and in parts of all other South American countries. One injection gives immunity in ten days, and some countries will not allow travel to these areas until ten days after vaccination. Immunity may last for four years, after which another injection is necessary.

Measles: Measles is a more common disease in the first year of life in many countries. If traveling to such areas be sure to give vaccine even before six months of age if necessary.

* Plague, cholera and yellow fever vaccine are not readily available except through the U.S. Public Health Service and in military clinics at points of embarkation.

QUESTIONS & ANSWERS

Q. *Is immunization against infection practiced all over the world?*

A. Not everywhere, and not to the same degree in all countries.

Q. *Can I have my child immunized without paying a private doctor's fee?*

A. Yes. In most parts of the world the child can be immunized in hospital clinics or through the local health department. (Always ask about charges before immunization.)

Q. *Do older children and adults have to be immunized against disease?*

A. Positively yes. Older children should be if they have not been before. Immunization against polio, measles, tetanus and smallpox are musts. When rubella vaccine becomes available it, too, will be a must. Mumps vaccine should also be given to pubescent children and young adults, especially nonimmune males. In the case of diphtheria, a test can be made. If the child proves to be susceptible, the injections are necessary. Adults should be immunized against diphtheria if they are likely to be exposed to it and are susceptible. It is wise for all children and adults to be immunized against tetanus, and everyone should be vaccinated against smallpox. It is not very important for older children to be immunized against whooping cough, since it is less dangerous for them. Anyone, young or old, should be immunized against any disease prevalent in his community or occurring in epidemic form among both children and adults. And he should be immunized against diseases which are prevalent in places where he plans to travel.

Q. *Does it matter which brand of vaccine or toxoid is used?*

A. Not generally. All preparations made by licensed pharmaceutical firms must measure up to standard specifications established by the U.S. Public Health Service before being released to the public. They are all effective and they are all dated.

Q. *Should a pregnant woman be immunized to diseases she has not had so that her infant will be immune when he is born?*

A. I do not think so, usually. In particular circumstances it may be very useful and at times very important to do, but this is an individual matter you should discuss with your doctor.

Q. *May my child visit a friend who has polio (diphtheria, whooping cough, German measles, typhoid) if he has been immunized against these diseases?*

A. No. It is not wise, and it may not be safe to let him expose himself deliberately to any of these. Immunity is a complicated and relative affair. He may be immune to diphtheria, yet the immunity may not be strong enough to ward off the disease if he is heavily infected. During the last war, some of our soldiers who had been injected against typhoid fever and vaccinated against smallpox every year nevertheless developed these diseases. This does not happen often, but you should avoid being exposed to disease whenever it is possible, except when it is especially recommended, as in the case of German measles for young girls.

Q. *Is it wise to expose my children to measles deliberately?*

A. No. It is preferable to immunize your child with measles vaccine. The results are more certain, more uniform and safer than having measles. It is so rare to have measles a second time that it would be quite safe for a child to visit a friend with measles if the diagnosis is definite. If there is any doubt as to whether the child has measles, avoid visiting.

Q. *May my child have routine immunizations in the summer when there is polio in the community?*

A. Yes. The child should receive the first oral polio vaccine at two months, whatever the time of year. During an outbreak of polio, vaccination with one type of polio vaccine may replace the type causing the outbreak. After

the polio immunization, the other may be started, particularly if there is an outbreak of diphtheria, whooping
cough or smallpox in the community. Should your child
be exposed to any of these diseases, suitable protective
measures should be promptly taken.

Q. *My child goes to a summer camp at the end of June. When
should he get his immunizations?*

A. At least six weeks before he leaves for camp if he is having
the initial injections, or two or three weeks for boosters.

Q. *Wouldn't they be effective if he had them two or three
days before he left?*

A. It takes about six weeks for the effect to reach its peak,
sometimes longer. Booster doses usually stimulate a higher
level of immunity in a week or two. So if you wait until
two or three days before he leaves, he may not be adequately immune when he gets there.

Q. *Does a Schick test serve the same purpose as a diphtheria
injection?*

A. No, it is not a substitute for immunization. In a person who
has immunity it may serve as a booster injection. In most
circumstances a booster dose of toxoid is preferable since
it stimulates greater immunity. By no means should one
rely on a Schick test to produce adequate immunity in a
person who was not previously immunized.

ACTIVE IMMUNIZATION

Q. *Is it better to get the diphtheria, tetanus and whooping
cough (pertussis) injections together or separately?*

A. I prefer to give them together, since it reduces the number
of injections from nine to three. Children do not like
injections, nine visits to the doctor are expensive and time-
consuming, and as a result the parents are less likely to
bring the child for all of the nine necessary visits. Most
important of all, the immunity which results from the
three injections of combined vaccine and toxoids is at
least as great and usually greater for each of the three
diseases than if each immunization were given separately.
There seems to be more antibody production when two,

three or four vaccines are injected at the same time. This is not true of more than four, however.

Q. *Is it ever better to give the injections separately?*

A. Yes, if there is a severe reaction to the combined vaccines. The reaction is usually caused by the whooping cough vaccine and this can be left out of the combination and given separately in smaller doses, or discontinued altogether.

It is often necessary to give a single booster of tetanus toxoid in case of injury. In case of exposure to diphtheria or whooping cough, a booster dose of that particular toxoid or vaccine is all the child may need.

Q. *Is the reaction the same to all three injections?*

A. Not necessarily. Sometimes there is little reaction to one of the injections and more to another.

Q. *If the reaction to the first injection is very severe, does it mean the others will be, too?*

A. They may be, but not always.

Q. *My child developed a hard lump on his arm where the injection was given. Does that happen often? And will it go away?*

A. It happens sometimes and it may last for several months. It is not painful or harmful and is a minor difficulty considering the great value of the immunity acquired from the injection.

Q. *Are some vaccines less likely to produce these lumps than others?*

A. Yes, the clear toxoid preparations are less likely to, but doctors usually prefer to use the toxoids prepared with alum because the immunity the child gets from them lasts longer.

Q. *I was vaccinated against smallpox as a child, but do I need it again?*

A. Yes.

Q. *How often should I be vaccinated against smallpox?*

A. Every five to seven years, if you live in an area quite free of smallpox. Every one to three years where it is more common. Local regulations vary. When you travel abroad, you may not reenter the United States without having been vaccinated within three years.

Q. *I was vaccinated successfully a year ago. Now there are some cases of smallpox in the town where I live. Must I be vaccinated again?*

A. Yes, be vaccinated again immediately.

Q. *Will I get the same reaction to the next smallpox vaccination that I had the first time?*

A. Probably not. The vaccination will take more quickly, last a shorter time, be milder and be less likely to produce a blister or a scar.

Q. *When I was vaccinated the second time, there was no scar. Does that mean it did not take?*

A. It took if it produced a red pimple. The pimple usually itches. But if there was no evidence of a take at all, have it repeated with fresh vaccine.

Q. *Is the Sabin polio vaccine available everywhere?*

A. Yes, except in remote parts of the world.

Q. *How many doses of Salk vaccine are required?*

A. Three injections given at intervals of 4 to 6 weeks, beginning at two months of age.

Q. *How often are boosters required?*

A. One year after the three injections, again annually or at least every two years thereafter, if Salk vaccine is to be continued.

Q. *Can one give the live vaccine after using the Salk vaccine?*

A. Yes, this is recommended.

Q. *Under such circumstances how many doses of live vaccine should be given?*

A. Three. Either three doses of trivalent or triple Sabin type vaccine, beginning at two to three months of age and repeated at four- to eight-week intervals, a fourth dose in a year, and again upon entering school. The alternate method which is more widely recommended is as follows: Give Type I live vaccine at the time of the first D.P.T.

vaccine at two months of age. Give Type III at the time of the second D.P.T. and a dose of Type II at the time of the third D.P.T. A year later give a dose of the triple or trivalent Sabin type vaccine and repeat this before entering school.

The end results of both methods are about the same: over 90 per cent of the vaccinated become immune to Type I, and nearer 100 per cent to Type II and III.

Q. *Can you be immunized against boils?*

A. Yes. The results vary and are unpredictable in any one patient. This is usually tried after other treatment has failed.

Q. *Do you think vaccination against boils is advisable?*

A. Yes, but only occasionally if antibiotics have not been successful.

Q. *What about the vaccines against influenza?*

A. They may be useful when there is an epidemic. They are recommended for older people and those of any age who have chronic lung or heart disease.

OTHER VACCINES

Virus vaccines have been successfuly used to prevent infection with some adenoviruses, influenza viruses, etc., but vaccines are not yet available to prevent infection with some of the other troublesome viruses.

Bacteria are often found in the nose and throat of patients with colds. A vaccine made of these bacteria is known as catarrhal vaccine, and if prepared from the bacteria recovered from the patient's nose and throat it is known as autogenous vaccine. There is little proof that these vaccines prevent colds. Most doctors doubt it. Others feel that the vaccine helps children who are allergic and get asthma with their colds.

Q. *Is there any other vaccine used regularly for children?*

A. Not in the United States, but in other parts of the world, vaccines against diseases prevalent locally are used as a regular injection. For instance, the inhabitants of other countries are routinely immunized against typhoid, yellow fever, cholera, bubonic plague and, in many places, tuberculosis.

Q. *Is there an immunizing agent for scarlet fever?*

A. Yes, but it is not needed because antibiotics stop and prevent the disease.

Q. *Is there a test for immunity to scarlet fever?*

A. Yes, the Dick Test, but the test material is hard to get.

Q. *Is there an immunizing injection for erysipelas and for streptococcus sore throat?*

A. No. They are both caused by the various types of streptococcus germ which are readily eliminated by penicillin or other antibiotics.

Q. *Can you be immunized against chicken pox?*

A. No, not really, but very large doses of gamma globulin may modify the disease in those exposed to it.

Q. *Can you be immunized against mumps?*

A. Yes. The vaccine has been proven to be effective.

Q. *When do you immunize people against mumps?*

A. At any time after the first eight months of age. In particular before age twelve, in the prepuberty and adolescent period and in young adults who have no record of having had mumps. I recommend immunization before school begins.

Q. *Can you be immunized against rubella (German measles)?*

A. Vaccines against rubella look very promising, but may not be available for routine use for some time. They are being tested at present.

Q. *If and when these vaccines against German measles are available, should they be given to all children?*

A. Yes, and to all women prior to their becoming pregnant, if they have not had the disease.

Q. *Can you be immunized against colds?*

A. There is no vaccine which will prevent "colds." Ordinarily the term "cold" is used to indicate an upper-respiratory infection, a stuffy or a running nose, a scratchy throat with or without a cough. However, the so-called cold can become complicated by bronchitis, bronchiolitis and even pneumonia, and may be caused by one of many agents—viruses in particular. Efforts to produce vaccines against the viruses which cause colds are being made in many laboratories.

Q. *Are measles and mumps encephalitis helped by gamma globulin?*

A. No. If given to modify measles, encephalitis rarely, if ever, occurs, but it is not helpful as treatment for the encephalitis after it has developed.

Q. *Is gamma globulin effective for any other diseases?*

A. It prevents infectious hepatitis, it prevents polio in experimental animals and there is evidence that it may prevent polio in humans if enough of it is given before the infection takes place. Special gamma globulin can be produced which are helpful in many other diseases. Large doses may prevent chicken pox.

PASSIVE IMMUNIZATION

Q. *Is the gamma globulin which is used to prevent measles or to make it milder the same kind used for infectious hepatitis and polio?*

A. Yes.

Q. *Are there any other gamma globulins?*

A. Yes. Special gamma globulin is sometimes prepared from the blood of people who have recently recovered from an infection, for example, whooping cough, tetanus, mumps. These are called hyperimmune GG.

Q. *Is gamma globulin always effective against measles?*

A. Usually, if it is given before the disease develops in order to make it milder, but it is only about 85 per cent effective if it is given to prevent measles entirely.

Q. *Does it do any good to give gamma globulin for measles after the rash appears?*

A. Not usually. Large doses given on the first or second days of the disease, before the rash appears, may lighten and shorten the disease.

Q. *Will live vaccine prevent measles after exposure?*

A. If given on the first or possibly on the second day of exposure, it may result in milder measles.

PASSIVE IMMUNITY TRANSMITTED BY THE MOTHER

Q. *If an infant has immunity to a disease at birth, is that immunity strong enough so that he can avoid the infection altogether?*

A. Yes, for some time. As the immunity grows weaker, the infant may develop a mild form of the disease if he is exposed again, and later as the immunity decreases, he may develop the ordinary form of the disease.

Q. *If an older child has measles, should his three-month-old infant sister be given gamma globulin to protect her against it?*

A. Yes, a small dose should be given in the hope that it will either protect her entirely or that she will get a modified form of the disease which usually gives lasting immunity. At three months the level of immunity acquired from the mother is often not high enough to completely protect the infant from intimate exposure.

Q. *Why are infants immune to some diseases and not to others?*

A. Infants are not immune to diseases to which their mothers are susceptible, and even if the mother is immune, the antibodies for some diseases do not seem to cross over from the mother to her infant. The molecule size of the antibiotics may be too large to pass across the placenta.

Q. *Do newborn infants get tuberculosis?*

A. Yes. When the mother has active tuberculosis, as many as 25 per cent of newborn infants may become infected, presumably while being born or soon after birth.

Q. *Do newborn infants get chicken pox?*

A. Yes, if they are exposed to it.

Q. *Are newborn infants ever born with an infection?*

A. Yes. Infants have been born with syphilis, pneumonia, malaria, German measles, toxoplasmosis, chicken pox, measles, and tuberculosis.

Q. *If an infant is born with an infection, how did he get it?*

A. The mother must have had the disease shortly before the infant was born and the infant contracted it from the mother by way of the placenta and bloodstream, or as with thrush or Herpes simplex virus infection, the infant contracts the infection at the time of birth from the mother's vagina. In the case of German measles the mother was infected early in pregnancy.

Q. *If an infant has no immunity to measles or mumps and is exposed to either of them, can he be infected and develop a long-lasting immunity without showing many symptoms?*

A. Yes. We assume that the infection can stimulate immunity to a high degree even though the infant is not very sick. This is sometimes offered as an explanation of why some people seem to have a "natural" immunity to some diseases.

Q. *Is it possible and advisable to give vaccine injections to a pregnant woman so that she will develop immunity and pass on some of it to her infant?*

A. It is possible, and occasionally it is advisable. But generally I prefer not to give vaccine or toxin injections to a pregnant woman unless there is an epidemic of some disease for which vaccination is successful. In that case it would really be for the protection of the mother, although indirectly it might benefit the child.

SKIN TESTS

Q. *Are there any other skin tests for detecting diseases besides the ones you have mentioned?*

A. Yes, there are many more. For example, tests similar to the tuberculin test can be made to detect some fungus diseases like histoplasmosis and coccidioidomycosis. They show whether or not the patient is or has been infected with the particular fungus. There is also a skin test for trichinosis, an infection acquired by eating undercooked pork, and for toxoplasmosis and other infections.

Q. *Are skin tests always reliable?*

A. They vary. Tests for infections or immunity are generally quite reliable. The tuberculin test is usually reliable when read by an experienced person. If the test is called positive, it should be repeated. If called negative, a stronger test should be done if tuberculosis is believed to be active. The Schick test is very reliable except in the newborn period and when done during an acute illness such as pneumonia. Tests for allergy are notoriously unreliable in babies under one year, although they are usually accurate in older children. Some tests may indicate sensitivity to the test material when it really does not exist, or the test may be negative although the patient is really sensitive to the substance. Regardless of the reaction to any test, when it is made on a sick child to try to determine the presence of an infection, the result has to be interpreted by the doctor in relation to the symptoms of the disease which are present at the time. Tests are very useful aids to diagnosis.

Q. *Are skin tests made by injecting the material into the skin more reliable than scratch tests and patch tests?*

A. In general, yes. The amount of material injected is more accurately measured than when you rely on the skin to absorb the material through a scratch or from a patch.

Q. *Are skin tests ever injurious?*

A. Usually no, but occasionally yes. In some diseases, especially tuberculosis, it is safer to make the test with a small amount of material first since a large amount may produce an unpleasant reaction. If the child has a negative reaction to a small amount of tuberculin, a larger amount of it can be used safely in the next test. Excessive amounts of diphtheria or scarlet fever toxins may cause inflammation at the site of the injection, but rarely do they produce general reactions. In fact, sometimes a Schick test boosts the immunity of a partially immune person to a high enough level to ward off infection.

Skin tests for allergy have been known to cause very severe general reactions of shock when the material is injected into the skin, but this almost never happens if the material is applied to a scratch on the skin. You should not worry about reaction to skin tests. The doctor knows these facts and always considers them carefully when he makes a test.

6: Hygiene

PRENATAL HYGIENE

Hygiene against infection should begin long before the child is born. In the chapter on German measles I stress that if a woman develops the disease within the first three months of pregnancy her baby may be born with physical defects. Other diseases in the early period of pregnancy may lead to abortion, stillbirth and possibly abnormalities like those we find with German measles. Less significant in most cases, but potentially serious, is that infants may be born with such diseases as chicken pox, measles, smallpox, malaria and toxoplasmosis, or develop them in a week or two after birth, if the mother was ill with one of them during the last few days or weeks of her pregnancy. Therefore it is very important that pregnant women avoid undue exposure to disease. Indeed, this is true for everyone unless the doctor advises deliberate exposure to a disease. There are sometimes special reasons for this, such as exposing a young girl to German measles to avoid the possibility of her catching it during her pregnancy, or exposing a child to measles as a cure for nephrosis. This, however, should never be done without the doctor's advice and supervision.

HYGIENE OF NEWBORN INFANTS

If the mother is ill with a cold or some other disease, the question of breast feeding should be decided by the physician.

Pneumonia, toxemia of pregnancy, active tuberculosis, poliomyelitis and other serious diseases might preclude nursing, while less serious conditions might not. If the condition is one which lasts only a few days, the mother's milk may be expressed and fed to the infant until her infection is controlled, for the milk will not infect the infant. It is being close to the mother which will.

In hospitals great efforts are made to protect the newborn from infection. For example, precautions are taken in delivery rooms and in nurseries for the newborn to avoid unnecessary contact with persons other than the nurses, the doctor and the mother. In hospitals the doctor must wear a clean gown over his street clothes and a mask, and must wash his hands thoroughly before handling the infant. No person except those who are directly responsible for the care of the infants is permitted to enter the nursery. Where "rooming in" is practiced, the mother and father may look after the child, and also the maternal grandmother may be allowed to visit. This protection of infants from unnecessary contact with people who might carry infectious agents from outside should be continued after the infant is brought home. Visitors should be limited as to number, and if possible they should admire the baby without touching him. A person who has, or who has just recovered from, an infection should not come into an infant's room. It is often impracticable, but I have recommended that, where possible, there should be a window in the door of the baby's room so that visitors may see him behind glass as they do in hospitals. If this cannot be done, a large sheet of cellophane might be put over the crib to protect the baby from contact with his visitors and from their breaths.

FEEDING HYGIENE FOR BABIES

Milk, water and any other food given to infants should be sterilized so that infections will not be introduced through the mouth and intestines. The terminal sterilization method is the best one. This is the method in which the milk, formula or water is poured into clean, but unsterilized nursing bottles and covered with nipples and caps; then the bottles and their contents are boiled in a covered pot for twenty-five minutes. This sterilizes everything at once and you run no risk of contaminating the milk while putting the nipples on the bottles. Certified milk, cereal, fruit and so forth which are precooked and packaged or cooked at home need not be sterilized. Nor should orange juice and vitamin mixtures be boiled. Boiling destroys vitamin C. Unless it is supplied in other forms, the infant may develop scurvy.

Since one of the most common and most dangerous diseases of the newborn and young child is infectious diarrhea, the precautions which follow are very important: If you do not use the terminal sterilization method, bottle nipples should be sterilized and kept in a covered, sterilized container. A nipple should be taken out with sterile tongs or with clean fingers. If fingers are used, they should not touch the other nipples or the inside of the container. If they do, resterilize the nipples and container. If you are breast feeding the baby, wash your breasts with soap and water just before each feeding.

As the baby becomes old enough to hold pieces of food in his hands (after about six months), sterilization of utensils may be discontinued, provided they are thoroughly washed just before they are used. Nursing bottles should be rinsed with very hot water just before use even after sterilization is discontinued. When you stop sterilizing the bottles, the milk should not be stored in them any longer.

FOOD HYGIENE

Milk: Milk is rarely completely free of bacteria, except after boiling or pasteurization, even under the most ideal conditions of preparation. The bacterial count of milk depends on the degree of hygiene used in milking the cows, in shipping the milk to market, refrigeration, bottling and distribution to the consumer. Depending on these factors, the milk will contain more or less bacteria, sometimes dangerous ones. Do not allow milk, even Grade A milk or boiled milk, to remain at room temperature or it will breed a large number of bacteria and possibly bacterial toxins which might make the child ill if he drinks it. When traveling, if you cannot get pasteurized milk, bring raw milk to a boil and keep it boiling for five minutes. Refrigerate it almost immediately after bottling.

Several brands of sterilized milk formulas are now available in separate bottles; some contain four ounces of formula, some eight ounces. These are used in many hospitals and at home. They are especially useful for traveling.

Water, Vegetables and Fruit: Avoid drinking from brooks and streams. Wash raw fruit before eating it. If you know that fruit you pick from a tree has not been sprayed with insecticides, it is safe to eat it; but if you do not know, wash it first. When you travel in countries (and there are many) where human excreta are used for fertilizer, avoid eating raw salads, vegetables or fruits which grow on the ground. Wash and peel fruit. Do not drink raw water where there is any doubt of its cleanliness and safety. Amoebiasis, intestinal parasites, typhoid fever and dysentery are some of the diseases spread by water and food. Water can be purified by boiling it for five minutes, or ten drops of a chlorine bleach mixed in a gallon of water will purify it after five minutes.

Shellfish, Cream and Custards: Do not eat uncooked shellfish except when you know they have been picked from safe waters and have been adequately refrigerated, and thus avoid typhoid fever and infectious hepatitis. Do not eat creamed or custard foods, except those you prepare yourself, unless they are bought from reliable shops, and avoid salmonellosis and other food poisoning. Do not keep foods containing cream or mayonnaise, eggs or smoked meats and fish—even those you prepare yourself—at room temperature for longer than absolutely necessary, never all day or overnight, especially in the summertime.

CLEANLINESS

No chapter on hygiene would be complete without the usual advice to wash your hands before eating or preparing food and after toilet, and to avoid the use of common drinking cups and toilet articles. Keep your kitchen, sickroom and toilet as free of flies as possible and thereby avoid diseases which may be spread by flies. Do not permit your children to play in sewage areas. Sewage may contain typhoid germs, polio viruses and other harmful agents.

ANIMAL HYGIENE

Do not pet stray dogs and cats, particularly in strange lands, and avoid such diseases as typhus, scabies, ringworm and other infections. Have your own dog vaccinated against rabies. Do not keep parakeets or other birds in your home unless they are certified to be healthy. They may carry psittacosis. Get rid of rats or mice if you find them around your home.

HYGIENE THROUGH IMMUNIZATION

The earliest vaccination given after birth is B.C.G. vaccine against tuberculosis. It is given immediately after birth to the infant whose mother has active tuberculosis, and routinely in countries with a high incidence of TB. This and other types of immunization are discussed in the chapter on immunization.

HYGIENE IN THE CARE OF A SICK CHILD

When you are caring for a sick child, follow the doctor's or nurse's directions about cleanliness and care of the patient. In general, the following measures may be suggested by them, depending on the kind of illness.

The Sickroom: The temperature of the sickroom should usually be about the same as the normal temperature of the house, comfortably warm and not drafty. In illnesses such as croup, you will need to make the air in the room more humid by keeping a kettle steaming on a hot plate or stove or by putting flat pans of water on the radiator. If possible, the room should be aired when the patient is not in it, or if he must be kept in bed, he should be well covered. The light should be normal except in cases of inflamed eyes, which are bothered by bright light. Then the shades may be drawn or a screen put in front of the windows.

When the doctor says that the child must have a separate room with separate bathroom facilities in order to be completely isolated from the rest of the family, he means that the child should be able to get to the bathroom without going through a hall or a room used by others in the family, and that the bathroom should be used by the sick child only. In the case of a small child, this can usually be managed by having a portable toilet in the sickroom as well as washing facilities.

After the illness is over, there are various ways of cleaning the room, according to the nature of the illness. In the virus diseases, extensive cleaning is unnecessary because viruses are killed very easily by air. The room should be cleaned as it ordinarily would be and well aired, after which it will be safe for a well child. In the case of bacterial diseases, the cleaning should be more complete. Horizontal surfaces should be washed with soap and water or disinfected with a solution of one of the cresylic acid disinfectants. The solution is made by mixing two ounces of CN or Lysol with one gallon of water. The room should be aired for half a day. The bed should be stripped and aired. Some bacteria are more resistant than others—streptococci, for instance. In the case of one of these diseases, it may be necessary also to wash down the walls and the furniture.

Bedding: To sterilize sheets, you should boil them for twenty minutes. If you are sending them to a commercial laundry, keep them in a paper bag separate from the other laundry, sealed and marked "contaminated." Inquire of your laundry whether it will accept such work. Some laundries will not, in which case you will have to do the sterilizing at home. Blankets should be dry-cleaned or washed, preferably with a detergent. It is a good idea to cover pillows with plastic cases under the regular cases so that they will not become heavily contaminated and can be taken out and aired when you want to clean them. If you must send pillows and blankets to a laundry or dry cleaner they should also be wrapped in paper and marked "contaminated" when the disease is one requiring strict isolation technique.

Dishes and Utensils: In many illnesses, it is not important to treat the dishes and utensils in any special way, but in some the doctor will tell you that the child must have separate ones. This can be done by having a separate set which is always kept in the sickroom and will therefore not have to be sterilized after each use. Or you can sterilize the child's dishes by boiling them in water for five minutes before putting them with the family dishes. The simplest, though not the least expensive, method is to get disposable dishes and utensils which can be burned or discarded. This is also simpler with handkerchiefs, towels and napkins.

Disposal: In city apartments it is often impossible to burn disposable objects such as paper towels, paper plates, contaminated toys and leftover food. You should have a paper bag in the sickroom for disposal of these. When the bag is to be discarded, it should be sealed and marked "contaminated" and put out for collection with the other garbage.

The Excreta: When the doctor asks for a stool or urine specimen, the child should use a bedpan, urinal or chamber pot which has been newly washed. You can get a special container from the drugstore, or the doctor will give you one, for the stool, but an ordinary clean jar with a tight top will do. Urine may be put in any clean bottle as long as it is large enough. A four-ounce bottle is a good size. The container should be marked with the child's name and the date and hour the specimen was taken.

In intestinal diseases which require sterilization of the excreta, the measures you must take depend on where you live. In large cities, such as New York, which are near the ocean or a large river, sewage is piped into water which is not used for drinking water and it is unnecessary to do anything but flush the contents of the bedpan down the toilet. In smaller communities, however, this is not usually the case. If you dispose of the excreta without sterilizing them first, you will be contaminating the sewage which may, in turn, contaminate the water supply. Your doctor will know about this, or the local health department will. If the excreta must be sterilized, make a large amount of disinfectant solution by adding two ounces of CN or Lysol to one gallon of water. It need not be newly mixed for each use, so make enough to last for a while. Keep it away from small children. You pour enough of this solution into the bedpan to cover the excreta (about as much as there are excreta) and let it stand for one hour before flushing it down the toilet. You then wash the bedpan with soap. It is not necessary to sterilize it after each use if it is used by only one patient.

If your doctor tells you to handle the stools carefully, as he may, during convalescence from polio or infectious hepatitis, he means that you should avoid contaminating your hands with the stool and should wash them very carefully after taking care of the bedpan or anything else which has come in contact with the stool. If you are not careful, you may be infected with the disease.

Toys and Books: Do not give your child playthings which cannot be washed or dry-cleaned when he has a disease requiring thorough disinfection, because they may have to be destroyed if they become heavily contaminated. After the disease is over, the washable objects may be washed with soap or a detergent and water or with the disinfectant solution recommended for washing the room. Nonwashable objects may be sent to the dry cleaner or cleaned at home if you have the facilities. If they are sent out, they should be wrapped and marked "contaminated." Books may be aired, preferably in the sun, for half a day, unless they have been heavily contaminated with discharges, in which case they should be disposed of. Letters the patient writes while he is ill should be aired before they are sent.

Thermometers: Rectal and oral thermometers should be washed before and after use with soap and *cool* water. You may also wipe them off with alcohol if you like, but this is not a substitute for washing. They should never be put back in a case without being washed or the case will be contaminated.

Bathroom Privileges: This merely means that the child may get out of bed to go to the bathroom rather than using a bedpan or urinal.

Bathing a Sick Child: During some mild infections with little or no fever, the child may take a quick tub bath in a warm bathroom, but see that he does not become chilled. When you must give him a bed bath, do it in a warm room. Some people like to put a rubber sheet or a shower curtain under the child while they are bathing him, but this is not necessary if you are careful. Cover him with a blanket and take his clothes off under the blanket. Put a bath towel under his head and wash, rinse and dry his face and neck. Then move the protective towel so that it is under his arm, wash, rinse and dry that arm, and so forth until you have washed each part of his body separately. In this way only one part at a time will be exposed to the air and he will not become chilled. A little rubbing alcohol and powder feel pleasant after a bath and are stimulating.

If a child has fever, it is better to postpone shampooing his hair until he is well, but in some of the longer illnesses, it is necessary to do it occasionally. There are numerous dry shampoos which can be brushed into the hair and brushed out again carrying dirt and excessive oil with them. Short hair is not too difficult to wash in bed with the help of a basin for wetting and rinsing. Long hair is harder, but it can be done. Dry the hair quickly afterward with a hand dryer or an electric heater. Frequent brushing will keep hair clean enough so that it will not be necessary to shampoo it as often as you would for a well child.

Steam Inhalations: If the doctor wants your child to have steam inhalations, as he might in croup or sinusitis, there are several ways to do it. If your water runs very hot, you might take the child into the bathroom with you and turn on the shower as hot as possible. This will steam up the whole bathroom very quickly. Lacking a shower, you could close the drains of the tub and basin and run hot water into them for as long as the child needs steam. If your kitchen is small, you could put several open pots of water on the stove to boil. If the child is older and needs regular inhalations, he could lean over a basin with hot water running in it and have his head and the basin covered by a large towel or a sheet. With a little child or a baby you must sit under the sheet, too. With a child who is confined to bed, you can make the bed into a steam tent. If it is a crib, make a tent by putting a sheet over the rails and direct the steam from a boiling kettle into an opening left on the side. With a bed, make the tent out of an umbrella and a sheet and get steam into it the same way. But don't, *even for a minute,* leave a young child or a baby alone near steaming water or boiling kettles.

Mouthwash Solutions: If your doctor tells you to wash your child's mouth with salt solution or bicarbonate of soda solution, make it by adding a half teaspoon of either to an ordinary glass of water.

Boric Acid Solution: The proper solution of boric acid, which is often used for eye inflammations and wet dressings, is the amount of powder which will dissolve in water at room temperature. You can dissolve a larger amount by using boiling water, but this solution will be stronger than necessary. Do not leave either the powder or the solution within reach of small children. They are poisonous when taken internally. It is wiser to omit boric acid from your medical supplies.

Strict Isolation Technique: When your doctor tells you to practice strict isolation technique, he means that the patient must not leave the sickroom, that he may not use the family bathroom, that anyone going into the sickroom must put on a gown and sometimes a cap or kerchief to cover his hair. All people entering the room must wash immediately after entering and before leaving. Bedding, clothes, dishes, utensils, leftover food, toys, disposable objects such as towels and tissues, and excreta must be either sterilized or destroyed, and the room and its furniture must be washed after the illness is over or after the child has gone to a hospital.

Isolation and Quarantine: Isolation of a patient may mean many things according to the disease, your doctor's opinions and the local health regulations. A child who is isolated because of whooping cough, for instance, may go outdoors. Sometimes the child is isolated from the public, but not from his family. Sometimes he is isolated from everyone except the person who is caring for him.

Quarantine of contacts is also variable according to local health rules. In some communities, not only the patient is isolated but all susceptible members of the household are, also. Sometimes quarantine merely means that a child who has been exposed to a disease cannot go to school until the incubation period is over.

Restful Convalescence: Many infections require a period of convalescence after the acute disease is over. If your doctor says your child should have the benefit of this period, he usually means that he may be up and around, but that he should not be very active. He will need a lot of rest and a chance to regain his appetite, if he has lost it. He often may be outdoors, but he should not be in crowds because after any illness he will be more susceptible to other infections.

Reporting a Disease: If your child has a disease which is reportable to the health department, your doctor will report it. But you should notify the child's school so that other parents may be warned that their children have been exposed. You should call the parents of any children who are not classmates with whom your child has been playing during the time he was contagious. (For information on when a disease becomes contagious, see the chapter on individual diseases.)

MENTAL HYGIENE

When a child develops an infection which is either severe or prolonged, his feelings and behavior and even the length of the illness may be profoundly influenced by the attitudes of his parents, nurse or doctor. His emotional reactions may influence many symptoms of disease. This does not mean that a child with polio will harbor the virus in his body for a longer time, or that his paralysis will be more extensive or more permanent if he is worried or unhappy. We do know, however, that a child who is in good physical condition resists or overcomes infection more easily than one who is not. For instance, we believe that polio is made more serious by fatigue. If a child is worried about himself, he may very well be sleepless and become tired. A worried child often cannot eat, and in almost any infection good nutrition is a factor in recovery.

There is also plenty of evidence that physical symptoms such as pain, breathing difficulty, change in pulse rate, flushing of the skin, itching and hot or chilly sensations can be the result of emotional response. In the case of a sick child, the symptoms might be a reaction to an overheard and misunderstood conversation between his mother and the doctor.

A child with chicken pox might become more itchy and irritable. A child with asthma might suddenly have great trouble with his breathing. A child with rheumatic fever might complain much more of the joint pain and might put an extra strain on his heart by developing a more rapid pulse. A child with an intestinal infection might have a sudden cramp and a desire to move his bowels. A child with whooping cough or pneumonia might cough more and vomit. A child with polio who has some paralysis of the throat, but is able to swallow his secretions, might suddenly have more trouble swallowing. Any of these reactions, if it is repeated over and over again, may very well aggravate an illness.

Conversely, a feeling of security, comfort and normality will help a child through an illness. A baby with an earache feels less pain when he is held by his mother. A child who is nauseated often can forget about it if his mind is diverted from his trouble. A child with asthma will relax and wheeze less if he is not frightened about himself. A child with any long chronic illness is much more cooperative about treatment when he is relaxed and happy and unafraid. All of these things go a long way toward speeding his recovery.

It is imperative that parents try to control their emotions in the presence of a sick child. They must be careful of what they say about the illness, its severity, its outcome and the dangers associated with it. Children, particularly those who are sick for long periods of time, learn a surprising amount from overheard conversations and since they rarely have any basis of knowledge, they often misunderstand what they have heard. Even a very small child can sense anxiety in his parents, and although he may not know what it is about, he will become anxious himself. Parents should also be careful not to talk about kinds of treatment and the person who is to administer it, unless they are talking directly to the child for his own information.

When Your Child Must Go to a Hospital: You must stress that a hospital is a place where the child can be treated and cared for in a way that is not possible at home. Do not deceive him by telling him he is not going to a hospital. Do not weep when you tell him what a good place it is for a sick child. When you leave him there, tell him the truth about when you expect to return. Do not say you will be right back unless you mean it. A disappointed child will brood, he will not cooperate with the nurse and he may be worse off as a result. He will also resent and lose faith in his parents, and thus become less cooperative after he comes home.

You should leave the nurses and doctors alone with the child when treatments are given, when an injection is given or when blood must be drawn. He is more likely to cooperate when his parents are not with him. The average child will get along very well in a hospital with his nurses, doctors and neighbors if he does not have his parents to lean on. He often will take food and medicine he would not touch at home because the child in the next bed takes them.

Most doctors recommend putting children in wards or rooms with other children unless they must be isolated. It is good for a child's morale to see that there are other children in the same fix, and the example of other children's cooperation helps a new child to conform. There is also the point that a ward is much more interesting because of the company.

Do not tell your child that the doctor or nurse will not hurt him. If possible, skip the unpleasant aspects of treatment when you are talking about them. But if the child questions you about the hospital procedures, answer him as simply and truthfully as you can. Do not go into too much detail.

Obey the hospital visiting rules and do not insist on more visiting than is allowed. The present trend is to allow as much visiting as possible, and excessive visiting might interfere with the nurses' and doctors' ability to treat the child. In some cases it may be important for you to stay with the child as much as you can, even overnight. Decide this with your doctor and the nurse. Hospital rules are flexible enough to allow for the necessary exceptions.

THE IMPACT OF HYGIENE
ON DISEASE

The hygienic measures I have discussed in this chapter have been most effective in reducing to a minimum the incidence of diseases like typhoid, bacillary dysentery, salmonellosis, brucellosis and tuberculosis. Diarrhea in infancy, a frequent and often fatal disease early in the century, has been reduced from its position as the leading cause of death in the first year of life to approximately number ten on the list. This has been accomplished almost entirely by the careful handling of milk by dairies, processors and distributors. Intestinal worm infestation occurs in 50 per cent to 75 per cent of all children in parts of the world where hygiene is poor. Where good hygiene is practiced in connection with fertilizers, sewage disposal and careful preparation of foods, worm infestation has become a rather infrequent occurrence, with the exception of pinworms.

Special measures for special situations such as a polio epidemic are discussed in the chapters on those specific diseases as well as hygiene, quarantine of contacts, isolation of patients and prevention of disease by immunization and drugs. More detailed information on preventive measures are also included in the chapters on immunization and the wonder drugs.

Common Childhood Diseases

7: Chicken Pox (Varicella)

Chicken pox is one of the most common of the communicable diseases of childhood. It is known everywhere, and occurs most often in winter and spring in the temperate zones. It occurs throughout the year in warmer climates. Like measles, there are more cases every other year than in the in-between years. About 70 per cent of children who have reached the age of fifteen have already had it. Chicken pox has been observed in newborn infants whose mothers had the disease just before their birth. It may occur any time after birth —even in old age. Like the other childhood diseases, it is most common in the early school years, earlier where housing is very crowded or where several young children live together, as in nurseries, infants' and children's homes and in boarding schools. About ten thousand cases are reported each year in the city of New York. Probably twice as many occur as are reported. Chicken pox is caused by a virus.

Contagion: The disease is easily spread from child to child either by direct contact or by a susceptible person being close to one who has it. The virus is propelled through the air when the patient speaks, coughs or sneezes. Dry scales are not infectious.

Incubation Period: The incubation period of chicken pox is usually fourteen to sixteen days, but it may be as long as twenty-one days.

Symptoms: The disease begins with fever, usually up to 101°, but sometimes as high as 104° or 105°. It is generally

milder in children than in adults. The child may not feel ill
at all, or may feel a little uncomfortable, or he may be quite
miserable. The rash appears late on the first day or on the
second day of illness, starting as pink blotches. At the
beginning, very few spots are seen—occasionally only one or
two—but by the end of a couple of days they are usually very
numerous. In the centers of the pink spots tiny blisters appear.
They vary in size from an eighth to a quarter of an inch in
diameter. The blisters become larger and are filled with clear
fluid at first, then they sink in the center (become umbili-
cated) and finally they become crusted. The blisters come out
in crops, fresh ones each day. In diagnosing a case of chicken
pox the doctor looks for blisters and crusts in all stages of
development. This is helpful when there is a question of
whether the disease is chicken pox or smallpox, because in
smallpox the lesions are all in about the same stage of development at the same time. In a light case of chicken pox the
blisters may be very few, but in a more severe case they will
probably be numerous, not only on the skin, but also in the
mouth, on the tongue, in the throat, on the scalp, on the eyelids and in the vagina. They usually appear last on the palms
of the hands and the soles of the feet. These are the areas
to examine in deciding when the disease has reached its last
stages of being contagious.

Treatment: The fever lasts two or three days, sometimes
longer. The rash itches a great deal and needs treatment so
that the child will not scratch and break the blisters. The
child's fingernails should be cut short and his hands kept
clean by frequent washing to avoid infecting the blisters.
There are several drugs like calamine lotion to apply to the
skin, and some, especially the antihistamines, to be taken
internally to reduce the itching.

You should keep the child in bed while there is fever of
102° or higher, and for a day or so longer. It is all right to
give a sponge bath, but you should take care not to rub the
blisters open. When the child's temperature is normal and
the scabs are dry, he may find a shower or tub bath comforting. The skin should be patted dry, not rubbed.

Chicken pox requires no special treatment with serum,

antibiotics or sulfa drugs unless there are complications. Give the child whatever he wants to eat and let him have bathroom privileges if he is not too sick.

Complications: Chicken pox usually is a mild disease which rarely produces serious complications if you are careful about cleanliness. The most common ones are due to secondary infection of the skin with bacteria. These are usually caused by infecting the blisters by scratching. If the blisters are scratched and broken and thus become infected, they may leave small scars which look like shallow pits. These scars are rarely as disfiguring as the scars of smallpox, but a few on the face can be disturbing to a child, especially to a girl. Chicken pox may cause encephalitis in rare cases.

Prevention: There is no available drug or serum which will regularly prevent chicken pox. Large doses of convalescent serum or gamma globulin may be effective in some cases, but they are not considered so for practical purposes and are not recommended. There are no skin tests or other methods to determine whether or not a person is immune to the disease. One attack gives lifelong immunity. Exceptions to this rule are very rare. I have never seen a second attack of chicken pox in any of my patients, but it is said to happen.

It is possible to identify the virus of chicken pox through laboratory techniques usually available only for scientific study. The only reason for identifying the virus is when the question arises as to whether the patient has chicken pox or the more serious disease, smallpox.

Isolation and Quarantine: People exposed to chicken pox are usually not quarantined and it is not recommended by the U.S. Public Health Service or by the American Academy of Pediatrics. Patients with chicken pox are considered infectious one day before the rash appears and until the individual skin lesions are dried. Usually this is a total of five to seven days. The U.S. Public Health Service believes it unnecessary to isolate chicken pox patients until all the scabs have fallen off. However, in some schools, children are not allowed to return until all the scabs are gone. You must abide by the local regulations of your community or school.

Hygiene: Cleaning the room well and airing it for an hour is usually enough to make it safe for others who have not had the disease. The laundry may be treated the same as that of the rest of the family. Dishes and utensils may be washed with the family dishes. It is so rare for the disease to be spread through contaminated clothes, dishes and eating utensils that it is not worth considering the possibility.

QUESTIONS & ANSWERS

Q. *How did chicken pox get its name?*

A. The name is believed to come from the Latin word *cicer.* It means chick-pea and was probably used because the chicken pox blister resembles a chick-pea in shape.

Q. *Is there a skin test for chicken pox?*

A. No.

Q. *My child has come down with chicken pox at a summer camp. May I take him home, even though the camp is in a different state?*

A. You must abide by the health department regulations for transportation in a public vehicle and interstate travel. Within a state a person with an infectious disease may not travel on a public vehicle, but he may travel in an ambulance or a private car. If it is a matter of taking a person from one state to another, you must have the consent of the health authorities of both states.

Q. *Must you be in actual contact with a child with chicken pox to become infected?*

A. No. Being close to him may be enough. The droplets of moisture expelled from his mouth when he speaks or through his nose when he breathes may contain the chicken pox virus. If you are close enough to be reached by these droplets, you may inhale them and become infected. Of course, the blister fluid contains the living virus and you could be infected by contact with this fluid.

Q. *Are the crusts infectious?*

A. No.

Q. *Is chicken pox related to smallpox?*

A. No, but sometimes it is hard to tell them apart.

Q. *Can chicken pox be confused with diseases other than smallpox?*

A. Yes. There are several diseases—shingles, cold sores, rickettsial pox and others such as hives—which may be confused with chicken pox. It is usually easy to diagnose, but occasionally identification is very difficult.

Q. *Can I diagnose chicken pox myself, or do I need a doctor to do it?*

A. You may be able to because you know your child has been exposed to it two or three weeks before and therefore anticipate it. But it is better to rely on the doctor's opinion than your own, since it may be very important in the future to know definitely whether or not your child has had chicken pox.

Q. *Are chicken pox and shingles different forms of the same disease?*

A. No. Chicken pox may follow shingles or shingles follow chicken pox in a home, but they are different diseases. The viruses which cause them are similar in size and shape when seen through an electronmicroscope and are believed to be identical. A person who has had chicken pox is immune to chicken pox, but not to shingles, and vice versa. I have seen shingles in three children who had had chicken pox.

Q. *My child developed chicken pox at boarding school. Should I take him home?*

A. I would leave him at the school infirmary until he has recovered and then let him resume his school activities.

Q. *Is chicken pox dangerous to a pregnant woman or to the developing fetus?*

A. It doesn't seem to injure either of them. Our knowledge of the effect of chicken pox on the unborn infant is not based on extensive experience. It is generally wiser to avoid any infection during pregnancy, especially during the first three months.

Q. *Is gamma globulin or convalescent serum effective for the prevention or treatment of chicken pox?*

A. For practical purposes, no, although very large doses may be effective. It may reduce the amount of rash.

Q. *Is there any toxoid or vaccine by which children can be made immune to chicken pox?*

A. Not now, but vaccines are being evaluated. Possibly one will become available in the next few years.

Q. *Can you prevent or cure chicken pox with any drug?*

A. No, we can neither prevent nor cure it.

Q. *Is it wise to expose a child to chicken pox to avoid his having it as an adult?*

A. While chicken pox is usually more severe in an adult, it is not necessary to have it at all, so it should be avoided.

Q. *Why do the regulations for isolation and quarantine vary in different cities and states in the case of chicken pox?*

A. They also vary for other diseases. While the disease is essentially the same everywhere and the suggestions of the U.S. Public Health Service are clear, local health officers do differ in their opinions medically, and their wishes usually prevail in their respective communities.

8: Diphtheria

Diphtheria is an acute infectious disease which has been known all over the world since the days of the ancient Hebrews, before the time of Christ. It has been with us ever since. It was completely and thoroughly described as a separate disease by Pierre Bretonneau in 1826. It is caused by a germ called the Klebs-Loeffler bacillus. In the temperate zones it occurs more commonly in the winter and early spring. People get it from infancy to old age.

Diphtheria was once a very common disease. In 1900 there were over twelve thousand cases in the city of New York, and of those not treated actively, 25 per cent died.

Today diphtheria is nonexistent in New York, although the population has doubled. It is still very common in countries where immunization of infants is not done or only for a few.

In 1919–1923 when I was a medical student, there was never any difficulty in finding cases of diphtheria to demonstrate to us. Today, when I teach, it is impossible to find a case of diphtheria to show to my students. Great credit for the drop in diphtheria is due to Dr. Bela Schick, who discovered the test which tells whether or not a person is immune, to Dr. Gaston Ramon, who developed diphtheria toxoid, and to Dr. W. Hallock Park, who introduced immunization on a large scale.

Contagion: Diphtheria is spread from the mouth of an infected person to one who is close by. The droplets can be transmitted by merely speaking or by coughing or sneezing. Occasionally it is spread by contaminated milk. About 10 per cent of patients have become infected by members of their families.

Incubation Period: Those who contract diphtheria incubate it for a period of two to five days, usually three or four days, before becoming ill.

Symptoms: The illness usually begins with a feeling of malaise, headache, sore throat and chilly sensation, and fever of 101° to 102°, and in more severe cases, 103° to 104°. Adults do not have a sore throat as often as children do. The throat is red at first, then grayish white spots develop on the tonsils. As the disease develops, the throat feels worse and becomes swollen, and the spots on the tonsils become larger and may spread to other parts of the throat. After another day these spots run together and give the appearance of a grayish-white, or dirty yellowish-white membrane. To the experienced person, the appearance of the throat, the membrane and the peculiar smell suggest diphtheria. The inflammation and swelling of the uvula and tonsils may be suggestive of the disease even when a membrane is absent.

Diphtheria usually involves only the throat and tonsils, but in 2 to 3 per cent of the cases, the back of the nose is involved too. When the nose alone is affected, the child is not as sick. A bloody discharge from the nose is very suggestive of the disease. It may also spread to the voice box (larynx). In little children, as many as 25 per cent of the patients may have this laryngeal type of diphtheria because the distance to the larynx is so short that it is more easily involved than in older children. When this happens, the child becomes hoarse, then loses his voice almost completely. It is particularly dangerous because the swelling and membrane in the larynx may result in marked narrowing with severe breathing difficulty, even to the point of suffocation. In rare instances, the membrane spreads down the windpipe and into the bronchial tubes.

Diphtheria may occur in other parts of the body. It occasionally involves the conjunctiva of the eye (the whites and lining of the eyelids) and the vagina, and it frequently infects wounds and ulcers of the skin. This last is known as wound or skin diphtheria. These localized forms are not usually as severe or as dangerous, but may be very serious.

Nature of the Disease: Wherever the diphtheria germ settles, it invades the tissues and liberates a very poisonous substance called diphtheria toxin. This toxin destroys the cells lining the throat or the tonsils, the cells lining a wound, or wherever the germ happens to be. As the toxin destroys these cells, the body reacts by pouring out serum and white blood corpuscles and fibrin (the part of the blood which makes it clot) in the place where the toxin is. The result is that the serum, the fibrin, the destroyed cells, the diphtheria germs and white blood cells which appear as defense against the germs combine in a congealed mass and produce the membrane. When the doctor tries to peel off the membrane, the surface under it bleeds a little. This is characteristic of diphtheria in contrast to other throat infections such as follicular tonsillitis. The membrane usually lasts seven or eight days, though this period may be shortened somewhat by early treatment with antitoxin and antibiotics. It is important to know that in about 10 to 15 per cent of diphtheria cases, the membrane does not develop at all, which makes diagnosis difficult.

Treatment: Diphtheria is best treated in a hospital.

In any locality where diphtheria is still present it is important that any sick person complaining of a sore throat and difficulty in swallowing be put to bed and examined by a doctor quickly. If the patient does have diphtheria, his chances of recovery vary between 75 and 99 per cent depending on how soon he is treated with diphtheria antitoxin. If given the antitoxin on the first day of illness, almost every child recovers. If treated on or after the fifth day, the chances of recovery drop to about 75 per cent. No antibiotic and no other medication can take the place of diphtheria antitoxin, but penicillin in large doses may be helpful.

Before antitoxin is injected, it is necessary to test the child for sensitivity to horse serum since the antitoxin is usually produced in horses. If the child is sensitive to horse serum, it would be dangerous to inject the antitoxin without first taking special precautions.

Keep the child in bed for at least three weeks, longer if he develops a complication of the heart or nervous system. Adults are kept in bed for six weeks. The patient is given a liquid or soft diet at first and a regular diet as improvement takes place. The patient is not allowed out of bed, even for toilet. He is given daily bed baths. Penicillin or one of the other antibiotics is given for about seven to ten days, or until the infection has been cured. The antibiotics have no effect on the diphtheria toxin, but they kill the germs which produce it, and therefore prevent the production of more toxin. The complications are treated as indicated by their nature and severity.

Chronic carriers of diphtheria germs are isolated and treated with antibiotics until they lose the infection. If antibiotics fail to accomplish this, removal of tonsils is usually effective.

Convalescence: The child's activity should be resumed slowly. He may return to school one or two weeks after being discharged from the hospital, but he should not climb more than a few stairs or join in strenuous games for another two weeks. A child convalescing from diphtheria is not usually aware of injury to his heart, and if he does perform hard work before he is completely recovered, he may suffer serious consequences. With careful return to activity, there is usually no permanent heart damage.

Complications: This heart involvement is the most common complication of diphtheria. It is usually more severe and more serious in adults than in children, but it may be very serious at any age. Some degree of heart involvement occurs in over 50 per cent of diphtheria patients. It usually calls for absolute rest in bed until recovery. The child is not allowed to feed himself. You feed him liquids at first, a soft diet as he improves. You wash him in bed. You do not allow him exciting radio or television programs. The restrictions are lifted only by doctor's directions. Make every effort to keep him from arguing or crying. Even such exertion and excitement may be harmful in diphtheritic heart disease.

Another complication of diphtheria is nerve paralysis. This may occur as early as the end of the first week of the disease, but more often occurs in the third to the fifth week. It may involve the arms and legs, but the paralysis most often seen is the one of the soft palate and throat. It makes the child talk as if he were speaking through his nose. When he drinks water, some of it may go through his nose as he tries to swallow.

The second most common paralysis is that of the eye

muscles. The child suddenly becomes cross-eyed. The chest muscles and diaphragm may be involved. This paralysis is sometimes so much like the paralysis of polio that it is almost impossible to tell them apart. Diphtheria may produce a loss of reflexes as in polio. While it may be hard to tell the difference between diphtheria and polio paralyses, it is possible to do so by carefully reviewing the history of the illness.

Diphtheria toxin also injures the kidneys, but seldom seriously. It is unusual to have even chronic heart or kidney disease as a result of diphtheria, and fortunately, almost everyone recovers from the paralysis. Indeed, this is in striking contrast to polio. It is rare to see paralysis from diphtheria last more than six months after the disease, whereas in polio a weakness or paralysis may continue throughout life.

Immunity: Over the last twenty-five years, diphtheria has become rare in the United States and in other countries where immunization of children is a general practice. This has resulted in a diminution of the number of carriers and, as a consequence, a drop in the percentage of adults who are immune as compared to the time when the disease was common. While the overall incidence of the disease is very much lower in the United States, a higher percentage of the patients are young adults than used to be the case.

When a woman who is immune to diphtheria has a baby, her infant will also be immune for a few months. Twenty-five years ago about 85 per cent of mothers in cosmopolitan areas in the United States were immune to diphtheria because they were constantly exposed to carriers. Ten years ago only about 65 per cent of these mothers were immune. Therefore, about 35 per cent of the newborn infants were susceptible to diphtheria. The immunity which is transmitted from mother to infant becomes weaker progressively after birth. It is not reliable beyond the first three months. If a child of three or four months were exposed to diphtheria, it would be necessary to protect him with an injection of antitoxin or with antibiotics. Since some infants are born without any immunity, and since in others the passive immunity acquired from the mother may diminish very rapidly, it is safer to start immunization against diphtheria when the infant is two or three months old.

Children seem to develop greater immunity as they get older

as a result of being exposed to carriers. By the time they reach adolescence, from 65 to 85 per cent have become immune. The percentage is greater whenever and wherever the disease is prevalent, and where carriers are numerous, and the lower percentage prevails where diphtheria is less common. People who come in contact with these carriers become infected, but only a few of them develop diphtheria. Others harbor the germ, have a few or no symptoms of the disease, and develop immunity which lasts for a long time, even for life. Some people are repeatedly exposed to carriers. The repetition reinforces the immunity. Each reinfection acts like a booster injection of toxoid and keeps the immunity at a high level.

The Schick Test: Fortunately, we do not have to depend on natural immunity to diphtheria. It is possible to be immunized. There is a well-known test called the Schick test which indicates whether a person is immune to diphtheria. The test is described in the section on tests.

Prevention: In the United States, immunization is usually started some time between the second and third month of age, occasionally earlier. Three injections of diphtheria toxoid, often combined with tetanus toxoid and whooping cough vaccine, are injected at monthly intervals. These injections are reinforced by booster injections one year and three years after the last of the original series, and then every two years until entering school, and again if exposed to diphtheria. Some doctors prefer to continue giving toxoid every two or three years until the tenth or twelfth year.

In the case of a child over five or six, or an adult, if the Schick test is positive, he should be immunized. However, he should not be given the usual dose of toxoid that is given to a younger child or a baby without first trying a test dose to make sure there are no ill effects. These ill effects are usually found only in older children or adults who have had previous injections of diphtheria toxoid, and since many of them do not remember whether or not they have had the injections in the past, the test dose is usually given before the regular injections. Older children and adults may be sensitive to one of the ingredients of the toxoid preparation and may get severe local reactions at the site of the injection, and high fever from the usual dose of toxoid, or even a small test dose. If the test results in a severe local or general reaction, no further injections are necessary. The person has some latent immunity and the test will serve as a booster. A new type of toxoid (adult toxoid) is now available.

In the city of New York a child must show evidence of having been immunized before he enters school. If he has not had the injections, the school asks his parents to have it done. If they have no private doctor, it can be done through the clinics of the health department or in most of the hospitals in the city.

Fortunately, we can protect people temporarily against an exposure to diphtheria and also give them a long-term immunity. If a person is exposed and has not been immunized, it becomes important for him to get temporary protection by an injection of antitoxin. This gives him a ready-made immunity for two or three weeks, which is longer than the incubation period, and therefore protects him quite well from developing the disease. Some doctors prefer antibiotics, which kill the germ before it can liberate much toxin, provided they can be in touch with the patient daily and give antitoxin immediately in case any evidence of diphtheria appears.

If an exposed child has been previously immunized, or if he is known to be immune because of a negative Schick test, it is not necessary to give him the antitoxin, but it is wise to give a booster dose of toxoid. The toxoid will stimulate a rise in immunity within a few days to a safer protective level. If a child has been exposed to diphtheria and has been given antitoxin, he should also be actively immunized by three injections of toxoid. This should be started two or three weeks later, when the antitoxin has worn off. Frequently the first dose of toxoid is given with the antitoxin.

Isolation and Quarantine: In most communities, the board of health posts a placard on the outside door of the patient's house or apartment to indicate that there is danger for anyone who enters, and that no one should enter unless it is absolutely necessary.

The patient is isolated until at least two cultures taken from the infected area show that all the diphtheria germs have left him or are not virulent. Sometimes the diphtheria germs found in the throat are not of the virulent variety—that is, they do not produce the toxin which is what injures the patient. Under such circumstances the patient is considered harmless to others and may be given his freedom.

If a child is exposed to an active case of diphtheria, it is important that he be watched closely and that he be kept out of school for at least five days. If he has been given toxoid injections and has a negative Schick test, the school authorities may allow him to come to school.

Hygiene: When a child has diphtheria, you should boil his clothes and laundry, and his dishes should be boiled or kept apart from the rest of the family's. It is not necessary to disinfect his urine or stool. No one should go in and out of the sickroom unless he has particular dealings with the patient. Anyone who must go in and out should wear a gown while in the room, and wash his hands after taking off the gown and before coming out of the room. The visitor's hair should be covered and he should be careful not to let the patient cough directly toward him or breathe right in his face. At the end of the illness, the room should be thoroughly cleaned. The toys the child played with should be destroyed if they cannot be washed with soap or dry-cleaned.

QUESTIONS & ANSWERS

Q.   *Is diphtheria the same all over the world?*

A.   Yes.

Q.   *Does diphtheria attack all ages equally?*

A.   No. Since most infants have some immunity for the first three to six months and some for the first nine months, it is relatively uncommon at that age. After nine months it is more common. It reaches its peak somewhere between the third and fifth year. Although about a quarter of the cases occur between two and five years, about half of the deaths are in that age group, so it is a more serious disease for young children than it is later. In areas where diphtheria is relatively rare, it occurs more frequently in young adults who have not had a chance to develop immunity in childhood.

Q. *Why do we worry so much about diphtheria if it has become a relatively rare disease?*

A. We are concerned about it because it is a very serious disease whenever it does occur and because it has become relatively rare only in parts of the world where children have been immunized. If we let down on immunization of our children, it is reasonably certain that the disease will become more common again, just as it is in other countries where immunization is not generally practiced.

Each year we have small outbreaks in various parts of the United States. In one large European city over five hundred cases of diphtheria were seen in one large clinic in one year. In some South American and Eastern countries it is still prevalent. With ever-increasing travel it is important for us to have immunity to the disease.

Q. *You say diphtheria was known long ago. Was the disease the same? And what did doctors do about it?*

A. Diphtheria seems to have been the same as it is now. Older doctors who practiced before Von Behring discovered antitoxin in 1898 have told me that it was a horrible disease, one which they dreaded. Before antitoxin there was nothing the doctor could do for the patient. There were no antibiotics or antiserum, nor did they know of the Schick test or about immunization. Many of the tombstones in our New England cemeteries stand witness to epidemics of diphtheria which took large numbers of children from colonial families.

Q. *Is diphtheria more common where people live in crowded quarters?*

A. Yes.

Q. *Is it more dangerous for city children or for those who live in rural areas?*

A. Actually, diphtheria is a more dangerous disease for people who come from rural areas because they have had less chance of becoming immunized by exposure to carriers, and because in many rural areas immunization is not practiced regularly. In the army, soldiers from the country are more likely to be susceptible than soldiers from cities.

Q. *Is diphtheria ever contracted through food?*

A. Yes, most often through liquid food, for instance, milk.

Q. *Are all diphtheria germs alike?*

A. No. There are several different types: (1) those which produce no harmful toxin—these are known as nonvirulent; (2) the *Mitis* strain which produces little toxin; (3) the *Gravis* strain which produces a great deal of toxin, and is therefore more dangerous; (4) the *Intermedius* strain, those germs which produce more toxin than the *Mitis* strain and less than the *Gravis* strain.

Q. *What is malignant diphtheria?*

A. It is a very severe form of the disease usually caused by the *Gravis* strain of diphtheria germs which produces a great deal of toxin. The patient is very sick. He quickly becomes prostrate, the temperature is very high. He may have pneumonia or a bull neck caused by the intensive swelling of the lymph glands in the neck and the surrounding tissue. The membrane is very extensive and spreads rapidly. This form of diphtheria is highly fatal and fortunately not very common.

Q. *Is a diphtheria epidemic caused by one type of bacteria?*

A. Not usually, but sometimes there will be a larger number of cases caused by the *Gravis* strain, and in other outbreaks the less serious *Mitis* strain will be responsible more frequently.

Q. *Does the immunity conferred by three injections of the toxoid last for life?*

A. No. It weakens, and a booster injection is required a year after the initial three injections, and perhaps every two or three years thereafter until about ten or twelve years of age.

Q. *Should anyone besides infants and children be immunized?*

A. Yes. Schoolteachers, nurses, doctors and all other people who are likely to be exposed to diphtheria ought to be

Schick tested, and if found positive, they ought to be immunized.

Q. *If my child complains of a sore throat, do I have to worry about diphtheria?*

A. You do if your child has not been immunized against the disease and if you are in an area where the disease is common. If he has been immunized and has received the necessary booster injections, it is quite unlikely that the sore throat could be caused by diphtheria.

Q. *How can a doctor be sure that he is seeing diphtheria when he examines a child with a sore throat?*

A. He suspects diphtheria when he sees a sore throat with swelling and membrane on the tonsils. If he does suspect it, he will make a culture of the throat or membrane. If he suspects strongly enough that it is diphtheria, he will treat the patient for diphtheria without waiting for the results of the culture because the difficulties increase with each day of the illness. For example, if diphtheria is treated the very first day, the chance of a fatal outcome is less than 1 per cent. The rate of danger increases rapidly so that in patients who have not been treated until the fifth day or later the mortality is almost 25 per cent. The overall mortality is about 4 to 5 per cent. It is still a very serious disease, and deaths need not occur if the doctor sees the child quickly and treats the disease actively.

Q. *What is a culture?*

A. A culture is made by removing bacteria from the throat or the membrane with a cotton swab. These bacteria are applied to a tube or plate of nutrient substance upon which they grow. After they have multiplied for several hours to several days, the bacteria are examined to determine which they are. Sometimes just an examination of the material clinging to the cotton swab will reveal the presence of the diphtheria bacillus.

Q. *Are laboratories always prepared to find out whether the specimen shows diphtheria?*

A. Yes. The city and state departments of health and most hospitals and private laboratories are always alert to the diphtheria problem.

Q. *Can diphtheria be treated at home?*

A. Yes, but hospitalization is much safer for the child and his family and much easier on the mother.

Q. *Can antibiotics be used instead of diphtheria antitoxin?*

A. No. The antibiotics are not a substitute. They do not counteract the toxin released by the diphtheria germs. They do kill the germs and get rid of them, but unfortunately, the toxin which the germs liberate acts even before you recognize the disease. It is therefore necessary to neutralize as much of the toxin in the body as possible and to use antibiotics at the same time to get rid of the germs so that no more toxin can be produced.

Q. *If a child has diphtheria and develops difficulty in breathing, what can you do?*

A. It is an emergency situation which requires immediate medical attention. The doctor will try to suction the membrane from the laryx. If this gives no relief, sometimes it is necessary to make an opening in the windpipe and insert a tube below the larynx through which the child can breathe until the disease is over.

Q. *Can any doctor do this?*

A. Any doctor should be prepared to do this operation (a tracheotomy) in an emergency. If there is time, however, a doctor who does this kind of work regularly is called to help out.

Q. *What sort of diet should a patient with diphtheria have?*

A. A soft diet with foods that are easy to digest. If swallowing is difficult, a liquid diet may be easier for the patient.

Q. *Should a child with diphtheria have television or a radio in his room?*

A. He should rest in bed and avoid excitement. After the child improves, he may have television or a radio provided the doctor thinks he can stand the excitement.

Q. *Why is it necessary to be so careful with a diphtheria patient?*

A. Because diphtheria attacks the heart. The toxin gets to the heart muscles and to the nerves which control the heartbeat and injures them, and one of the commonest causes of death from diphtheria is heart failure. Excitement strains the heart.

Q. *How frequently does nerve paralysis occur in diphtheria?*

A. In 10 to 20 per cent of the cases.

Q. *Can I take care of my child with diphtheria and at the same time care for the rest of the family?*

A. I would not encourage it. It is too risky. You might carry diphtheria germs to other members of the family. Diphtheria is best treated in a hospital.

Q. *Is it all right for my maid to clean my son's room while he has diphtheria?*

A. Preferably not. She may, however, if she is immune to diphtheria and protects herself with a gown and face mask. If she does not know whether she is immune, she should not enter the boy's room.

Q. *Shouldn't everyone in a household where there is diphtheria have Schick tests and booster shots?*

A. Yes, and they should have throat cultures made and followed.

Q. *Is placarding practical any more?*

A. No.

9: German Measles (Rubella)

German measles is a mild, contagious virus disease prevalent all over the world. It has become very important since it was discovered that infants born of mothers who have had German measles in the first three months of pregnancy may be defective. It occurs in all ages except the very young infant whose mother has had the disease, but most frequently between the ages of three and twelve. It is a well-known disease in army camps where young susceptible adults who come from rural communities live together, and there are occasional epidemics in colleges and boarding schools. The disease is often confused with measles, scarlet fever and roseola, but it is absolutely separate and distinct. A child who has had German measles does not develop immunity to any of the other diseases, nor does a child who has had measles develop immunity to German measles. An attack of German measles results in immunity to German measles alone. A single attack apparently gives lifelong immunity. People who claim to have had German measles one, two, three or four times have probably had, at various times, measles, German measles, roseola, scarlet fever, erythema infectiosum or some other virus disease accompanied by a rash (e.g., entero virus, Coxsackie virus, infectious mononucleosis).

Contagion: While it is moderately contagious, it is not as contagious as measles or chicken pox. Susceptible people are apparently infected by droplets of moisture from the nose and throat of a person who has the disease.

Incubation Period: The incubation period is usually about seventeen to eighteen days, but can be as short as thirteen or as long as twenty-one days.

Symptoms: A child sick with German measles may feel nothing but soreness and little bumps behind the ears or at the back of the head. These are swollen lymph nodes. When the child moves his head from side to side, the discomfort caused by stretching the skin over these glands makes him feel as if he has a stiff neck. The lymph nodes become swollen and tender any time between one and three days before the rash appears. Usually there is little or no fever until one to three days before the rash appears or on the day of the rash. Then the temperature is low-grade in most children, but occasionally it reaches a high level and lasts as long as three or four days, rarely longer. This is equally true of adults. The fever is usually at its height at the time of the rash. The disease usually lasts three or four days, but may go on for six or seven days during which time it remains infectious.

The rash begins on the face and spreads over the whole body within a day and lasts for two or three days longer. It consists of flat, pink spots usually separate, though some of them run together and look like larger spots. Usually the rash looks like that of measles or roseola, but occasionally it resembles the rash of scarlet fever, being fine and producing an effect of blushing. In those cases you can find on the arms or wrists or some part of the body the typical rash which looks like the rash of measles. Other signs and symptoms are occasionally a cough and, not infrequently, redness of the throat and the soft palate, sore throat, a feeling of malaise, even occasional chills with a high fever and headache. One may have German measles without a rash, and this is probably more common than German measles with a rash, as studies of immunity indicate.

Treatment: A child with German measles requires no special treatment. If the fever is high or if the patient feels quite ill, he should stay in bed until he feels better. He may have bathroom privileges. He may eat a regular diet. Antibiotics are unnecessary and serum or gamma globulin treatment are of no particular value.

Complications: Unlike measles, German measles is rarely complicated by ear infections or pneumonia. It hardly ever leaves any lasting ill effects, though in rare cases inflammation of the brain (encephalitis) develops as a complication. The patient usually survives the encephalitis, but some patients may have some permanent aftereffects.

When it involves a pregnant woman it does injure the embryo in some way, so that about 20 per cent of infants born under such conditions have defects of the brain, eyes, ears, heart, intestines, or any combination of these.

Prevention: Although German measles has been known for over a hundred years, it was not until some twenty-five years ago that it was found that the disease may be very serious if it occurs in women during the early months of pregnancy. Children, especially girls, should be permitted to contract German measles in order to avoid the possibility of getting it later during pregnancy. There is no preparation which regularly or surely prevents the disease in those exposed to it, but gamma globulin in large quantities may eliminate the rash, but not the infection.

Vaccines made of the rubella (German measles) virus are now being evaluated. Results are such that we may expect to have vaccine available to the public within the next few months, possibly sooner.

Isolation and Quarantine: In the light of our present knowledge about the spread of the diseases, the present regulations should be changed.

Hygiene: The patient's clothes, bedding and dishes are treated no differently from those of the rest of the family.

QUESTIONS & ANSWERS

Q. *Why do you say that the present rules of isolation and quarantine should be changed?*

A. It is now known that the virus of German measles can be recovered from patients with German measles—as long as a week before the rash appears and for several days after the rash and fever have left. This suggests that our present recommendation for isolation and quarantine must be changed. For example, people, especially pregnant women, who have not had rubella should avoid contact with children from about a week after the child has been exposed to the disease and for four to five days after he has recovered from the disease, or for a period of about two weeks. In fact, in case of a woman in the first three months of pregnancy, she should avoid contact with an exposed susceptible child, from a week after exposure for a period of two weeks, since he might have the disease without a rash or fever. Swollen glands behind the ears and the back of the head may be a clue that he is ill.

Q. *Is German measles the same disease as ordinary measles?*

A. No.

Q. *My doctor said I had German measles last year, and now he says I have it again. Is that possible?*

A. It is most unlikely. It is more likely that you had a different disease last year or have a different disease now. There are several diseases with rash resembling that of rubella.

Q. *Wouldn't it be better for girls to have German measles before they grow up?*

A. Yes, it certainly seems better to get it over with before they are married.

Q. *Should I deliberately expose my eight-year-old daughter to German measles?*

A. I would, until an effective vaccine becomes available, but only if your doctor advises it.

Q. *Is there any way of giving a child German measles artificially if all attempts to expose her naturally have failed?*

A. In recent years attempts have been made to give young susceptible children German measles by giving them injections of blood obtained from people with active cases of German measles. It would be especially desirable for girls to become immune. Several things have been learned from these studies:

First, it was shown that a susceptible child could be infected this way or by having his nose sprayed with infected blood plasma.

Second, it was shown that most of the children who developed German measles by this method had become immune when another injection was tried later, though some of them did get the disease when they were exposed naturally.

Third, these studies made it obvious that some of the children who were artificially infected developed immunity to German measles without developing a rash. Now that we know a child can have the disease with no rash, we have altered our thinking about the extent of its contagiousness, because many people must have been infected and become immune without obviously having the disease.

Q. *What other diseases can be confused with German measles?*

A. Measles, roseola infantum, scarlet fever, allergic rashes, drug rashes and those caused by other virus infections, e.g., some of the Echo viruses, etc.

Another is Fifth Disease, or erythema infectiosum. It is a contagious disease characterized by a rash on the cheeks which resembles a fresh sunburn or a slapped face. The rash spreads over the entire body and usually looks different and lasts longer than the rash of German measles. Fever is usually low grade—older people may have joint pain. The infection spreads to contacts. It occurs in epidemics, but more recently it has been present in some areas for two or three consecutive summers.

Q. *Must I keep my child in a darkened room when he has German measles?*

A. No, it is not necessary.

Q. *Is there any special diet for a child with German measles?*

A. He may have a regular diet.

Q. *Is there any special treatment for German measles?*

A. Nothing more than keeping the patient comfortable.

Q. *Does German measles affect the eyes?*

A. Usually not.

Q. *Is German measles always harmless?*

A. No. Encephalitis, inflammation of the brain, occurs infrequently. And it may be harmful to the embryo in the first three months of development.

Q. *What is the rubella syndrome we read so much about in newspapers, magazines, etc.?*

A. It is the condition observed in newborn infants of mothers who had German measles in the first three months of pregnancy. The infant may be small or premature and have a "purpuric" rash—purple spots of bleeding into the skin—disturbances of the brain, eye, hearing, heart abnormalities in various combinations and other abnormalities. Blood platelets are temporarily reduced to low levels. Such infants may infect the hospital nurses and may harbor the virus for many months, even up to eighteen to twenty-four months.

Q. *Is the mother injured by German measles?*

A. Apparently not. The injury to the baby seems to occur as a result of the virus passing through the mother and affecting the developing infant.

Q. *Do infants of one or two months suffer ill effects from German measles?*

A. No, usually not. It is only the developing fetus, the unborn infant in the early stage of development, that seems to be affected.

Q. *What should a woman who is six weeks pregnant do if she catches German measles?*

A. She should talk it over with her obstetrician and her family doctor and be guided by their advice.

Q. *What can you do about German measles in a pregnant woman?*

A. Once it has developed, there is nothing you can do. If, however, a woman who is one, two or three months pregnant knows she has been exposed to it, her doctor might give her injections of large doses of gamma globulin in an attempt to keep the disease from developing, or recommend abortion.

Q. *Is gamma globulin always effective?*

A. No, not always. Recent studies indicate that the gamma globulin does not prevent infection, but the infected person may develop the disease without a rash. Such a woman could transmit the virus of gamma globulin to the unborn infant and cause the rubella syndrome. Even though we have no definite idea of how effective the gamma globulin will be in any one person, it is worth trying.

10: Hepatitis

Hepatitis means inflammation of the liver. There are several causes for this inflammation, such as mechanical obstruction and some kinds of poisoning, but the ones we are discussing here are the ones which are infections and are caused by viruses. When the liver, which secretes bile, fails to function properly as it does when it is inflamed, one of the results is that bile pigments enter the bloodstream. When sufficient bile pigment gets into the blood, it causes the skin and whites of the eyes to become yellow and the urine to become amber-colored. All of this indicates jaundice. While it is impossible to distinguish between infectious hepatitis and serum hepatitis by the course of the disease, there are some distinguishing differences.

INFECTIOUS HEPATITIS
(CATARRHAL JAUNDICE)

This disease is known everywhere. It occurs most often in the late autumn and winter, but we find it throughout the year, especially when it occurs in epidemic form. Before World War II it was called catarrhal jaundice and was frequently observed in hospitals. The disease occurs both sporadically and in epidemics, the epidemics usually being reported from institutions and rural areas, and from some sections of large cities, such as New York. It is more prevalent where there is any concentration of people. Epidemics are known to have occurred as far back as the Napoleonic wars, and they have recurred with each war since then. Usually the civilian population near a military establishment also becomes contaminated. Since the disease has become reportable to health departments, there seems to have been a considerable increase in the number of cases, making it a serious problem.

Infectious hepatitis is most common in older children and young adults and its incidence declines with advancing years. It is not very common in young children, except in institutions, particularly those for retarded infants. Newborn babies have been found to have it when their mothers had it during pregnancy. It is not the same thing, however, as congenital jaundice which is caused by defective development of the bile ducts. There is usually permanent immunity after an attack, and in the cases where there is recurrence, these are believed to be part of the original attack and not another one, or due to other viruses, serum hepatitis, cytomegalic inclusion disease or other infections.

Contagion: The virus which causes infectious hepatitis is usually transmitted by contact with the stool of patients with the disease. In experiments made with volunteers, the disease has been transmitted by injecting them with blood from a hepatitis patient or by having them swallow material filtered from contaminated stool. The virus is quite resistant to the usual types of sterilization, and there is evidence that the infection can be passed on when the virus lives on hypodermic needles and in hypodermic syringes which have been in contact with contaminated blood. Some outbreaks have originated in contaminated food, water or milk, but mostly the disease spreads in family contacts.

Infectious hepatitis usually remains communicable for several weeks, but it can be transmitted as long as the virus is in the stool of the patient, and this is sometimes more than six months.

Incubation Period: The incubation period varies between fifteen and forty-five days and is usually about twenty-five days.

Symptoms: The disease may be so mild as to go unnoticed, for in spite of its former name, it does not always cause jaundice. Probably there are more cases like this than more serious ones. It may be moderate, with a temperature of 100° to 102°, or very severe, starting with fever of 104° to 106°. There is usually headache, along with abdominal pain, nausea, vomiting, occasionally diarrhea and usually malaise and lassitude. After a period of up to fourteen days the child develops jaundice. The whites of his eyes and his skin become yellow, his urine becomes very dark, and his stools may be a pale chalklike color. The jaundice usually lasts for about ten days to two weeks, sometimes a month or six weeks. The high temperature stays up for four or five days, but there may be low-grade fever of 100° to 100.5° for months more. The general feeling of fatigue and lack of appetite may last longer than the jaundice or the fever.

The average child with hepatitis is ill for four to six weeks in all, but in some instances the disease may go on for two months or more. The usual outcome is a complete cure with no return of the disease, but occasionally the infection is more severe and more persistent, and there may be a relapse after the child is thought to be cured.

Treatment: A child with infectious hepatitis should be in a hospital unless it is possible for him to be in a separate room with separate bathroom facilities at home. There is no effective medicinal treatment. The only treatment we know is for the symptoms. Good general care, bed rest, a diet high in proteins, starches and sugars and relatively low in fat, and extra mixed vitamins are helpful. Antibiotics are not effective. Sleeping drugs should be avoided since the liver is unable to remove their toxic properties when it is not functioning properly. After the child's temperature becomes normal, he may be given bathroom privileges.

Convalescence: When it becomes obvious that the child is recovering, when his temperature is normal, the jaundice is gone, and laboratory tests indicate that liver function is improved or normal and the blood and urine are free of bile, he may be allowed limited activity. During the first two to four weeks after he has recovered, he should not be allowed excesses—strenuous sports, overeating and so forth.

Complications: Infectious hepatitis affects the liver mostly, and permanent liver injury is the only complication. This is rare in children, though it happens more often in adults.

Prevention: A child who is exposed to infectious hepatitis should be given an injection of gamma globulin to try to prevent the disease from developing. Gamma globulin is effective for only two to five weeks, so that if he is exposed again after three or four weeks the injections should be repeated. There is no method known of giving permanent immunity. No vaccine by which active immunity can be stimulated is presently available. The only other preventive is good personal hygiene.

Isolation and Quarantine: The child is isolated while he has fever and jaundice. In some hospitals this period is extended until other evidences of infection have disappeared. People who have been exposed are not quarantined.

Hygiene: While the child is ill, his stools and nose and throat discharges should be disinfected, and the stools should be handled carefully for several weeks after the fever and jaundice have disappeared and the child seems well.

SERUM HEPATITIS
(HOMOLOGOUS SERUM JAUNDICE)

The symptoms and course of the disease in serum hepatitis are indistinguishable from infectious hepatitis except for a longer period of incubation. When the doctor makes a diagnosis of serum hepatitis, it is usually because the child has received a blood transfusion or an injection of human blood or a blood product one to six months before the beginning of the symptoms. In most cases of this kind, an investigation will show that the blood donor had had jaundice or had been exposed to hepatitis. If his blood was injected into several people, probably more than one of them developed jaundice. Some studies have shown that as many as 2 to 3 per cent of transfused people develop hepatitis whether or not the donors could be found to have had it themselves. While serum hepatitis and infectious hepatitis are so similar clinically, there are some distinguishing differences:

	Infectious Hepatitis	Serum Hepatitis
Incubation period:	25 days (15 minimum and 45 maximum)	45–150 days 29 days minimum
Manner of infection:	Contact with infected patient or by injection	Injection of human blood or blood products or use of contaminated needle
Prevention:	Gamma globulin is effective	Gamma globulin is not effective
Outcome:	Usually favorable	Generally favorable, but less often than in infectious hepatitis

QUESTIONS & ANSWERS

Q. *Is infectious hepatitis very contagious?*

A. Less so than measles or mumps, but probably much more so than we suspect because of the large number of patients who do not develop jaundice and thus miss diagnosis.

Q. *Is the liver alone involved in this disease?*

A. It is the seat of most of the trouble, but the spleen and lymph glands may be enlarged, and the entire body is involved to some extent.

Q. *If the child does not have jaundice, does it mean the liver is not involved?*

A. No. We have tests which show that the liver is not functioning normally even when there is no jaundice. There are probably more cases of hepatitis without jaundice than with it.

Q. *Are there any diseases which resemble hepatitis?*

A. Yes. In adults, infectious mononucleosis can be very similar. In children, jaundice with infectious mononucleosis is less common. Any disease which causes fever and jaundice has to be considered in the diagnosis of infectious hepati-

tis. These diseases vary with local conditions. For instance,
where malaria is common, it would have to be considered
more seriously than where it is not. Other infections may
also cause jaundice.

Q. *Is the hospital the best place to treat infectious hepatitis?*

A. Not necessarily, unless the child requires fluid injections
into the bloodstream or if the facilities at home are poor
for adequate care of the child and separation from other
members of the family.

Q. *If my boy stays at home, how shall I take care of his
dishes and linen?*

A. The dishes should be boiled. Or use paper dishes and destroy them. The laundry, too, should be boiled for at least
twenty minutes.

Q. *Are there any other precautions?*

A. Yes. He should have a separate room and facility to dispose of his urine and stool without possible contact with
others in the home. His stool should be disinfected as long
as he is ill, and his nose and throat discharges should be
disinfected for the first three or four days.

Q. *If my other children had injections of gamma globulin,
would the patient have to be moved to a hospital?*

A. No.

Q. *Would the other children be protected by the gamma
globulin while he is at home?*

A. Probably, but it is not an absolutely sure thing.

Q. *If my child with infectious hepatitis will not eat, what
should I do?*

A. Try milk and other liquids, puddings, ice cream and other
soft foods.

Q. *Would eggs be bad for the liver?*

A. No, he probably would not eat enough of them to make
any difference.

Q. *May he have cream if he wants it?*

A. Yes.

Q. *Isn't the fat harmful?*

A. If he does not develop indigestion from it, no harm will be done.

Q. *How do I give a high carbohydrate diet?*

A. Give him extra fruit juices, cookies and hard candy. Keep them by his bed or chair so that he can have them any time he wants them.

Q. *How can I give him a high protein diet?*

A. Offer him eggs for breakfast, meat at lunch and dinner, cheese and skim milk and sponge cake at or between meals.

Q. *What if he refuses these foods?*

A. Let him eat what he can.

Q. *Are antibiotics or sulfa drugs helpful?*

A. No, and some sulfa drugs are harmful to the liver and should not be given, even when a different infection starts during infectious hepatitis.

Q. *Are all of your answers equally true for both kinds of hepatitis?*

A. Yes.

Q. *Are both kinds of hepatitis caused by the same virus transmitted in different ways?*

A. No. The viruses are different, but related.

Q. *If a child has jaundice with hepatitis, how can you tell whether it is due to infected human blood or exposure to infectious hepatitis?*

A. You can't without very difficult studies which are almost impossible to have made. A history of an injection of blood or a blood product may reveal which it is.

Q. *If my child had a transfusion four months ago and was exposed to infectious hepatitis one month ago and now has hepatitis, how can I tell which caused it?*

A. You cannot tell without involved, time-consuming studies, and even then there is no uncertainty.

Q. *If a child receives a transfusion of blood from a person with infectious hepatitis, will he develop serum hepatitis or infectious hepatitis?*

A. He may develop infectious hepatitis because that is what the donor had. Both types can be transmitted through infected blood.

Q. *If this child recovers and gets another transfusion and again develops hepatitis, which will it be this time?*

A. This one will almost surely be serum hepatitis because he will have become immune to the virus of infectious hepatitis after the first transfusion.

Q. *You mean that a person can have both?*

A. Yes. In fact, he might even get both at the same time.

Q. *Would he then become immune to both?*

A. Yes, probably.

Q. *Isn't this subject very confused?*

A. It certainly is. Its solution is yet to be discovered. .

Q. *Is there a skin test for infectious hepatitis?*

A. Yes, but we do not know how accurate it is.

Q. *Is there any vaccine to give permanent immunity to either kind of hepatitis?*

A. No, but efforts are being made to develop one.

Q. *Is there any drug treatment for either one?*

A. No.

Q. *When my boy has recovered from infectious hepatitis, has no fever, no jaundice and has a good appetite, may he go back to school?*

A. He may go back after he has had no symptoms for two weeks. He needs at least two weeks of convalescence before he becomes very active.

Q. *How can one avoid serum hepatitis?*

A. The only way is to avoid hypodermic injections, transfusions or injections of human blood or blood products whenever possible. But this does not mean that you should refuse to let an infant who has been exposed to measles have an injection of gamma globulin. When blood or blood products are indicated, do not interfere with the doctor's recommendations because of the possibility of jaundice. Less than 1 per cent and up to 3 per cent of those being transfused with whole blood may get hepatitis.

Q. *Is it true that infectious hepatitis is on the increase?*

A. It seems to be, in the United States, as of this time.

Q. *Is infectious hepatitis in dogs the same as it is in man?*

A. No.

Q. *I had hepatitis ten years ago. Why am I still rejected as a blood donor?*

A. Because it is possible, though unlikely, that you may still be a carrier of the virus causing the disease.

11: Infectious Mononucleosis (Glandular Fever)

Some thirty-five or forty years ago the bizarre disease now known as infectious mononucleosis was seldom recognized in children, and only rarely in adults. I have diagnosed the disease in a child nine months old, but it is not often observed in very young children or older adults. It is most common in older children, adolescents and young adults. Infectious mononucleosis is probably the same disease which used to be called glandular fever or Pfeiffer's disease.

Although we believe it is produced by a virus, its exact cause has not been discovered, nor has a cure for it been found. We do not know whether a single attack results in lasting immunity. We do know that it does not in some cases, because the disease may linger for weeks, months, and in rare instances, for a year or longer. During this period, the disease may quiet down, then flare up as if it were a new attack. I have never seen a case of infectious mononucleosis several years after recovery from the first attack, although such cases have been recorded.

Contagion: It is called infectious, but we do not often see more than one case in a family at the same time. However, I have seen the disease in a six-year-old boy whose father had had it six weeks before. The father was in contact with, and may have been infected by, an intimate friend next door who had had it. Though not particularly contagious in families, infectious mononucleosis often occurs in outbreaks in colleges, affecting many students, perhaps more than those who are sick enough to report for medical care. It is quite possible that many people who come in contact with it get it in a very mild form, too mild to be reported to a doctor, or to be recognized if the patient is examined.

The source of infection is probably discharges from the noses and throats of infected people, and kissing is strongly suspected of being responsible for the spread in many cases.

Incubation Period: An exact incubation period is not known, but it is believed to be about fourteen days, probably longer in some instances.

Symptoms: A sore throat, fever, swollen glands in the neck, and possibly in the armpits, groin and elsewhere in the body, puffy eyelids, sometimes a rash over the whole body, and, in a small percentage of cases, yellow jaundice suggests infectious mononucleosis. This is especially true if it occurs in adolescents and young adults.

In younger children the intensity and pattern of the disease differ considerably, being very severe in some and very mild in others. It may be so mild as not to be suspected except that the child feels below par and the parents try to find a reason for it. In cases where the disease lasts a long time, and in cases where the child has apparently recovered and a relapse occurs, infectious mononucleosis may vary from time to time in the same person. There may be one or more relapses, and when there are, they may be milder or just as severe as the first acute phase of the illness.

The fever of infectious mononucleosis may be low grade, 100° to 101°, and last for weeks or months, and in rare cases for a year or longer. It may be very high, 103° to 105°, and last a week or two, then become normal or remain at a lower level for a longer time. As in many other infections, the temperature may be normal for part of the day and become slightly elevated in the evening.

Infectious mononucleosis occurs without a sore throat in many cases. If there is a sore throat, however, it may be very mild or very severe. A membrane may be present on the tonsils similar to, and sometimes hard to distinguish from, the membrane seen in diphtheria. The disease should be suspected in a child whose sore throat fails to improve after treatment with antibiotics for several days, especially if a membrane is present and diphtheria can be ruled out as the cause.

The swollen glands may be very large or only slightly enlarged. They are usually painless, but not always. They are often accompanied by an enlarged spleen and sometimes an enlarged liver. Even when it is not enlarged, the liver is affected in a great many patients. In about 5 to 10 per cent of adults with infectious mononucleosis, jaundice occurs as a result of the liver disturbance, though this happens less frequently in children.

There is sometimes a rash, but not in every patient. Usually it looks like a scarlet fever or German measles rash, but it may be one of several different types. The same patient may have one kind of rash at the beginning of the disease and another with a relapse. Infectious mononucleosis also may involve the nervous system, the brain, the stomach and intestines, and as a result there may be symptoms of drowsiness, headache, stiff neck, abdominal pain and diarrhea.

Diagnosis: The blood count is quite indicative of this condition. The doctor is helped in making the correct diagnosis by finding certain characteristic changes in the blood cells under a microscope.

Another characteristic finding is a test of the blood, the heterophil test. This test is very helpful when positive, since it establishes the presence of the disease. A negative test does not prove that infectious mononucleosis is absent, since this test is not positive in all cases and may be positive at one stage of the illness and negative later. A newer and simpler test (mono test) is a good indicator of the disease, but should be corroborated by the heterophil test.

Treatment: A child ill with infectious mononucleosis should be kept in bed during the acute phase of the disease, or while there is sore throat and fever, and while there is a rash, swollen glands, enlarged liver or spleen, or jaundice. It is not necessary to restrict the child's activity until all of these have become normal, but only until they become stationary on a very much improved level.

If the child continues to have a low-grade fever, 99.5° to 100.5° daily, and if the lymph glands are still slightly enlarged after the acute phase of the illness has passed, you may let him out of bed and allow him limited play. If the low-grade fever continues for longer than four weeks, you may let him go back to school, provided he seems equal to it and does not tire too easily.

Treatment with antibiotics seems to be of no use. There are no useful serums or antitoxins. A well-balanced diet, vitamins and adequate rest are important. We can only treat the symptoms, and if there is a high fever or painful glands, aspirin may be helpful.

Complications: All patients with infectious mononucleosis recover except for the extremely rare case in whom the nervous system is irreparably damaged.

Prevention: There is no vaccine or serum which either prevents, cures or helps the disease. Unnecessary contact with a person who has it should be discouraged.

Isolation and Quarantine: The patient does not have to be isolated. Children who have been in contact with him are not quarantined. Exposed children may go to school and to the movies and other public places. They may go on with their normal routine without restrictions.

Hygiene: The patient's clothes, linens and dishes may be washed with those of the rest of the family. He may use the bathroom except when he is too ill to get out of bed.

QUESTIONS & ANSWERS

Q. *Are there many forms of infectious mononucleosis?*

A. It may affect people differently, but as far as we know, it is the same disease.

Q. *Does the disease differ in different parts of the world?*

A.   No.

Q.   *If I visit a friend with infectious mononucleosis, will I get it and can I carry it to my children?*

A.   No one can answer that with certainty. If you are in close contact with your friend, you may get it, but the likelihood of your getting an attack which makes you sick is rather small. The chance of your carrying it from your friend to your children is even smaller. But since we are not sure that you will not catch it, and since we do not know for sure whether it is a disease transmitted by carriers, it might be safer if you do not visit your friend until she has recovered. At least do not kiss her, especially on the mouth.

Q.   *When a child has infectious mononucleosis that lasts months, or even a year, does he remain infectious all that time?*

A.   Probably.

Q.   *Should a child with infectious mononucleosis be treated in a hospital?*

A.   Not usually, but some cases look so much like diphtheria that the child is sent to the hospital on the chance that it might be.

Q.   *Is it true that many doctors have found that some antibiotics cure infectious mononucleosis?*

A.   There have been some claims, but no proof of them. I have not been able to confirm the favorable results of treatment with antibiotics.

Q.   *Do the swollen glands ever become abscessed?*

A.   Not because of infectious mononucleosis.

Q.   *Does infectious mononucleosis ever result in serious damage to the patient?*

A.   Almost all patients recover completely, except for the very rare fatal case in which the nervous system is damaged beyond repair.

Q.   *Is the heterophil test always diagnostic?*

A.   Yes, if it is positive and done properly. Many laboratories do not do the "absorption test" unless requested to do so.

If the first test is negative, nothing more need be done. If strongly positive, even after the patient's blood serum has been diluted more than fiftyfold, the absorption test must be done to determine whether it is because of infectious mononucleosis, rather than serum sickness, or something else. Many illnesses are diagnosed as infectious mononucleosis because this absorption test is omitted. This may result in incorrect treatment for the actual condition present.

12: Measles (Rubeola)

Measles, until a few years ago the most common childhood disease except for the common cold, is destined to be reduced to an uncommon status if the available vaccines are given to most of the childhood population above nine months of age. From approximately three to four million cases per year in the United States, of which some six hundred thousand were reported, the recent U.S. Public Health Service report indicated a reduction to about two hundred thousand cases of measles annually reported.

In crowded sections of large cities we often find measles in infants and very young children, but in sections where there are many private homes it is more often a disease of the early school ages. You can get measles at any time from birth to old age, but infants born of mothers who have had measles have some immunity for the first six weeks to six months. If the mother has not had measles, the baby can get it at any time.

One attack of measles usually gives immunity for life. Second attacks do happen, but they are very rare, even if the first attack occurred in infancy.

Measles is caused by a virus. It comes in epidemics which recur every two or three years. In New York City, for instance, there have been as many as fifty thousand to a hundred thousand cases in an epidemic year, and only five or six thousand cases in other years. This number has already been reduced tremendously by the widespread use of vaccine to about 20 per cent of what it was.

Contagion: A child catches measles by coming into contact with droplets of moisture from the nose and throat of a person who has it, when the patient coughs, sneezes, talks or even breathes. It is one of the most contagious of the communicable diseases.

Incubation Period: The disease begins eleven days after exposure, sometimes in as few as seven or as many as fourteen days.

Prevention: Let your doctor know if your child has been exposed to measles. He may want to give him gamma globulin or some substitute which will make the disease milder if he should get it. If the child is less than two years old, or is older but ill with some other disease, or undernourished and in a weakened condition, the doctor may want to prevent measles entirely. The gamma globulin does not give permanent immunity. It gives a temporary one of two to four weeks. If a small amount is given within eight days—preferably within five or six days—of exposure to measles, it can modify the disease by making it milder. And if enough gamma globulin is given within five or six days of exposure, it may even prevent measles entirely. When measles is modified by gamma globulin or a substitute, the complications are reduced tremendously and the possibility of mortality is practically eliminated.

An injection of live vaccine on the first day of exposure may prevent measles or at least make it very mild. This has the advantage of producing lasting immunity. It must be done early to be effective.

Symptoms: Measles begins like a common cold. The child feels tired, uncomfortable and feverish. A cough and running nose develop and the eyes become inflamed and sensitive to light. The cough is hard and dry and is not helped by any of the usual medicines, and the fever usually becomes higher each day. It is during this period that the disease is most contagious. The rash starts at the end of the third or the beginning of the fourth day, first behind the ears or at the hairline. It spreads downward, covering the entire body in about thirty-six hours. In the beginning the spots are pink, about an eighth to a quarter of an inch in diameter. As the rash spreads, some of the spots run together, making it look blotchy. It often itches. The child feels sickest, the temperature is highest and the cough worst during the day or two of the development of the rash.

Remember that if your child has been exposed to measles and has been given gamma globulin to make it milder, it may be very different from the usual case. The fever may last a short time, a day or two. The rash may be scant, the coughing occasional. You will be watching for symptoms and you should call the doctor the moment the child shows any evidence of being ill. In a few cases the incubation period is longer than usual. It is shorter after an injection of live-measles-virus vaccine.

Diagnosis: In about 95 per cent of the cases Koplik spots (tiny red spots with white centers) appear in the mouth and can be seen on the cheeks and the gums near the molar teeth. Until these spots appear it is not possible to diagnose measles with certainty, except by special laboratory tests. They appear before the rash comes out, and they are difficult to see unless you know just what to look for. Do not try to diagnose and treat measles without a doctor. Without proper treatment the disease may become serious. Before we had antibiotics and sulfa drugs, measles was fatal to about 20 per cent of the infants who got it in the first year of life, and to about 6 per cent of children who got it in the first three years. Since the introduction of antibiotics and sulfa drugs, the mortality in New York City, for instance, has been reduced to 0.08 per cent. Even if the measles is mild and there is little or no danger of serious trouble, it is important to have a doctor make sure it is measles so that the child may be kept in bed away from other children, especially in schools.

It is very important for future reference to know whether or not the child has had measles, since there is almost no chance of getting it again once you have had it. It is particularly important to have the doctor identify the modified form since it also produces long-lasting immunity and may not be recognized by an inexperienced person. If you know the child has had measles, further injections of gamma globulin are unnecessary even if he is exposed again and again. Your child does not have to have measles to grow up, but if he is exposed to it, see what can be done to make it milder, and if he gets it, see what can be done to make it safe. All of this will soon be merely of historical interest since immunization with live measles vaccine seems to render the child immune for years (now known to be eight years) and possibly for life.

Treatment: While the child's eyes are feeling sensitive to light, a pair of dark glasses or dimmed lights in the room may be helpful. None of the usual medicines stops the cough completely, but the doctor may prescribe something that will help. The child wants to sleep and to be left alone. He should be encouraged to take fluids, but it doesn't matter if he eats little solid food. The doctor may give him one of the antibiotics or sulfa drugs to avoid complications or to treat the disease if it has already developed. Do not let anyone with a cold or a sore throat near a child with measles. It is these cold germs which cause the complications.

Convalescence: In the average case of measles, the temperature becomes normal about two days after the rash is completely out. The rash fades quickly, but leaves staining of the skin which may become so vivid at times, especially after a warm bath, as to suggest that the rash has returned. The skin peels in very fine, branlike flakes. For a week after the measles, the child is more susceptible to common infections, so convalescence should be restful.

Complications: Measles is a serious disease unless treated adequately. It is especially dangerous in young infants because of the complications which may result, particularly pneumonia and bronchitis, infected middle ear, sinus infection, lymph gland inflammations and occasionally encephalitis. You should suspect a complication if the child continues to have fever more than two days after the rash is completely out, or if the temperature becomes normal for a day or two and then rises, or if he complains of pain in the ear, chest or abdomen.

Isolation and Quarantine: A child who has measles is infectious, and is isolated for a total of seven to eight days, from three or four days before the rash appears until the temperature is normal and the rash begins to fade. The child may be freed from isolation at this time. If the child is exposed to measles, he is not infectious unless he develops it. Since this usually takes ten or eleven days after the first moment of exposure, he need not be quarantined for at least seven days. Most schools want exposed children kept away from the seventh to the fourteenth day after exposure, so it is important to notify the school that the child has been exposed. By the end of this time it will be obvious whether or not he has caught it.

Hygiene: To make the child's room safe for people who have not had measles, it need only be thoroughly cleaned and aired.

QUESTIONS & ANSWERS

Q. *How many different kinds of measles are there?*

A. Only one. German measles is called by that name because sometimes the rashes are similar, but German measles is a totally different disease.

Q. *Is measles the same all over the world?*

A. Yes, but the severity and complications differ somewhat with the climate, with its prevalence, with the season of the year and with other factors. Measles can be mild, in which case the child does not feel very ill and the temperature stays below 102°. It may be severe and the patient is very sick, has a high fever, and a heavy cough. The severe form is more likely to have complications, although they sometimes come with the very mild form, too.

Q. *Does everyone have to have measles?*

A. No, and most people will never have ordinary measles if they are vaccinated with live measles vaccine.

Q. *What causes measles?*

A. A virus.

Q. *Do domestic animals like cats and dogs get measles?*

A. No. Distemper is rather like measles, but it is not the same disease. The rinderpest virus is also very similar to that which causes measles.

Q. *Can you get measles more than once?*

A. Yes, but rarely. Many people claim to have had it two or three times. but usually this is due to incorrect diagnosis, probably made without a doctor. An occasional case has been seen after the patient has had the modified type or reaction to the live vaccine.

Q. *If a child is exposed to measles and does not get it, does that mean he is immune and will never get it?*

A. No. About 83 per cent of children get it after an intimate exposure such as being with a brother or sister who has it. About half of those who failed to get it the first time get it on the second exposure. Most of the rest get it later.

Q. *Should I deliberately expose my children to get it over with?*

A. No, have your child given live measles vaccine.

Q. *If you get modified measles, are you immune for life?*

A. Probably yes. Modification of measles has been practiced on a large scale for only thirty-five years. It may be too early to answer that question with certainty. We know of only a fraction of 1 per cent of children who had had modified measles and developed the disease in regular form sometime later. Possibly there are more such cases which have not been recorded.

Q. *Can a person who has had measles carry it?*

A. Yes, but he will not infect others until he develops symptoms of the disease.

Q. *Can a person who has not had measles carry it right after he is exposed?*

A. No. The measles virus can be carried for only a few moments.

Q. *Is a person contagious during the incubation period if he has been exposed?*

A. No, not until the first symptoms of the disease begin—usually about ten days after infection.

Q. *How do you know when you have been exposed?*

A. If you have been with a person who develops the measles rash three or four days later, consider yourself exposed.

Q. *How long an exposure is necessary to catch measles?*

A. A single breath from the sick person is enough, but the longer your exposure, the greater the chance of getting it.

Q. *Do you have to be in actual contact with a measles patient to get it?*

A. You have to be close enough to be reached by the patient's breath.

Q. *Is it transmitted only by the breath?*

A. Yes, almost always. The patient passes the virus in tiny droplets from his nose and throat. Any susceptible person near by may be infected. It is only very rarely passed on by contaminated clothes or utensils.

Q. *For how long after measles starts is it contagious?*

A. Seven to eight days from the beginning of the first symptoms.

Q. *For how long before the rash comes is measles contagious?*

A. Usually three or four days. Rarely, a day or two longer.

Q. *If you give gamma globulin, will it give a child lifelong immunity?*

A. No, the effect of GG lasts only for two to four weeks. If the child doesn't get modified measles and is exposed again two or three weeks after the injection, it will be necessary to give another dose of GG—preferably he should be given live vaccine if he has not had measles.

Q. *In a modified case of measles, how long is the child contagious?*

A. Modified measles is usually contagious for a shorter time, because the whole course of the disease is shortened. But the child can spread the disease as long as he is ill, especially while he is coughing.

Q. *Why is it so important to give gamma globulin to infants who are exposed?*

A. Measles is a very dangerous disease in the first two years of life. The death rate can be quite high. If gamma globulin is given, there is almost no mortality and the complications are reduced to only 1 to 2 per cent. Avoid the need for GG by immunizing the child at ten to twelve months of age with live measles vaccine.

Q. *I have had measles. Since the immunity transmitted from me to my baby lasts six weeks to six months, should I do anything if the baby is exposed during that time?*

A. Probably not until the baby is three months old. After that, it may be safer to give him a very small dose of gamma globulin because his immunity may be less strong by then.

Q. *Can you be vaccinated against measles for permanent immunity?*

A. Yes. Vaccination is now available throughout the United States and in many other countries. The live measles vaccine is almost 100 per cent effective and should be given to all over nine months of age who have not yet had the disease.

Q. *Is there such a thing as internal measles?*

A. Measles does involve the inner parts of the body, such as the bronchial tubes, the tonsils and the appendix.

Q. *Can you have measles without a rash?*

A. Yes, if it has been modified by gamma globulin, or is the result of live measles vaccine.

Q. *What are black measles?*

A. A very severe and rare form in which the rash is accompanied by black-and-blue spots. But most often what is called black measles turns out to be some other condition, which is accompanied by a hemorrhagic skin rash, such as epidemic spinal meningitis or purpura, a blood disease.

Q. *Does the rash always behave the same?*

A. Usually, but not always. It may take a little longer to come out completely, and in very severe forms of measles it may come out within twelve to twenty-four hours. It also varies in its intensity and its depth of color.

Q. *Can a mother diagnose measles?*

A. Yes, sometimes. But she might label many other diseases with a rash as measles. Her diagnosis should always be confirmed by the doctor's.

Q. *Does fever or heat bring out the measles rash?*

A. No. The rash develops whether the temperature is high or low. The idea that the patient should be kept very warm or given a hot bath to bring out the rash is an old wives' tale.

Q. *Must the patient be kept warm?*

A. Yes, comfortably so. The room should be about 72°.

Q. *How can you stop the cough?*

A. There is no way of stopping it completely, but it may be helped with medicine prescribed by the doctor.

Q. *What can you do for the itch that comes with measles?*

A. A sponge bath with cornstarch or oatmeal flour may be helpful or calamine lotion or some similar product. The doctor may prescribe other medicine such as the antihistamine drugs if the itch is very annoying.

Q. *Are antibiotics or sulfa drugs used in the treatment of measles?*

A. It depends on the presence or absence of complications, on the age of the child, and on the point of view of your doctor. You should never use these drugs yourself without consulting him.

Q. *Shall I let my child with measles go to the bathroom?*

A. Yes, if it is close by and he is not very sick. Otherwise a bedpan and urinal are preferable.

Q. *Will an injection of gamma globulin after the disease has begun do any good?*

A. Possibly, but it is only practical under unusual circumstances because a large amount has to be given before the rash appears in order to be effective.

Q. *Can a child with measles eat what he likes?*

A. Yes, if he wants food.

Q. *Should there be any special care of the eyes?*

A. If light annoys the child, and it usually does, let him wear dark glasses or dim the room. Don't black it out altogether, though, because light kills the measles virus.

Q. *Are the eyes affected permanently in measles?*

A. No.

Q. *Will reading hurt my child's eyes?*

A. While he is very sick he probably will not want to read. When he feels well enough, he may.

Q. *How soon may I let him watch television?*

A. As soon as his eyes are no longer sensitive to light. Probably this will be a day or two after the rash disappears.

Q. *May I bathe the child?*

A. Only sponge him. He may be chilled in a tub bath.

Q. *How soon may he go out of doors?*

A. When he is completely well and has been so for a few days.

Q. *May he travel in a school bus as soon as he is well?*

A. Yes.

Q. *May he lead a normal life right after measles?*

A. For a week or two he may be more susceptible to infections, so you should be careful about exposing him to crowds, and he should rest more than usual.

Q. *If a pregnant woman gets measles, is anything likely to happen to the infant?*

A. No. It is German measles that has a bad effect on the unborn infant.

Q. *Is it better to have measles during childhood?*

A. Yes, after five years of age. It is more dangerous in infancy and old age as most infections are. Preferably he should be given the live vaccine when he is ten or twelve months old, or as soon thereafter as possible.

Q. *If a child develops a running ear as a result of measles, does he remain contagious?*

A. No longer than he does if the ear does not run.

Q. *What can you do to prevent complications before measles has started?*

A. Your doctor may give the child gamma globulin to modify it.

Q. *What can you do to prevent complications after measles has started?*

A. Your doctor may choose to give the child some of the antibiotics or sulfa drugs if any sign of a complication appears.

Q. *How can you tell whether the measles is complicated?*

A.   A pain in the ear or the chest or the abdomen indicates a complication; so does fever if it continues more than two or three days after the rash is out completely, or if the temperature drops, stays normal for a day or two, then rises, or the patient starts coughing again.

Q.   *My maid's child has measles. Can she go home and then come back here without bringing measles to my family?*

A.   If she has had measles, she can't carry it to your family. If she has not, and has been with her child during the measles, she may not develop the measles until two weeks after her child is completely well. If she has not caught it by that time she is safe for your family.

Q.   *My child has been exposed to measles. May he keep on going to school?*

A.   Some schools allow it for the first seven days after the first day of exposure, after which he would have to stay home for a week after the last day of exposure. Others will not let him come for two weeks after the last day of exposure. You will have to abide by the ruling of the health department in your community and by the ruling of your school doctor.

Q.   *May a child have visitors while he has measles?*

A.   Yes, if the visitors have already had it.

Q.   *How soon after the measles rash is gone may my child go to the movies?*

A.   That depends on his temperature and general condition. If he has had no fever for a week after the rash has disappeared and his eyes are clear, he may go to the movies.

Q.   *If a child has measles, do all his clothes and toys become infected, and how can you get rid of the germs?*

A.   His things will be free of the measles virus if they are left exposed to the air for an hour.

Q.   *Should the child's urine and stool be treated with an antiseptic?*

A.   No.

Q.   *After a child has had measles, how do you make the room safe for one who hasn't had it?*

A. It is probably safe after about an hour without your doing anything, but clean and air the room thoroughly, and leave the window open for an hour. The bed linen and the patient's clothes will, of course, have to be laundered.

Q. *May letters written by a child while he has the measles be sent through the mail?*

A. Yes.

Q. *May clothes worn by a child with measles be sent to a laundry?*

A. Yes.

Q. *Must eating utensils and dishes be boiled?*

A. No. Washing with soap and water is good enough.

Q. *Will measles be completely eradicated through the use of a vaccine?*

A. It is conceivable if children everywhere in the world were to be immunized with live measles vaccine.

Q. *Is it safe for everyone to be vaccinated with live measles vaccine?*

A. Not quite. Persons with convulsive tendencies, those with leukemia, lymphoma, cancer, active tuberculosis, pregnant women who have not had measles, and others acutely or chronically ill should not take the live measles vaccine alone.

Q. *Should they not be protected?*

A. Yes, of course, they need protection. They should be given both gamma globulin and live-virus vaccine.

Q. *Is the measles which follows the live vaccine contagious?*

A. No, not at all. Most children do not look or act ill.

Q. *May a child who has just received the live measles vaccine attend school?*

A. Yes, if he does not have fever.

Q. *Even if he has a rash?*

A. At that time he may also have fever. In any event, he may not be permitted to attend school, since it is quite possible that the rash is due to some other infection—and not to the vaccine.

Q. *Will gamma globulin be needed once the child has been vaccinated?*

A. Some recommend a small dose of gamma globulin at the time of giving the measles vaccine, because it makes the reaction to the vaccine much milder. If the child has not had the vaccine and is exposed to measles, the GG will be helpful. A danger in giving GG at the time of vaccination with live measles vaccine is that just a small increase of the GG may block the development of immunity from the vaccine.

Q. *What kind of measles results from the vaccine?*

A. The killed measles vaccine causes no more illness than an injection of diphtheria toxoid, and in a few cases fever for a day or two and slight swelling at the site of injection. This vaccine is no longer recommended in the United States. The live vaccine produces fever most commonly on the sixth to eighth day. It may begin as early as the fifth day and as late as the fourteenth day after receiving the vaccine, and lasts one to three days. Fever of 101° to 102° occurs frequently in 50 per cent or more, 103° or higher occurs in 15 per cent to 30 per cent, depending on the vaccine. Some vaccines are less likely to produce high fever and rash. The rash may occur in 10 per cent to 50 per cent depending on the vaccine. It is usually very mild and lasts one to three days.

Q. *What are the complications following the live vaccine?*

A. Almost none.

Q. *Is the vaccine immunity permanent?*

A. Most children who had the vaccine at age five or six and up to eight years of age are still immune. Few have subsequently gotten regular measles. The immunity seems to be permanent in most children.

Q. *It seems as if measles can be eliminated. And to think that my grandmother believed that one has to have measles to grow up. Is that not true?*

A. Yes, that is what grandma believed. We know more about it now. The vaccine, if used universally, can make measles as rare as poliomyelitis, and more children will grow up without the damage resulting from measles. Grandma, like so many other wonderful people, was in tune with her generation, but, of course, not with modern developments.

Q. *Who discovered the measles vaccine?*

A. A great and wonderful person and scientist, a Nobel Prize winner—Dr. John F. Enders, of Harvard University. Of course, he was the leader of a fine group of associates who helped develop it.

Q. *Do you recommend any special type of live measles vaccine?*

A. There are several, all quite good and very effective. Some are supposed to cause less fever and less rash than others. These are known as further-attenuated vaccines. Many researchers are trying to produce vaccines which are both effective and less productive of reactions. When these are available, they will undoubtedly be more popular. One has recently been developed—Moraten. The early trials indicate that it is very good.

13: Mumps
(Epidemic Parotitis)

Mumps is one of the most common diseases of childhood. It is prevalent everywhere. Wherever there are groups of children and young people living together, mumps is likely to occur in outbreaks. Children's institutions, boarding schools and army camps are especially liable to have epidemics. Although mumps has been found in newborn babies and elderly people, it is most common between five and nine years. Second and third children are likely to have it earlier because their older siblings bring it home, and children living in crowded areas catch it earlier than others. About 50 per cent of children fifteen years old have had it, and possibly the percentage is even greater since we know that immunity to the disease is even more widespread than that. About a hundred and fifty thousand cases of mumps are reported each year in the United States. Since the disease often is not recognized, the actual number of cases is probably more than double the number reported. It is most common in winter and spring in temperate climates, but there are some cases all year. It is caused by a virus.

Mumps is usually thought of as an infection settling in the salivary glands. These are the parotid glands just below the ears, the submaxillary glands under the lower jaw, and the sublingual glands under the chin. Actually, mumps is a more general infection, and it involves not only the salivary glands, but the testicles or ovaries, the pancreas, the nervous system, and occasionally even the heart. The mumps virus can be found in the patient's blood, which means that it is possible for it to spread through the entire system.

Some doctors consider the sex gland involvement a complication, while others think of it as a part of the disease, affecting these parts of the body more in some cases than others. The sex glands hardly ever seem to be seriously involved in children before puberty. In my forty-three years of active pediatric practice, I have seen obvious swelling of the testicles only six or eight times in boys who had not reached puberty, and a few more boys of four to seven years have complained of pain in the testicles for a day or two during mumps without visible swelling.

Some doctors also consider involvement of the nervous system a regular part of the disease rather than a complication. In most cases where the nervous system is involved, the patient recovers without evident ill effects. Fortunately, involvement of neither the sex glands nor the nervous system is as serious as most people seem to think. It is possible to become sterile because of mumps, but it doesn't happen very often— only in about 5 per cent of those who have orchitis (inflammation of the testis) or oophoritis (inflammation of the ovaries). For the past twenty-five years we have realized that people can have mumps without obvious swelling of the salivary glands. We are sure of this for two reasons. First, adolescents and adults who have been exposed to mumps have shown no evidence of illness until the sex glands have become swollen and painful, or until the patients have become dizzy, had headaches and other symptoms which indicate a nervous system involvement. Second, we now have accurate laboratory methods for finding out whether a person has recently had mumps. These tests have shown that those who had had only sex gland or nervous system symptoms had really been infected with the mumps virus, and that other people who had been exposed to mumps had developed immunity to it without being aware of illness. Furthermore, many patients who were thought to have had polio or other serious forms of nervous system disease, and who had recovered, are shown by these tests to have had nervous system involvement caused by the mumps virus.

These tests have enabled us to say that infants born of mothers who have had mumps have immune substance for

about two or three months, and that many more adults have
had mumps infections in the past than we used to think. This
may account for the apparently very low number of people
who catch visible mumps when they are exposed, for, unlike
measles, which always comes with a rash, mumps may not be
noticed. By these tests we have also been able to find out
that every swelling of a salivary gland is not necessarily
mumps.

Although many people say that second attacks of mumps are
rare, I have found in my own practice that they are not so rare.
In one army station hospital I questioned many mumps patients
and to my surprise learned that many of them had had mumps
as children when their brothers or sisters had had it. I have
treated children with their first attacks and then again when
they caught it on being exposed again several years later. My
last such patient had had his first attack before puberty and
the second one at nineteen. With the second attack he had
both testicular and nervous-system involvement. While this is
not the usual thing, it is important to point out, for it shows that
adults should avoid unnecessary exposure to mumps even
though they have had it as children. Of course, other viruses
may produce similar illness. It is therefore uncertain that a
"second attack" can be positively identified as mumps.

Contagion: Mumps is very contagious, but less so than
measles or chicken pox. It is spread by droplets from the
throat of the patient to the susceptible people who come in
contact with him. The virus dies so quickly when exposed to
the air that it is unlikely that anyone would catch it by
handling contaminated clothes or dishes or bedding.

Incubation Period: The incubation period of mumps varies
a good deal. It may be anywhere from eleven to twenty-six
days. Usually the disease begins eighteen days after exposure.

Symptoms: The first sign of mumps may be painful swelling
of the parotid glands in front of and below the ear. As they become swollen and tender, they hurt more when the child opens
his mouth. He may complain of discomfort in the mouth when
he eats acid food such as citrus fruit or pickles, but this is not
as foolproof a test for mumps as many people think, because
acid foods do not bother some mumps patients at all. The child

usually has a fever ranging from 100° to 104°, usually between 100° and 102°, for a day before any swelling of the face is noticed, and for two to four days after the swelling starts. The beginning of mumps may be mistaken for the beginning of a cold or the grippe, with the same general discomfort. The swelling of the glands, on one or both sides, increases in the first two or three days, then becomes less until about the fifth to seventh day when it can no longer be seen or felt. Both sides may be swollen at once, or one or more glands in one place may swell and recede before others begin, or only one side may ever swell. Just when the illness seems to be finished, other symptoms may appear indicating that other parts of the body have been infected such as the sex glands or the nervous system. These symptoms usually appear in the second week of the illness.

Treatment: When mumps begins, you should put the child to bed or make him rest until all signs of active disease have disappeared, that is, until there has been no fever for a day or two, lessening of swelling or tenderness of the salivary glands, and no evidence of other involvement. This may be hard to do with a lively youngster whose temperature has become normal, but it is easier if an armchair or a couch is used for part of the day instead of a bed. Radio and television help. You should call the doctor early in the disease to make the diagnosis and outline the treatment of the patient.

Treatment usually consists of simple devices for controlling the fever and the pain in the swollen glands. Camphorated oil or cold compresses on the child's swollen cheeks may be comforting. Don't give him tart foods if he complains of pain when he eats them. If they don't bother him, give him a regular diet. Some doctors prefer a diet that is low in fat, with very little butter, cream, bacon or other fat foods because the pancreas, which secretes enzymes to digest the fat, may be involved in mumps. I, myself, doubt whether the diet matters much.

Various drugs and serums have been tried to speed up recovery, but none of them seems to be very effective.

Convalescence: Convalescence after mumps should continue for at least seven days, especially in children past puberty.

Complications: If we think of involvement of the sex glands and the nervous system as complications rather than part of the disease, complications are frequent. The testicles are involved in 5 to 15 per cent of male patients past puberty, and in occasional outbreaks as many as 35 per cent of adults have testicular involvement. This rarely happens before puberty. It is hard to estimate the number of female patients who have involvement of the ovaries. When sex gland inflammation occurs, the patient is kept in bed. The scrotum is supported in a suspensory sac. Male sex hormones, female sex hormones and other hormones have been tried. Some doctors think that cortisone helps, but there is little proof that any hormones do. If a child with mumps becomes very dizzy, usually around the end of the first week, it is evidence of involvement of the nervous system. He may have trouble lifting his head off the pillow. Then he may vomit and have a headache. The temperature may rise after being normal for one or several days. Usually this passes without any ill effects and needs no special treatment except complete rest for a few days. On rare occasions it is not so mild and results in deafness or some other nerve injury.

The heart may be affected by mumps, but rarely significantly in childhood; I mention it only for the sake of completeness. Even in adults this complication is rarely troublesome.

Prevention: In childhood, mumps is usually mild so that preventive measures may not seem to be indicated. If, however, the frequent complication of encephalitis is considered, prevention of mumps is important. Effective vaccine has been available in Eastern Europe and one has recently become available in the United States. It is being recommended for pubescent children, adolescents and young adults of childbearing age. I prefer to immunize children before they enter school, playgroups, day camps, etc., to avoid infecting older children and adults who have not had mumps. If a child or adult who has not had mumps is exposed, he may be given some gamma globulin especially prepared from the blood of persons convalescing from the disease.

Isolation and Quarantine: A child may spread mumps a day or two before the gland swelling appears and as long as there is any swelling—usually about five to seven days. He is isolated during this period. If another gland becomes involved, the child has to be isolated until he is completely recovered, possibly as long as fourteen days. Children who have been exposed to mumps are usually not quarantined, but quarantine measures are sometimes necessary if many cases break out in a school, nursery, children's home or army barracks, and it is considered necessary to try to stop the epidemic.

Hygiene: While the child has mumps, no special methods are necessary. Soap and water for bedding, clothes, dishes and utensils are enough. After the disease is over, you can clean the room as you normally would.

QUESTIONS & ANSWERS

Q. *Why don't babies get mumps if the immunity they get from their mothers lasts only a few months?*

A. Probably because they are more protected and do not become exposed to it.

Q. *Would a six-month-old baby get mumps if he were exposed to it?*

A. Probably, but it might be difficult to detect. Most infants have immunity for the first six months.

Q. *My child had mumps on one side last year. Is he apt to get it again?*

A. No. The immunity you get from a case of mumps has nothing to do with how many glands are swollen. You do not become immune on one side and remain susceptible on the other. It affects the whole body.

Q. *Can you carry mumps?*

A. Not unless you are about to come down with it yourself.

Q. *I have not had mumps. May I visit my cousin who has them? Will I bring it back to my child?*

A. No. You should not visit your cousin, since you may catch the disease and have it without any swelling of your glands. Even so, you could infect your child.

Q. *Is it dangerous to kiss or embrace a child who has mumps?*

A. Possibly, even if you have had it. Of course with an infant, it is impossible to avoid intimate contact and the likelihood of getting it again is quite small.

Q. *Will the use of a mask lessen the chances of catching mumps from my child?*

A. Yes, somewhat.

Q. *Is a person contagious during the phase of testicle swelling?*

A. Yes.

Q. *Is he contagious if he has involvement of the nervous system?*

A. Yes, probably.

Q. *My child was with a friend on March 7, 8 and 9. On March 10 his friend had typical mumps. When is my child likely to get it?*

A. About eighteen days from March 7, 8 or 9, that is, March 25 to 27. The extremes are from March 19 to April 1, but this is less likely.

Q. *My child has mumps. His glands are swollen, but he has no fever and doesn't feel sick. Should I keep him in bed?*

A. No. He may be up and about in his room or in the house if everyone in the house has already had mumps.

Q. *The gland swelling is gone, but my child still has fever. Why?*

A. Possibly another part of the body is involved or a complication has set in.

Q. *Is there any special diet that is best during mumps?*

A. No, but tart foods may cause some pain in the mouth. If they do, they should be left out of the diet. Some doctors restrict the amount of fats, but I don't believe this is necessary.

Q. *Is it all right to bathe my child while he has mumps?*

A. Yes.

Q. *May I wash my daughter's hair while she has mumps?*

A. It would be better not to, but there really is no good reason for not doing it.

Q. *Is there any medicine to make mumps milder?*

A. Nothing reliable.

Q. *Does gamma globulin affect the disease once it has started?*

A. Generally speaking, the answer is no.

Q. *Do the antibiotics help mumps?*

A. No.

Q. *How can I tell when my child has recovered?*

A. When the swellings are gone and the temperature has been normal for two or three days, and the child feels well.

Q. *What can I do to avoid the complications of mumps?*

A. Nothing more than taking good care of the child. Let him rest and do not let him be very active while he has fever.

Q. *Do hormones help the sex gland involvements of mumps?*

A. Some hormones have been tried and have failed to prevent it, but cortisone or other similar drugs may relieve the pain and swelling once it has developed.

Q. *What can be done for the nervous system involvement?*

A. There is no specific medicine or serum, but cortisone has been used with questionable success.

Q. *Are complications of the ovaries as frequent as those of the testicles?*

A. There are no accurate figures on this question.

Q. *Does gamma globulin prevent mumps?*

A. Possibly large doses of gamma globulin or convalescent serum might be effective.

Q. *Since mumps is less dangerous before puberty, should I deliberately expose my six-year-old son?*

A. No. A vaccine is now available which results in immunity in over 90 per cent of cases.

Q. *My child has been exposed to mumps. Should he be given gamma globulin or vaccine?*

A. If he is in good condition and has not reached puberty, you might just do nothing. If he has passed puberty, the hyperimmune gamma globulin might be worth trying. If the exposure lasted only one or two days, vaccine may be helpful.

Q. *Is it worthwhile to have a skin test to find out whether I am immune to mumps?*

A. It is not generally recommended, except when adults have been or are about to be exposed. Then the doctor is likely to make a skin test to find out whether or not he should give you an immunizing injection. It is not always reliable. An injection of live mumps virus vaccine might be more useful.

Q. *My son has been exposed to mumps. May he go to school during the eighteen-day incubation period?*

A. That depends on your local health department or school regulations.

Q. *May he go to a party on the eighteenth day of the incubation period?*

A. Not unless all the children at the party have already had mumps. This is when he may be infectious.

Q. *May he go to the movies during the time he is likely to develop mumps?*

A. No.

Q. *How soon after the gland swelling is gone may my child have company?*

A. If his friend has had mumps, he may visit at any time. If he has not, he may come seven days after the onset of the disease, or two or three days after the gland swelling is gone if there is no fever or other sign of active disease. To be absolutely safe, a child who has had swelling on only one side should have no susceptible visitors for a week after the gland swelling is gone, because the glands on the other side sometimes swell after the first ones have subsided. This indicates that the infection is still present.

Q. *A case of mumps broke out in my child's class at school. Should my child, who has not had mumps, be kept at home?*

A. No, he should be given the live-virus vaccine promptly and continue to attend school.

Q. *Is it important to separate a child with mumps from his sisters and brothers who have not had it?*

A. Yes, if you don't want the other children to get it. They have probably already been exposed, but the longer they are in contact with it, the more likely they are to get it. Give them vaccine immediately after the initial exposure.

Q. *Should my older boy, who is seventeen, be allowed to visit a friend who has mumps?*

A. No. Mumps at seventeen may be associated with sex gland involvements and is more dangerous than in early childhood.

Q. *My husband has not had mumps. May he play with our son who has it now?*

A. No. Your husband should avoid contact with the boy because there is an 85 per cent chance of his getting it. However, there is also an 85 per cent chance that he is immune.

Q. *Should the dishes used by a mumps patient be boiled?*

A. No. Washing with soap and water is enough.

Q. *May I send my child's clothes and bedding to the laundry while she has mumps?*

A. Yes.

Q. *Should I take special precautions with my child's laundry while she has mumps?*

A. No. Ordinary laundering or airing for several hours will get rid of the mumps virus. Use paper dishes and disposable plastic utensils.

Q. *How soon may my child's room be occupied by someone who has not had mumps?*

A. Probably within a few minutes after the room is thoroughly cleaned. To be absolutely sure, air the room for an hour after cleaning it before someone else sleeps in it.

Q. *Is it likely that effective mumps vaccine will soon be available?*

A. Good vaccine is already available.

Q. *Should all children be given mumps vaccine if they have not had mumps?*

A. Yes, with some reservation. It is definitely recommended for pubescent children, for adolescents (especially boys) and for young adults who have not had mumps. I think it useful in the preschool period, especially if there are pubescent or adolescent children or parents who have not had mumps. I know no contraindication for giving the vaccine to infants who are a year old or older.

   If given on the first or second day of exposure, it may be helpful, but we do not have adequate experience with this problem.

Q. *Why should the infants and younger children get the vaccine if it is not dangerous at those ages?*

A. Mumps is never really safe, but if the younger children get it they may infect those who are older, for whom the mumps is more dangerous.

14: Roseola Infantum (Exanthum Subitum)

Sometimes I am worried by seeing a baby with a fever of 103° to 105° for which there seems to be no explanation, and who does not look very ill. Most of the time the illness has proved to be roseola.

Roseola is a very common disease known everywhere, occurring most frequently in the fall, winter and spring. It usually occurs in the first year of life, rarely after the third year, although it has been seen in children up to six or eight. It is probably caused by a virus. To the best of our knowledge, one attack leaves permanent immunity, although recurrence of a similar type of infection a year or two later has occurred. In many such cases it is impossible to tell whether it is the same disease since it is often difficult to distinguish it from German measles, reaction to drugs and, occasionally, other diseases with rashes.

Incubation Period: The incubation period seems to be about two weeks.

Contagion: It is apparently not as contagious as some of the other diseases, since brothers and sisters in the same house do not catch it, though possibly the infection they get is very mild, without fever or rash. We do not know whether this can happen, as it does in German measles.

Symptoms: Early in the disease the child has a very high fever which lasts three or four days, the temperature then drops to normal, and after twelve to eighteen hours a rash appears. The rash usually consists of flat, pink spots covering the whole body. They are rather pale compared with a measles rash. Even though the temperature goes as high as 104° or 105°, the child does not look very sick except that he may be jittery. Occasionally he becomes so nervous that he has a convulsion. Usually his throat is not particularly red. Behind the ears and on the back of the head the lymph glands become enlarged, but they are not very tender. Lymph glands in other parts of the body may also be enlarged.

Diagnosis: The white blood cells drop in number, and one particular type, the leukocytes, is sharply reduced while another type, the lymphocytes, remains high or is increased. The unexplained high fever, the presence of enlarged lymph nodes at the back of the head, behind the ears and in the neck, the relative state of well-being in spite of the fever, and a low white blood cell count in an infant or young child are enough to suggest the diagnosis of roseola.

Treatment: The child should be kept in bed, comfortably warm. If he is old enough to use the bathroom, it is all right to let him do it. There is no special form of treatment. The temperature should be reduced with aspirin and sponges. Other medicines such as antibiotics are not effective. The child may eat as usual if he wants to.

Complications: The only complication I have seen in roseola was convulsions, and these are not at all rare, and may occur more than once. They almost never leave any injury. These may be avoided by keeping the temperature below 102° with aspirin.

Prevention: There is no preventive drug, vaccine or serum which protects against roseola. A skin test for diagnosis is not available.

Isolation and Quarantine: You need not isolate a child with roseola any more than you would isolate any sick child from well ones, and there is no quarantine of children who have been exposed.

QUESTIONS & ANSWERS

Q. *Is roseola known by any other name?*

A. Yes. It is frequently called *exanthum subitum* (unexpected eruption), and in Germany it is called *Vierte Krankheit,* or fourth disease.

Q. *Is roseola another form of German measles?*

A. No. They are separate diseases.

Q. *My child has had roseola three times. How do you explain that?*

A. I doubt very much whether it is possible. Probably one of the illnesses was German measles, possibly another was measles or a drug rash and the third roseola.

Q. *Does roseola resemble measles?*

A. No, except that the rash sometimes looks like a measles rash. Otherwise the course of the disease is quite different. Immunity to roseola does not immunize a child against either measles or German measles.

Q. *Do children with roseola cough or sneeze?*

A. No.

Q. *Do they have a sore throat?*

A. They are usually too young to complain of it if they do, but sometimes the doctor finds the throat is red.

Q. *Do the swollen lymph glands hurt the child?*

A. No, apparently not.

Q. *My child had all the first symptoms of roseola, but she never had the rash. Could it be roseola?*

A. Yes. Sometimes the rash lasts such a short time and is so faint that the mother does not see it, though usually it lasts for a day or two. Occasionally we observe an illness similar to roseola in every way except that no rash develops.

Q. *Is there anything special to do for a child with roseola?*

A. Yes. It is important to keep the temperature down by sponges or aspirin, since some doctors think the convulsions occur only because of the high fever.

Q. *Do the sulfa drugs or antibiotics help roseola?*

A. No.

Q. *Are there any complications or aftereffects of roseola?*

A. I have never seen any except an occasional convulsion, and that has left no aftereffects—none that we have detected.

Q. *Should a child with roseola be isolated?*

A. No.

Q. *Is a child quarantined if he has been exposed to roseola?*

A. No.

Q. *May an older child go to school during the time his baby brother has roseola?*

A. Yes. It is rare in children over two years of age.

15: Shingles
(Herpes Zoster)

Shingles is caused by a virus, one which appears to be identical to the chicken pox virus, when seen with the aid of an electron microscope. It is contagious and produces shingles in some and chicken pox in others, particularly those who have not had chicken pox.

The incubation period is usually thirteen to sixteen days, occasionally up to twenty-one days.

Shingles may occur in outbreaks as well as sporadically. It may occur more than once in the sense that children who have had chicken pox may acquire shingles later. While chicken pox causes a general eruption, herpes zoster usually erupts along a nerve path.

Symptoms: There may be a general sick feeling with fever. This is usually followed in a few days by the eruption, most often a chain of small red pimples. The pimples blister rapidly, the blisters become dry and they itch as they scab and heal, sometimes leaving scars. In dark-skinned people, the eruption may cause loss of pigment at the site of the blisters.

The eruption is usually on the back or chest or both, parallel with a rib, but it may occur on the forehead and in that case, it sometimes involves the eye. When the eruption is on the back, it usually starts near the spine and travels forward. There is no truth in the old wives' tale that if the eruption circles the body it is fatal.

The illness may last ten days to two weeks and make the

child quite uncomfortable. The area of the eruption is usually quite painful. In adults it often lasts much longer and causes excruciating pain.

Treatment: There is no special treatment, except the usual drugs to reduce fever and control pain. Antibiotics are not effective for the original disease, but may be useful for secondary infection. Cortisone seems to offer relief, but must never be taken except when it is prescribed by the doctor.

A child with shingles should be isolated, but contacts need not be quarantined. There is no vaccine or serum for prevention of shingles.

QUESTIONS & ANSWERS

Q. *If my husband has shingles, will my child surely get chicken pox?*

A. No. In fact, he is not very likely to, unless he has not had chicken pox.

Q. *If my son has shingles, should I report it to his school?*

A. It is not usually required, but it may be helpful to others if you do.

Q. *Should I keep my child away from a child who has been exposed to shingles?*

A. Not unless the child develops shingles or chicken pox.

Q. *Is there any special treatment for shingles?*

A. No. The only treatment is aimed at relieving the discomfort, but it does not cure the disease.

Q. *Some say antibiotics cure shingles. Do you think this is true?*

A. No. The proof offered for this claim does not justify it.

Q. *What about the various hormones?*

A. Some of them—the cortisone drugs—do seem to give relief, but they do not cure the disease.

Q. *Do many children get shingles?*

A. It is not really rare, but it certainly is not very common in children.

Q. *Can one have shingles and chicken pox at the same time?*

A. Probably not.

16: Smallpox (Variola)

This disease, once a scourge, is now quite uncommon in most parts of the world where vaccination against it is widely practiced. Not so long ago, there were fifteen to twenty thousand cases a year in the United States. Now the number is usually less than a hundred, and there were none in the last two years. This reduction has come about entirely because of vaccination and effective health measures, such as isolation of the patient and quarantine of contacts.

Smallpox may occur in a mild form with as little as 1 to 2 per cent mortality, or in epidemics with a death rate of as high as 30 per cent. The mild type is known as alastrim. The disease is caused by a virus.

Contagion: Smallpox is spread through contact, direct or indirect, with the lesions on the skin or mucous membranes of the patient. Airborne infection is said to be rare, but the smallpox virus can survive on the walls or on the floor of the room of a patient with the disease or with vaccinia (a widespread reaction to a vaccination) for a long time, and might possibly be the source of infection of a child with a skin rash, such as eczema or an open sore.

Incubation Period: The incubation period of smallpox is usually twelve days, but occasionally it is as short as seven or as long as sixteen days. Rarely, it takes twenty-one days for the disease to develop.

Symptoms: Smallpox starts with fever, headache and severe malaise. After one to five days an eruption appears, first on the face, then on the forearms, wrists and hands, then on the legs. It is apt to be very scanty on the trunk. The spots are raised and red. They blister, and later the clear fluid in the blisters becomes puslike. These pustules dry and scab, and after one to several weeks the scabs fall off leaving scarred pits in the skin, most abundantly on the face.

Treatment: There was no specific treatment for smallpox until a few years ago, when B-thiosemicarbazone became available. A child with the disease must be in a hospital because of the very strict isolation required. There he will be given specific drugs. Therapy should be used in any case of smallpox or severe reaction to vaccination. Hyperimmune gamma globulin is also quite effective in the treatment of vaccinia and is available at special locations known to your doctor. Treatment should include B-thiosemicarbazone as well as drugs to lower the fever, antibiotics for secondary infection of the pocks, good feeding, sedatives and good nursing care.

Isolation and Quarantine: The patient is isolated until all the scabs have fallen off. He is not allowed to have visitors. The greatest care is taken to avoid the spread of infection. All contacts of smallpox patients must be quarantined for sixteen days after the last exposure unless they are revaccinated promptly. In that case, quarantine may be suspended at the point where the vaccination reaction reaches its height. In some parts of the world, the sixteen-day quarantine is enforced even if the person does get revaccinated. During quarantine the person must be observed closely so that if the disease develops, it may be diagnosed at the earliest possible moment.

Prevention: Smallpox can be prevented by vaccination. All infants should be vaccinated late in the first year except where the disease is prevalent. In some areas, vaccination is done on the day of birth, or in the first week or month of life. The methods and recommendations for frequency of vaccination are discussed fully in the chapter on immunization. Smallpox is the classic example of a disease which can be prevented and which has been eliminated from much of the world. A person who is exposed to it or who is about to travel in areas where smallpox is prevalent is revaccinated even though he has been successfully vaccinated within the past year. If he leaves the United States, he will not be allowed to reenter the country unless he has been vaccinated within a period of three years.

There are stringent international controls on smallpox, such as quarantine of a ship if smallpox breaks out aboard it.

Hygiene: The hygienic measures designed to prevent the spread of smallpox are rigidly enforced. All contaminated items that can be discarded are destroyed by burning. Those which can be saved are boiled or sterilized by high-pressure steam. The premises must be thoroughly cleaned and disinfected after the patient has been taken to the hospital.

QUESTIONS & ANSWERS

Q. *Is smallpox always dangerous and severe?*

A. It varies. In some epidemics the outcome is very much worse than in others. In some countries the disease seems less severe in general than in others.

Q. *If my child is vaccinated in the United States, is it safe for him to travel to countries where smallpox is still prevalent?*

A. Yes, in most instances. In some rare cases a vaccinated person does catch smallpox when he is exposed to it, so keep away from smallpox even though you have been vaccinated.

Q. *I have heard that in some countries the doctor, when he vaccinates, scratches several areas and produces up to four sores instead of one as we do in this country. Does this give greater immunity?*

A. Most doctors believe that if the reaction to a single scratch is a lively one with a blister and redness around it, the immunity is just as great as that caused by multiple scratches, but some doctors think otherwise.

Q. *Is it possible for a vaccination to have serious consequences?*

A. Yes, but this is so rare that it would be foolhardy not to be vaccinated because of the possibility. In the past few years, since an effective drug has become available for the treatment of smallpox, a few have expressed the belief that the reaction to vaccination is more dangerous than omitting vaccination altogether in the United States where smallpox rarely occurs. However, I am not ready to abandon a procedure which has wiped out the disease in the United States, and I recommend highly the procedure of vaccinating infants and revaccinating the children before they enter school.

Q. *Doctors' opinions seem to vary a great deal as to the proper interval between vaccinations. How often should it be done?*

A. Immunity from a smallpox vaccination may last many years, even for life, but as in other immunizations, boosters are necessary to keep the immunity at a high level. In most cases this can be accomplished by repeating the vaccination every five to seven years. If there is any risk of actual exposure to smallpox, however, it is safer to vaccinate every one to three years.

Q. *When a person has a large number of scars on his face, does it always mean that he has had smallpox?*

A. I know of no other disease that causes so many scars on the face, except the scarring from a bad case of acne. Smallpox scars, however, are usually round, small and pitted, and are distributed all over the face. Acne scars are more irregular, sometimes resembling a burn scar and usually confined to certain areas.

Q. *Did you say that vaccination should be done after one year of age?*

A. Yes, for infants born in areas where the disease is rare. Vaccination after the first year is less likely to produce complications.

Q. *You do feel that vaccination is necessary?*

A. Yes, I feel it safer to prevent the disease rather than have to treat the infection. In over forty years I have had no serious complication in any patient I vaccinated.

17: Tuberculosis

The National Tuberculosis Association estimates that in 1954 there were some four hundred thousand cases of active tuberculosis in the United States, and approximately eight hundred thousand cases of inactive or arrested tuberculosis. The major problem, however, is with the hundred and fifty thousand people who have active tuberculosis and are not aware of it or have not reported it to a physician or the health authorities. This large group spreads the infection to others through daily contacts. Each year about a hundred thousand people in the United States will catch tuberculosis.

The disease is caused by the tubercle bacillus.

The mortality has declined steadily over the past three or four decades and new drugs have caused a sharp drop in infant and childhood deaths from tuberculosis. It has been possible to close many tuberculosis hospitals in the United States because the drugs are so effective. But tuberculosis continues to be one of the most important diseases of childhood (and adulthood), and it is one of the most difficult to treat successfully. It is still one of the leading causes of death in many underdeveloped countries.

The incidence of the disease varies greatly in different parts of the world and in different sections of the same country, state and city. In the city of New York, it varies even in different neighborhoods. The largest number of cases in New York City come from the crowded Negro and Puerto Rican sections where some of the inhabitants have inadequate food, inadequate housing and poor hygiene. In these groups, it is not only more frequent, but occurs at an earlier age. At the age of thirteen, for instance, about twenty years ago 35 per cent of children in these surroundings had been infected with tuberculosis as opposed to 15 per cent of thirteen-year-olds in better environments. The rate is now much lower in all groups.

According to the National Tuberculosis Association, tuberculosis in the United States is not only more frequent, but more serious among American Indians, Americans of Spanish descent and Negroes. The mortality in these groups is several times as high as in the rest of the population, but the incidence goes down when living conditions are improved, so probably the difference in incidence has little to do with race and can be blamed almost entirely on difference in economic levels.

Tuberculosis increases in frequency with age and is more common in urban areas than in rural ones. In impoverished areas throughout the world it is also very prevalent in rural areas. Climate is probably not as important a factor as it was once considered. The incidence of the disease is higher in girls than in boys during the latter part of childhood and adolescence. At other times of life there is no appreciable difference between the sexes. Tuberculosis may, in rare instances, be congenital, the mother infecting the infant before birth, but this does not mean that it is inherited. There is no evidence to suggest that one inherits the disease or even the tendency to develop it.

Susceptibility and Resistance: There seems to be a greater susceptibility to tuberculosis in infancy and again at adolescence. The most important factors in resistance to tuberculosis are the state of health, state of nutrition and the absence of fatigue. Tuberculosis has always become more widespread during periods of famine or malnutrition and is more likely to take hold in a person who is generally run-down. A child who is ill has less resistance to tuberculosis. Measles, whooping cough and influenza are particularly likely to lower the bars to a new infection with tuberculosis or to allow a flare-up of an old one which had been quiet up to that time.

Skin Tests: A child can be tested to establish the presence of a recent or old tuberculous infection. This is done by a simple skin test known as the tuberculin or Mantoux test. Another skin test known as the patch test is a slightly less reliable modification of this. Newer tests, the Tine test, the health test and others are good if done and interpreted by persons with experience. From six to ten weeks after infection with the tubercle bacillus, the skin test will show a positive reaction. A positive test in a baby under eighteen months old is almost absolute evidence of active disease since he is unlikely to have an old healed infection. After that time the test shows only that the child has been infected at some time in the past, and the test will be positive even if the infection is well healed. Many adults have positive tests. They have been infected without being aware of it. Almost all adults in countries where the disease is very common have positive tests; in the United States this is true for only 5 per cent of males seventeen to twenty years of age.

The discovery of a positive skin test is often frightening to parents. It should not be, because knowing at an early stage that there is or has been infection can save a great deal of trouble. The test may call attention to an infection which needs treatment, and the treatment can be started promptly. The infection may prove to be quiescent, and the child may pursue his normal activities. But if the test is positive for either reason, it calls for an immediate search for the source of infection. Careful examinations, including chest X-rays, should be made of all other members of the household. Often when a child is found to have tuberculosis, it is the first sign that a member of his family also has it and is spreading it. Treating this member of the family will avoid further spread of the disease.

The Nature of the Disease: In a child's first infection with tuberculosis, the bacteria usually enter through the mouth and nose, and descend to the roots of the lungs (the section where the windpipe enters the lung) where they cause swelling of the lymph glands. The infection spreads along the lymph channels into the lung itself and causes inflammation there. This infected area is typical of a "primary" infection. The infection can heal, leaving some significant scarring. It may cause pleurisy. It can cause a destruction of lung tissue, producing a cheesy (caseous) mass. It can spread into the bloodstream so that the tubercle bacilli are carried throughout the body, but especially throughout the lungs, causing innumerable small separate areas of inflammation (miliary tuberculosis). It may settle in the brain and cause tuberculous meningitis. It might also cause tuberculosis of the bones, of the skin or of the kidneys. Tuberculosis may involve practically any organ or tissue of the body. As a student, I was taught that tuberculosis, like syphilis, can produce a disease apparently similar to any other disease.

A thorough discussion of the many forms of tuberculosis encountered in children would have to be encyclopedic in size. I will discuss here only four forms: primary or childhood tuberculosis, reinfection or adult tuberculosis, miliary tuberculosis and tuberculous meningitis.

Contagion: Tuberculosis can be spread as long as the affected part of the body discharges live tubercle bacilli to the outside, as long as any lesion remains open. This may mean an open sore on the skin, a discharging sinus from a broken-down lymph gland in the neck, a discharging infection of the bone which has broken through the skin and, most often, lung tuberculosis which discharges bacteria into the bronchial tubes to be coughed out or spit up.

Incubation Period: The incubation period of tuberculosis is at least two weeks and probably longer in most cases.

PRIMARY TUBERCULOSIS

Most childhood tuberculosis is of the primary type, which means it is the child's first infection. The adult or reinfection type presupposes that a first infection has healed and a second one occurred later.

The characteristic primary infection may be attended by no symptoms at all or the child may have fever of 100° to 101°, cough, night sweating, weight loss and chronic fatigue and irritability. The diagnosis is made on the basis of a high index of suspicion and positive tuberculin test, chest X-ray and history of contact.

If the child is symptom-free and is discovered to have tuberculosis in the course of a routine tuberculin test, an X-ray of his chest should be made. Usually nothing of importance will be seen, or a small shadow representing a healed area may be discovered. In the primary type, these areas heal by calcification—that is, the infected areas become encased in lime deposited by the body. If, on the other hand, the child is acutely ill, the X-ray picture may reveal a more active, unhealed lesion which requires urgent treatment. Generally, primary tuberculosis heals, and except for the very young, the mortality is low. But this is not true everywhere. In some parts of the world, the mortality from primary tuberculosis is much higher than in others.

REINFECTION TUBERCULOSIS

This type usually occurs at puberty or later and only in someone who has previously been infected. Although it is called the "adult type," this term is becoming less and less correct since more young adults are becoming infected for the first time in adult life instead of during childhood. They therefore are likely to contract childhood or primary tuberculosis. By the same token, a child who has been infected when very young and develops active tuberculosis several years later has the adult or reinfection type even though he is not an adult.

This type of tuberculosis is usually characterized by chronic low-grade fever, cough with sputum (and occasionally spitting of blood), loss of weight, night sweats and fatigue. The chest X-ray most often shows involvement of the top part or apex of the lung. Unlike the lesions of the primary type which heal by calcification without having formed cavities, these infected areas often break down, leaving holes which heal by scar formation (fibrosis). If one of these cavities connects with one of the bronchial tubes, the patient coughs up sputum containing tubercle bacilli and he is particularly likely to infect others.

MILIARY TUBERCULOSIS

This form of tuberculosis is usually caused by the erosion of an infected lymph gland which releases tubercle bacilli into the blood stream. They are carried in the blood and form numerous small areas of involvement (tubercles) throughout the lungs. These areas are the size of millet seeds, hence the name, miliary. Because the spread is through the blood, other organs such as the liver, the spleen, the kidneys and the brain are often involved, as well as the lungs. This form of tuberculosis is very serious and used to be always fatal until streptomycin and the isoniazid drugs and other drugs used in conjunction with these came into use. Now the results are most encouraging and most patients recover completely after prolonged therapy. Dr. Edith M. Lincoln, a well-known authority on childhood tuberculosis, said in a report on treatment with the new drugs that in the six years between 1946, when streptomycin was first used, and 1952 only one child at Bellevue Hospital in New York died of miliary tuberculosis. This child had been brought to the hospital too late for treatment to be effective. During these six years the hospital treated just as many cases as had been treated formerly, but the treatment was infinitely more effective. Since then, preventive measures against tuberculosis and treatment of primary tuberculosis have become so effective that not a single child was admitted to Bellevue with miliary tuberculosis in 1955.

The child who has miliary tuberculosis is usually acutely ill with high fever and prostration. In spite of the fact that both lungs are almost always involved, he frequently has no symptoms referable to the respiratory tract such as coughing, spitting of blood, chest pain or shortness of breath. The diagnosis is made primarily by chest X-rays which show the characteristic tiny areas of disease throughout both lungs. Examination of the child's sputum or of the material washed from the child's stomach (since most children swallow their sputum) reveals the tubercle bacilli. The treatment of miliary tuberculosis requires prolonged hospitalization and intensive medication.

TUBERCULOUS MENINGITIS

This is an infection of the covering of the brain and spinal cord (the meninges) with tubercle bacilli. It usually precedes,

follows or accompanies miliary tuberculosis, but it sometimes
occurs in the course of the primary type. It is not uncommon,
particularly in infants and young children in areas where the
rate of tuberculosis is high. At one time as many as 40 per cent
of the children who died of tuberculosis did so after developing tuberculous meningitis which was then 100 per cent fatal.
Ever since the early treatment for tuberculosis was begun, we
see less TB meningitis, and it is hardly ever seen in some hospitals.

The symptoms are variable and the diagnosis is often difficult. The patient may suddenly become acutely ill with high
fever, stiff neck and back, convulsions and coma, or he may be
chronically ill with few specific complaints. Examination of the
spinal fluid is often very helpful, but sometimes it is impossible
to tell tuberculous meningitis from a virus encephalitis or an
early or partially treated bacterial meningitis at the time the
patient is admitted to the hospital. In these instances, the plan
of treatment will depend on the doctor's judgment. Most often
he will treat the patient for tuberculous meningitis if he has
the slightest suspicion that the patient might have this disease.

When streptomycin was introduced in the treatment of tuberculous meningitis in 1945 and 1946, the mortality dropped
from 100 per cent to about 50 per cent, but many of the survivors were left in very poor condition. Since the isoniazid
drugs have come into use recently in conjunction with streptomycin, the mortality has been reduced to 15 to 30 per cent, but
in order to get good recovery as well as survival, the patient
must receive treatment early. The earlier he is treated, the better are his chances of both survival and recovery. When the
disease is more advanced at the beginning of treatment, the
mortality is higher and the patient is more likely to be left
with serious defects, such as blindness, deafness, paralyses and
convulsive disorders.

Treatment: Since most primary tuberculosis is not easily
identified, most children's lesions heal without having been
discovered. If the primary infection is discovered, the child is
kept at home, withdrawn from school and play groups, and the
treatment is outlined by the doctor. If the child has no fever,
is not coughing and seems well, he may be permitted limited

activity. Hard play like running, football, basketball and so forth are not allowed. The child is given fresh air, some sunlight, a diet high in calories, vitamins and meat, milk, fish and eggs. He must have plenty of rest. X-rays of the chest and blood-sedimentation-rate tests may be used by the doctor along with the temperature curve as guides to how long treatment should last. Most doctors recommend the drug therapy for all cases of primary tuberculosis for at least one whole year.

Treatment for the reinfection type usually includes all available forms of drugs, bed rest and diet. Once started, drugs may have to be continued for a year or longer. Treatment is best started in a hospital, and after the disease is arrested, it may be continued at home. When treatment is carried out at home, there must be a separate room for the child, the mother must be able and diligent about giving the medicine recommended by the doctor, she must have ample time to look after the child and she must keep doctor's appointments for regular checkups.

Miliary tuberculosis and tuberculous meningitis require hospitalization and drug therapy immediately. Miliary tuberculosis can be cured in most infants and children if treatment is started early and continued as long as necessary, at least twelve months. Tuberculous meningitis may require several months in the hospital. When drug therapy is started early, the chances of survival are more than 75 per cent. Of these survivors, many more recover with fewer aftereffects than was formerly the case. Treatment is quite complicated and cannot be directed by anyone but a physician who is experienced in treatment of tuberculosis.

I shall omit any discussion of the surgical treatment of tuberculosis. This involves special problems which are too numerous and too technical to go into here, and are best decided by the physician and the surgeon.

Isolation and Quarantine: Tuberculosis must be reported to the local department of health. This will be done by your doctor. Any child with active tuberculosis in which the part of the body affected can discharge live bacilli to the outside should be isolated from children who have never been infected. Sanitarium or hospital care may be indicated, but in some cases the child is cared for at home with good results if the child can be controlled, treatment is carried out religiously and medical attention is obtained as needed.

Contacts of tuberculosis patients are not quarantined, but they are observed. A chest X-ray should be made and a tuberculin test done when the exposure is discovered. If they are negative, they should be repeated in six to eight weeks.

Prevention: Enough rest, adequate and nourishing food, lack of crowding and good hygiene are the best means of preventing tuberculosis. Routine annual skin testing of all preschool children and mass X-ray examination of all members of the community are the most effective ways of discovering unsuspected infections.

If tuberculosis is discovered in one member of a family, the doctor will report it to the health department. Either the doctor himself or the health department will X-ray the chests of every other member of the household. Tuberculin tests will be done on all children, and both the skin tests and the chest X-rays will be repeated in six months, again in a year and periodically thereafter. All members of the household who are discovered to have X-ray evidence of active disease should be treated. Those with healed lesions will be permitted complete freedom of activity.

Children who have positive skin tests but negative X-rays will probably be observed for fever, blood sedimentation rate and other possible signs of active disease which are not detectable by X-ray. The procedure used in skin testing for tuberculosis is described in detail in the section on skin tests.

B.C.G., a vaccine for prevention of tuberculosis, is discussed in the chapter on immunization.

QUESTIONS & ANSWERS

Q. *Is tuberculosis the same all over the world?*

A. Yes, in that the same germs cause the disease. The only difference is that in some parts of the world the bovine type, which infects cows and is transmitted by them, is still common.

Q. *Do birds have tuberculosis?*

A. Yes, they do. In very rare instances, they transmit it to man.

Q. *Is the tubercle bacillus which infects birds the same as the one which infects man?*

A. No. The bird type is known as the avian type.

Q. *Is tuberculosis more common in cold, damp climates?*

A. The climate is not in itself an important factor, but if along with a cold, damp climate there is inadequate heating or food, the combination makes tuberculosis more likely.

Q. *Are all forms of tuberculosis contagious?*

A. No, only those in which the tubercle bacilli can be discharged to the outside.

Q. *Can children catch tuberculosis from household pets or farm animals?*

A. It is conceivable, but not usual.

Q. *If a person with active tuberculosis visits my child, can my child catch it?*

A. Yes, even when the contact is not very long.

Q. *Is it safe for an adult just discharged from a tuberculosis hospital to visit my child?*

A. Only if he is not coughing and has no open sore or external draining sinus.

Q. *Is it safe to let him kiss my child?*

A. It may be, but I think it unwise unless he is definitely cured of the disease.

Q. *How could I tell if a person visiting my child had tuberculosis?*

A. You probably could not if the person himself was unaware of it, but if you do not allow anyone with a cough from any cause to visit your child, you will be almost sure to avoid his coming in contact with tuberculosis.

Q. *If I have a nurse for my child, should she be examined for tuberculosis?*

A. Yes, I think anyone working with children should have a
    chest X-ray to make sure she is well. It may happen that a
    healthy nurse catches tuberculosis from a sick child.

Q. *Do doctors and nurses in hospitals ever get tuberculosis
    from their patients?*

A. Yes. In fact medical students and nurses sometimes pick
    up the infection when they begin to see sick patients.

Q. *How do children catch tuberculosis—by being with adults
    who have it?*

A. Usually from the breath of the infected person. The bacilli
    are coughed or sneezed or spit out into the air, or some-
    times the child is kissed on the mouth and has even more
    direct contact.

Q. *If you become infected with tuberculosis, do the germs
    stay in the body forever?*

A. They may, but after healing, the germs may be encased
    in lime and therefore can do no harm.

Q. *Is tuberculosis curable?*

A. Yes, of course it is. In some parts of the world almost all
    adults have had tuberculosis and live through a normal life
    span after it is healed. One of the best bits of evidence
    that it is a curable disease is that a person treated very
    early will become negative to a tuberculin test and later
    upon reinfection again will become positive to a skin test
    for tuberculosis.

Q. *Is it true that the dark-skinned races such as Negroes and
    American Indians are more susceptible to tuberculosis?*

A. In the United States there is more tuberculosis among
    these groups than among whites, but this seems to be be-
    cause their living conditions are often inferior. Among
    Negroes and American Indians who live in good sur-
    roundings and have adequate food and good hygiene, the
    rate is no higher than among whites. It is true that there
    are groups in which the mortality from tuberculosis is
    higher although the susceptibility is not. The explanation
    offered for this is that there seems to be some inherent
    quality in these groups which makes the infection more
    serious. Negroes and American Indians and Puerto Ricans

are among them, but Scandinavians are also, as are many very blond peoples. On the other hand, Eastern European people seem to have a greater resistance to serious tuberculosis than most.

Q. *If my child has tuberculosis, will he be admitted to any hospital?*

A. No. Some hospitals do not have the facilities for the long-term care required for active tuberculosis.

Q. *What hospitals will take a case of active tuberculosis?*

A. Your doctor will know. If you have no doctor, call your local health department. When tuberculosis is discovered, it must be reported to the health authorities. As soon as they learn of it, one of their social workers will probably visit your home and make arrangements for care of the child and for X-ray examinations of all other members of the household.

Q. *Must a child go to a hospital if he has tuberculosis?*

A. No, only if he cannot get the proper treatment at home, or if he would endanger other children in the family.

Q. *Do children get tuberculosis in school?*

A. It is possible, and epidemics of tuberculosis have occurred in some schools, but usually schoolchildren are healthy. No child who has a cough should be going to school.

Q. *Do all doctors test for tuberculosis routinely?*

A. No, but many do. I think it is a good practice, especially in infancy and before the child enters school or any play group.

Q. *Is it wise for my child to have a chest X-ray at his routine visits to the doctor?*

A. Yes, but only if this has not been done before or if there is suspicion of a lung infection, or to exclude the possibility of a lung condition. It should not be done routinely.

Q. *If my child has had tuberculosis, how soon may he go back to school?*

A. As soon as the doctor considers him free of contagion and strong enough to undertake the school program.

Q. *How about summer camps?*

A. The same advice holds for camps as for schools.

Q. *If my child has tuberculosis, should I take him away to a warm, dry climate or to the mountains?*

A. It is not necessary to leave your own home provided that your child can get enough air and sunshine, enough rest, good food and the necessary care.

Q. *Should my child have injections against diphtheria and whooping cough while he has tuberculosis?*

A. If he has not had the first injections against these diseases and is not very sick, they should be given to avoid the possibility of his catching whooping cough which is very bad in the presence of tuberculosis.

Q. *What should be done if he is too sick for the injections?*

A. He should be carefully guarded against exposure to whooping cough and given the injections when he has recovered from tuberculosis.

Q. *What if he is actually exposed to whooping cough when he is very ill?*

A. This is unlikely, but if it should happen, I would give him an injection of hyperimmune gamma globulin or convalescent serum, which is quite effective in producing temporary immunity to whooping cough, and an antibiotic which is known to offset the whooping cough bacillus.

Q. *If he has already had his initial injections for whooping cough, should he have boosters while he has active tuberculosis?*

A. I think this should be handled in the same way as I have indicated for the initial injections, except that if he was actually exposed to whooping cough, I would give him the hyperimmune serum and, as soon as possible, a booster dose of the vaccine.

Q. *What about poliomyelitis and measles vaccine?*

A. Live poliomyelitis vaccine may be given as soon as the child has become free of fever and feels well; otherwise, the Salk or killed vaccine should be given and followed by the live or Sabin vaccine as soon as advised to do so. Live measles vaccine should be avoided during the period of TB activity, except when gamma globulin is also given, and preferably after several weeks of treatment with isoniazid, etc.

Q. *Is a lot of sunshine good for tuberculosis?*

A. Not for tuberculosis of the lung. It should be used in graded amounts governed by the doctor's advice.

Q. *Should all children receive B.C.G. vaccine?*

A. Yes, if you live where tuberculosis is prevalent or if there is active tuberculosis in the family. If the child is likely to be exposed to tuberculosis and his skin test shows that he has not yet been infected, B.C.G.may be helpful.

Q. *How else can you prevent tuberculosis?*

A. By avoiding contact with persons who have it, by drinking only pasteurized or boiled milk, by eating foods which are clean and by keeping your child in good physical condition. Good nutrition and cleanliness are the two best safeguards against tuberculosis.

Q. *Are the new drugs certain to cure tuberculosis?*

A. No. They may or may not be completely curative. They make it possible for the body to fight off the disease and they prevent serious complications from the spread of the disease.

Q. *Can you use the drugs to prevent tuberculosis?*

A. Yes, when there is great danger of infection, the drugs are helpful. Drugs may also prevent the spread of TB. For example, if a child has tuberculous glands, bone, etc., which require surgery treatment, antituberculosis drugs for two or three weeks before surgery may help prevent spread of the disease.

Q. *Is tuberculosis on the decline?*

A. While the mortality from tuberculosis is lower in the United States and in Scandinavian and European countries, it is still high in many parts of the world.

18: *Whooping Cough* (*Pertussis*)

Whooping cough is a very serious children's disease the world over. In the United States about three hundred thousand cases are reported every year. It occurs in all seasons and the disease may attack anyone from infancy to old age. Babies whose mothers have had whooping cough do not usually have enough immunity to withstand a heavy infection with the germs and are therefore in danger of catching it if they are exposed anytime after birth. Most of the cases are in children under ten years of age, and about half of these children are under five. While an attack gives immunity for a long time, second attacks in adults who have had it as children are not rare. Therefore, it is unwise to expose anyone at any age unnecessarily. It is particularly dangerous for children below the age of two. Ninety per cent of all deaths from whooping cough are in this age group. Whooping cough is caused by bacteria known as bacillus hemophilus pertussis.

Contagion: Whooping cough is highly contagious. When the exposure is intimate, as at home, it infects in the same way as measles or chicken pox. It is transmitted by coughs and sneezes and by contact with the discharges from the nose and throat and with the vomitus of the child who has it.

Incubation Period: The incubation period is usually from five to seven days, occasionally as long as fourteen, and in rare instances it extends to twenty-one days.

Symptoms: Whooping cough usually begins like a mild cold with a cough. The cough is hacking, comes frequently and is not easy to control. This stage stays about the same for ten to fourteen days, or the symptoms may get a little worse during that time. Then the coughing begins to come in spells or bouts. These may occur three or four times during the day and at night, or they may come so often that they deny the patient any rest at all, day or night. That coughing spell is unmistakable. It is caused by an attempt to get rid of thick mucus. The child has bursts of eight or ten rapid coughs in one breath which forces much of the air out of his lungs. Finally when his face is either red or blue from the effort and the lack of oxygen, a forcible noisy intake of air makes a crowing sound which is known as the whoop. Often the coughing spells are followed by vomiting. After a night of coughing and whooping, the child's face looks puffy, especially around the eyes and lips.

This period of whooping lasts two or three weeks and then the attacks become less severe and less frequent until the disease is over, usually in about six weeks. The whoop may start earlier than the end of the second week of the disease and occasionally comes without the previous appearance of any other symptoms. Some children have whooping cough in which the cough may be severe and come in bursts without the whoop. Sometimes the cough lasts longer than six weeks from the beginning of the disease—eight to twelve weeks, or even longer. But usually the bacteria which produce the disease are gone from the patient's throat by the end of the fifth week of illness, and they can rarely be found after the sixth week. If the child continues to cough after six weeks, it is due to the irritation of the voice box, windpipe and bronchial tubes, or it may have become a habit. The fact that the cough can be habit-forming is so well known that the stage after the bacteria can no longer be found and while the child is still coughing is sometimes called the neurotic stage.

Diagnosis: In the first week or so it is very difficult to tell whooping cough from a cold or a cough due to some other illness. You may suspect it because of the stubborn type of cough, the puffy face of the child who has had the choking spells, and the absence of other reasons for the cough. A blood count or an examination of the bacteria in the throat may be helpful in arriving at a diagnosis. The blood count does not suggest whooping cough until after the first ten days. The bacteria which cause whooping cough may be found in the nose or throat for the first three or four weeks of the disease.

Treatment: As soon as the child starts coughing, you should call the doctor. If you know that he has been exposed to whooping cough, the doctor should be told this long before the disease starts. He may want to give the child protective serum, a special type of gamma globulin or some antibiotic, and unless this is done early in the incubation period, the treatment may fail. The earlier treatment is started, the more likely it is to succeed. While we all agree that we have no sure, quick cure for whooping cough, we know that the child can be helped, and complications can be warded off or cured if they are already started.

It is not necessary to keep most children in bed. They may do better being up and around and out in the fresh air, though not, of course, with other children. If the child has fever or is very weak, however, bed rest may be important. And some children seem to cough less if they stay in bed. The child should be shielded from anyone with a cold. He is more likely to pick up other infections because of his lowered resistance.

Good nursing care is essential. Fresh air, small and frequent feedings, refeeding in about twenty minutes if a meal is vomited, oxygen when recommended by the doctor, making sure that the child really gets and retains the medicine ordered by the doctor, are all vital in the care of the child with whooping cough.

For several months after a child has had whooping cough, he may start coughing in typical spells every time he has a cold. This is not because he has had a relapse, but probably because there is still irritation or because he has developed the habit of coughing in that way whenever any irritation is present.

Complications: The child with whooping cough runs little or no fever. A temperature of 101° or more should make you think of a complication. The most common ones are bronchitis, pneumonia and, in infants, exhaustion and severe loss of weight. Any complication should be treated promptly and vigorously by any and all available means.

Prevention: Infants as young as two or three months can be immunized. Three injections of vaccine are usually given a month apart, though some doctors recommend giving the third injection four to six months after the second. I usually give the first injection at three months, the second at four months, the third at five months, and booster doses at one year, three years and five years after the first series. To some children I give another booster three years after this and again if they are exposed to the disease. When whooping cough is prevalent or where living conditions are crowded, the chance of catching whooping cough is greater, and immunization can be started as early as two months.

About 25 to 35 per cent of children who get whooping cough vaccine develop fever and pain and sometimes swelling at the site of the injection. In rare instances the reaction is very severe. If the reaction to whooping cough vaccine is so severe that it causes a temperature of 104° or more or a convulsion, the injections are sometimes discontinued or sometimes the doctor will try again with a much smaller dose of the vaccine. If this small dose causes no ill effect, repeated small doses may be given.

The immunity a child gets from the injections is not as lasting or as regularly effective as that which follows injections against diphtheria or tetanus, but vaccination against whooping cough is worthwhile and protects many. I have seen quite a few cases of whooping cough in children vaccinated six months to three years before. About half of the cases were just as severe and lasted just as long as the usual case, but the other half were very mild.

Isolation and Quarantine: While the child with whooping cough often gets along better if he is allowed out in the open air, he may not, of course, be taken on public vehicles or to public gatherings. He is barred from school from five to six weeks. If he is still coughing after five or six weeks, the question of return to school must be left up to the doctor and the school authorities.

If a child who has not been immunized is intimately exposed to whooping cough, he should be quarantined from the ninth or tenth day after the first exposure to fourteen days after his last exposure. During this time, he may not go to school, to the movies, or to any other public gatherings. He may not play with children who have not had whooping cough or who have not been vaccinated against it within the previous year. In some schools the child who has been exposed to whooping cough is allowed to go to school, and in that case a school nurse or doctor checks on his health each day when he gets to school. If he is not well in any way he is sent home.

Hygiene: While a child has whooping cough, his clothes, towels, nightclothes and bed linen should be thoroughly washed or dry-cleaned. Paper towels and handkerchiefs are useful since they can be burned. The dishes used by the child while he is sick should be carefully washed with soap and water. His room should be thoroughly cleaned and aired before being used by others.

QUESTIONS & ANSWERS

Q. *Is whooping cough a seasonal disease?*

A. Generally it is more common in winter and spring but an outbreak or epidemic may start in the spring and continue through July and August. Epidemics may start in institutions for children at any time and continue through most of a year.

Q. *How soon after having had whooping cough can you get it a second time?*

A. Second attacks most often occur in adults. For instance, when a parent or a grandparent who has had whooping cough as a child takes care of a child with whooping cough and is infected heavily and repeatedly, he might catch it. I do not mean to imply that second attacks are very common, though.

Q. *Must all infants and children be immunized against whooping cough?*

A. It is not required by law, and although some schools recommend it, they do not insist on it. If your doctor has not advised it, you must ask him for it. It is routinely given to all infants.

Q. *Does the immunity last long?*

A. Only a few years. Booster doses should be given one, three and five years after the initial injections, and some doctors advise it every three years thereafter until about fifteen years old.

Q. *Is the course of whooping cough fairly regular?*

A. Usually, but it may differ. Occasionally the disease begins as an ordinary cold. The cough may start with the typical whooping spells instead of a stubbornly resistant dry cough. The cough may never come in paroxysms at all and the whoop may be absent. In the ordinary case, the disease is divided into three phases of two weeks each: in the first, the cough increases to the stage of the whoop; in the second, the cough with the whoop is most severe and most frequent; and in the third, there is progressive recovery. Unusual cases, however, may be the same from the beginning to the phase of recovery, or the second phase may last three or four weeks. Sometimes the third phase lasts much longer than two weeks.

Q. *Is a second attack of whooping cough like the first?*

A. Yes, but it may be milder and more difficult to detect.

Q. *Is there any way of telling whether a child has become immune?*

A. Yes, there are several blood tests for this.

Q. *Is it possible to tell when the child is no longer contagious?*

A. If laboratory tests prove that there are no bacteria present in the nose and throat, the patient cannot spread the disease.

Q. *Should the patient be kept in bed?*

A. Not unless he has fever or is very tired and run-down.

Q. *Is it helpful to let him sleep on a porch?*

A. It may be, if the porch is sheltered and the weather is good.

Q. *My mother took me to the gas house when I had whooping cough to smell the fumes of burned coal. Is that helpful?*

A. The smell of smoking creosote may be soothing to the windpipe and larynx, but it does not cure whooping cough.

Q. *Should the patient's room be kept especially warm and moist?*

A. The room should be comfortable as to temperature and humidity. A very hot and dry room would be uncomfortable.

Q. *Is any cough medicine effective?*

A. Some work better than others, but none of them stops the disease or the cough entirely.

Q. *Should I urge my child to eat while he has whooping cough?*

A. Yes, but not too much at a time. It may cause him to cough and vomit more if you press the issue too much.

Q. *In the case of an infant, should I feed him more often?*

A. That depends on the vomiting. The usual feeding schedule should be followed if the baby does not vomit, but if he does, the feedings should be small and more frequent. If the child vomits a meal just eaten, he should be fed again in about twenty minutes. Infants who vomit a great deal may need more drastic treatment than refeeding because they lose so much fluid. The doctor may want to inject fluid into a vein or under the skin. A doctor can tell whether this is necessary. Hospital care may be required in these cases. It is difficult to find hospitals where whooping cough patients are admitted. City hospitals usually have facilities for contagious or infectious diseases.

Q. *Are all whooping cough patients better off in hospitals?*

A. Not if they can be cared for at home. A hospital is better under two conditions: (1) when the mother cannot adequately care for the child, or would have to neglect the other children to do so; (2) when the child needs the type of treatment only available in hospitals.

Q. *Since whooping cough is so serious in infants, should they be treated in hospitals?*

A. Not necessarily. Visiting nurses are very helpful and may be called on for any type of care, from medical treatment to relief of a tired mother.

Q. *Should oxygen be available in the home when a child has whooping cough?*

A. Yes, if the patient is an infant or a very young child. It is not usually necessary for older children.

Q. *Can oxygen treatment be carried out by the mother at home?*

A. Yes, if someone shows the mother how to use it.

Q. *Isn't home oxygen treatment very expensive?*

A. That depends on your ability to pay for it. If it is too expensive and your child needs oxygen, by all means take him to a hospital.

Q. *Do all children benefit from antibiotics?*

A. I believe not. The drugs may or may not destroy all of the whooping cough germs. Complications may require such treatment.

Q. *Should all patients be given convalescent serum or hyperimmune gamma globulin?*

A. No, but it may be helpful for infants and young children, for some older children who are very ill, or have complications, or have some other illness (such as tuberculosis) preceding the whooping cough.

Q. *If one of my children has whooping cough, may the others go to school or the movies?*

A. Yes. If the others have had whooping cough or have had injections against it within the past year, and are not coughing. But this has to be governed by the regulations of the local school and board of health.

Q. *Is the patient infectious throughout the disease when it lasts as long as two months?*

A. No, not usually after the first five weeks, and very rarely after the sixth week.

Q. *Can you avoid the complications of whooping cough?*

A. Yes, usually, if the child has good medical and nursing care.

Q. *Can the complications be cured if they develop?*

A. Most of them.

Q. *Why is the disease considered so dangerous for infants?*

A. Infants are more difficult to treat, especially when they are weakened by loss of rest, sleep and food. When an infant coughs up the plug of mucus, or vomits, he is more likely to aspirate it (pull it down into his lungs). If this vomitus or mucus is not coughed up, it may block off the passage of air into a part of the lung, resulting in collapse of that part and pneumonia. Pneumonia is more frequent and more severe in infants than in older children, though the mortality has been reduced sharply by the use of penicillin and oxygen, and by good nursing care and hyperimmune gamma globulin.

Q. *If whooping cough starts in a nursery group, how can its spread be limited?*

A. First, by separating those exposed from those not exposed and by isolating the sick child, and second, by injections of gamma globulin for those who have neither had the disease nor been vaccinated against it.

Q. *What can you do to keep a child who is in a weakened condition because of whooping cough from getting other infections?*

A. Keep him away from anyone with a cold, or who is coughing or sneezing, or who does not feel well. Give him plenty of rest and quiet, and try to get him to eat well. His vitamins should have been kept up through his illness and the dose repeated if it is vomited.

Q. *Is there only one kind of vaccine?*

A. There are several.

Q. *Are these injections advised for older children and adults?*

A. Not usually, but if an older child has been immunized several years before and is exposed, sometimes a booster is given.

Q. *If the child does not have a reaction to the vaccine, does it mean that it didn't take?*

A. No, only about a third of children develop reactions, but almost all of them develop immunity.

Q. *If my three-year-old is exposed to whooping cough should he be given an injection of serum?*

A. If he has already had injections against whooping cough, a booster dose of vaccine may be enough. It usually stimulates immunity in about a week. If he has not been immunized, an injection of gamma globulin should be given.

Q. *Is gamma globulin always effective?*

A. No. Not always.

Q. *When a child gets whooping cough in spite of having been immunized, does it change the course of the disease?*

A. Not necessarily. I have seen more than fifty cases of children who had been immunized six months to three years before. About half of the attacks were very mild; the others were moderate or severe.

Q. *How does the doctor make a diagnosis in these cases?*

A. In the usual way. The child coughs without having a cold or sore throat, the cough gets worse and does not respond to cough mixtures, and the whoop develops just as in children who have not been immunized. A blood count may be helpful, and finding the whooping cough germ in the child's throat is positive proof.

Q. *How long do you isolate a child with the very mild kind of whooping cough?*

A. For six weeks, unless the cough stops completely before that time.

Q. *My child has convulsions with high fever. Is it all right to give him whooping cough vaccine?*

A. It is wiser to call this to the attention of the doctor. He will probably recommend that vaccine be deferred. He may prefer to recommend hyperimmune gamma globulin if the child is exposed. Remember that whooping cough is most dangerous in infancy and not so dangerous later.

19: *Streptococcal Infections*

The Group A hemolytic streptococci cause many diseases. The most important of these are scarlet fever, streptococcus sore throat, erysipelas and puerperal sepsis (infection occurring during childbirth). This same group of streptococci, of which there are numerous members, also sometimes produces otitis media, sinusitis, cervical adenitis, pneumonia, mastoiditis, osteomyelitis and meningitis, as well as skin diseases other than erysipelas, especially cellulitis and some cases of impetigo. Indirectly these streptococci are responsible for rheumatic fever and acute nephritis.

Most of the infections caused by this family of microbes occur in spring, winter and fall. They are more common in temperate climates than in the tropics. With the exception of puerperal sepsis, they are more likely to occur in early childhood than after ten or twelve years of age, although erysipelas and streptococcus sore throat are quite common in adults also, particularly in military groups.

SCARLET FEVER (SCARLATINA)

Scarlet fever, often called scarlatina, is a childhood infection known everywhere, though it is less common than measles, chicken pox, whooping cough and mumps. About seventy-five thousand cases are reported in the United States each year. The disease varies in its severity and frequency, but it is always less frequent and less severe in tropical and semitropical climates than in temperate ones. In the United States most of the cases occur in the late winter and spring.

Infants whose mothers are immune to scarlet fever are immune for the first few months of life. Infants whose mothers are not immune may get it at any time after birth. The youngest patient with scarlet fever I have seen was seven months old. It probably would occur in younger infants if they were exposed, but they usually are not because they are more sheltered than older children. The disease is most common during the early school years. Like other infections, it strikes preschool children where living conditions are crowded. Also like other infections, it often breaks out in epidemics where children or young adults live together in large numbers.

Scarlet fever is caused by bacteria known as the beta hemolytic streptococci of Group A. We know some forty different members of this group of bacteria which are able to produce a similar disease. An outbreak is usually caused by only one of them, but as the epidemic progresses, it may be replaced by another. The germs causing scarlet fever are very much like those causing septic sore throat, erysipelas, and many cases of tonsillitis. Septic sore throat (strep throat) is actually scarlet fever without a rash. Historically scarlet fever, like other diseases, e.g., diphtheria and tuberculosis, occurred in cycles of great frequency and great severity.

In my own medical lifetime scarlet fever has changed; it is no longer so severe and does not commonly occur in epidemics as in the past. In the United States an average of 142,274 cases were reported in the years 1942 to 1946, 113,076 in 1946, 84,379 in 1947, 78,662 in 1948, and 74,913 in 1949. (The figures on the years before 1942 are higher than 1942.) By 1952 or 1953 scarlet fever was occurring more frequently and increasing in severity. For some years the complications, such as rheumatic fever, were mild, as was the scarlet fever. After a few years streptococcal disease increased sharply, and rheumatic fever occurred more frequently and in more severe form.

While sulfonamides were discovered in 1936, the use of sulfadiazine did not become widespread until 1941, and penicillin was not in general use until 1945. Undoubtedly these drugs played a very large part in reducing the frequency of scarlet fever as they did in other diseases caused by the hemolytic streptococcus, especially erysipelas, septic sore throat and childbed fever.

Scarlet fever has not been completely wiped out, however. Almost every year a new outbreak occurs somewhere for reasons not absolutely clear to us. Montreal had a large outbreak in 1949, Zurich the year before, and New York City in 1953. We still must be alert to the possibility of this disease reappearing in epidemic form at any time.

Contagion: The streptococcus usually enters the mouth and settles on the tonsils and throat where it causes inflammation. Scarlet fever is almost always spread directly between the patient and the people he comes in contact with, but the germ is spread widely in his room and can be carried by objects he has touched, such as clothes, bedclothes and dishes. Occasionally contaminated milk or food causes an outbreak of scarlet fever. The streptococcus may also enter through a wound or a burned area of the skin, and it is then called wound or burn scarlet fever. Of those exposed to scarlet fever, about 15 per cent develop the disease with a rash, but many more are infected and develop sore throat or tonsillitis or have no symptoms at all.

Incubation Period: The incubation period of scarlet fever is two to five days. Less often the disease begins as soon as one day or as late as seven days after exposure.

Symptoms: The disease may vary in its intensity from being hardly noticeable to being very severe with marked toxicity. The active illness lasts about a week. In the beginning the child complains of a sore throat and pain when he swallows. He is nauseated and may vomit, usually only once. He may feel achy and have a headache and feel chilly. Shaking chills are not frequent. His temperature rises, if he has a mild case, to 100.5° or 101.5°. If it is severe, the temperature is apt to be 103° to 105°. The rash usually begins on the neck, behind the ears and on the back at the end of the first day of illness, and spreads rapidly down the back and chest and on the arms and legs, abdomen and buttocks, especially in the folds of the skin, elbows, backs of knees and groin. Sometimes it is itchy. There is usually no rash on the face, but the cheeks are often flushed and there is a pale ring around the lips. The rash is fine, the tiny spots are slightly raised so that the skin feels a little rough and looks bright pink. Sometimes, however, instead of being vivid, it is hardly noticeable.

In uncomplicated cases the fever drops slowly, and in about five days it is normal and the rash is gone. In about 80 per cent of children the skin peels, beginning around the finger-nails and toenails or in parts where the rash was thickest. The tongue peels too, but this happens earlier in the disease.

Diagnosis: As the tongue begins to peel, it leaves a red surface with prominent small elevations, giving the tongue the appearance of a strawberry. This is where the name "strawberry tongue" comes from. Since it comes early in the disease, it may help the doctor to make his diagnosis. When scarlet fever is very mild, the first clue that the child has had it may be the peeling of the skin (desquamation).

Treatment: When a child becomes ill you should call the doctor. Usually it is not hard for him to recognize scarlet fever, although at times it may be confusing. You keep the child in bed, comfortably warm, and give him a bland diet free of extra salt and condiments. You give him aspirin as you would with almost any fever. This may also help the soreness of his throat. If his throat is still painful, the doctor may prescribe another drug which will make him more comfortable. An antibiotic or a sulfa drug should be given. This is the fastest way to rid the throat of the streptococcus that is causing the disease. The drug should be kept up for seven to ten days to make sure that there will be no return of the streptococcus.

Convalescence: If the child has had an uncomplicated case of scarlet fever and it has been treated with an antibiotic or sulfa drug, it is over when the fever is gone except for the peeling of the skin. The disease may still be contagious, how-ever, as long as there is a persistent discharge, such as a run-ning ear, from any body opening. If the disease was mild, the child is usually well enough to return to school or take up his other activities in seven to ten days. If the disease was severe, it is better to keep him away from school for several more days. I usually insist on a convalescent period of a week after the illness is over for such children.

If the child was not given drugs which destroy the streptococcus, he should be observed for two weeks after the rash has disappeared, since complications (especially kidney complications) may appear in the third week of the illness.

Complications: The complications which may be the result of scarlet fever are swollen glands in the neck, inflamed ears, inflamed sinuses, pneumonia, kidney disease (acute glomerular nephritis) and rheumatic fever, either a new attack or the awakening of an earlier rheumatic condition. The kidney involvement and rheumatic fever are the most serious complications, but fortunately the least frequent, and these can be avoided largely by early treatment with one of the sulfa drugs or with an antibiotic. In one test, seven hundred soldiers developed streptococcus infections and were treated with antibiotics or sulfa drugs. Only three developed rheumatic fever. In a similar number who were not treated with these drugs, twenty developed it.

Prevention: If a child who has not had scarlet fever is exposed to it, it is possible to prevent the disease from developing at all by starting active treatment early with suitable drugs before any of the symptoms have appeared. Since the incubation period is so short, you should not postpone telling your doctor about the exposure. Let him decide what should be done.

Scarlet fever can be prevented, too, by convalescent serum and other serums prepared to combat the streptococcus germ. But today these are not often used and are rarely needed because penicillin or other drugs are so effective, easy to get and relatively inexpensive.

It is possible to immunize children against scarlet fever by several injections of streptococcus toxin, but this immunity does not last very long and may be gone in six months. This immunization procedure used to be practiced widely, especially for nurses and doctors who were not immune to scarlet fever and were about to work in hospitals for contagious diseases, but it is rarely done today. If a susceptible person has to be exposed to scarlet fever, or if he has already been, it is possible to keep him from getting it by giving him small doses of sulfa or penicillin daily. In institutions where epidemics of scarlet fever or streptococcus sore throat get started, we can stop the spread of the infection by giving the drugs to everyone who has not shown symptoms. When a child gets scarlet fever, I give the well members of the household small amounts of sulfa or penicillin daily for five to seven days and they are thus able to avoid catching it. In the past few years, it has become evident that penicillin is preferable since some of the germs have become resistant to the sulfa drugs.

Immunity: The Dick test is a skin test which shows whether or not a person is immune to scarlet fever. You can have scarlet fever more than once. Presumably this is possible because different members of the hemolytic streptococcus family can produce the same disease and the immunity which follows one attack is an immunity to the particular member of the group of streptococci which caused the disease. Immunity to other members of the group may be quite low. A second infection by another member of the group is therefore possible. I have seen second attacks of scarlet fever in my practice more than twenty-five times in twenty-five years. Because there is more than one streptococcus responsible for scarlet fever, the material for the Dick test contains toxin produced by several of the strains of streptococcus which can produce it.

As I said earlier, one can have scarlet fever without a rash and one can become infected with the scarlet fever germ without becoming sick. For example, if a child has scarlet fever, someone else in the household, usually an adult taking care of him, may develop a severe sore throat or tonsillitis due to the same streptococcus germ which produced the scarlet fever in the child. Some may become infected, but not be sick at all. We know this is true because tests done on all members of a household before and after scarlet fever occurred showed that several members of the household were not immune to the scarlet fever germ when the child first developed it, but the tests repeated after he had recovered showed that not only had the child become immune, but so had most of the members of the household.

The same course of events occurs on a large scale in communities where there are scarlet fever epidemics. Many more people become infected and develop immunity without noticeably having the disease than people who actually become sick with sore throat or scarlet fever. This process of becoming infected and developing immunity without a noticeable illness is well known, not only in scarlet fever, but in mumps, polio, diphtheria and many others, too .

While this phenomenon of immunization is well established, no one should assume that he is immune to a disease simply because he has been exposed to it. Only some of the contacts become immune. And there is considerable question whether a person in contact with scarlet fever would become immune if he is given penicillin or sulfa to prevent the disease. One must be in contact with the germ for some time to build up an immunity to it, and if the germs are rapidly destroyed by drugs, the immunity might not develop. This could be determined by the Dick test in the case of scarlet fever.

Isolation and Quarantine: The child who is infected with the scarlet fever germ harbors it in his throat even before the disease starts. Therefore, immediately after exposure he should be given penicillin daily for ten days or an injection of a long-acting penicillin which will be effective for two to four weeks. After that, a throat culture will be useful to learn whether the child is free of the streptococcus. In some areas the child is isolated for seven days or for as long as the fever lasts.

In New York City a child who catches the disease is isolated for a period of seven days or for as long as the fever lasts, whichever is longer. This is done if there is no complication with pus formation, for example, running ear. If a complication with a discharge such as a running ear or a sinus infection develops, the child must be kept isolated unless it can be shown by laboratory tests that the germ which caused the scarlet fever is no longer present in the pus or secretions.

The regulations on length of isolation in New York City have been found more economical in uncomplicated cases, although it is understood that even after seven days there is a possibility of spreading the disease. But if a child is actively treated with antibiotics or sulfa drugs for the seven-day period of his illness, the chance of his spreading the disease after that time is very small. In other communities the isolation period varies from one to six weeks, and you must and should abide by your local regulations. Health conditions vary in different places and your local health authorities should be the judges of how best to manage the question of isolation and quarantine.

Hygiene: The child's bedding and clothes should be washed immediately after use with hot water and soap or soaked in a disinfectant solution for one to two hours before the usual washing. This last procedure is probably not necessary if washing is done in a machine. Soap is a very good antiseptic. It is most unlikely that the streptococcus could survive a thorough washing with soap and water. You should wash the child's toys and air his books, and mail should not be sent without airing it for several hours. When he is well, you should clean his room thoroughly and air it. The floors and other horizontal surfaces which collect dust, such as table tops and window sills, should be washed with soap. The germs that cause scarlet fever can live a long time. They are not as easily destroyed as the viruses of measles, mumps or chicken pox.

STREPTOCOCCUS SORE THROAT
(SEPTIC SORE THROAT)

This disease is essentially the same as scarlet fever, except that there is no rash. Like scarlet fever, it is caused by the Group A hemolytic streptococcus, but these streptococci lack the factor which is responsible for the rash, or in some cases the patient is immune to the toxin which causes the rash. The disease can spread very rapidly by means of contaminated milk or other foods, especially among people living in large groups such as schools and camps. I know of a group of a thousand men into which the disease was introduced by a person in the kitchen who had tonsillitis. Within five days, a hundred and twenty-five men reported ill with sore throats. Before a week had elapsed, about five hundred men had become ill. Luckily, the epidemic could be controlled quickly with sulfa drugs and penicillin, but pasteurizing milk and preventing sick people from handling food are important safeguards against such epidemics.

When a child is infected, he becomes immune to that particular streptococcus, but since there are numerous strains which cause the disease, infections like the first may follow.

It is often difficult to distinguish streptococcus sore throat from sore throat caused by other bacteria, but pain on swallowing, enlarged, red tonsils (often covered with white spots), swelling and vivid redness of the throat, fever, chills and general weakness are strongly suggestive of this disease. When this condition occurs in epidemic form, it usually means that a streptococcus is responsible, but it is necessary to identify the Group A hemolytic streptococcus by laboratory tests to make a definite diagnosis.

Occasionally a child develops scarlet fever and other members of the family later develop streptococcus sore throat without a rash. Or the order may be reversed, but the infection is the same. The prevention and treatment of the disease, the need for isolation and the complications are all similar to the measures for scarlet fever.

Many people treat sore throats very lightly, but from what I have said, you can see that it is just as important to keep a child at home and treat him when he has a sore throat as it is when a rash accompanies it, as in scarlet fever.

ERYSIPELAS (ST. ANTHONY'S FIRE)

Erysipelas is an infection of the deep layers of the skin caused by the Group A hemolytic streptococcus which is closely related to, but not identical with, the streptococcus which causes scarlet fever and the one which causes streptococcus sore throat. Erysipelas occurs at all ages, from the newborn to old age, but it is most common at both extremes. It is especially prone to break out around injured skin, around cuts and bruises, and places which are already infected by some other germ. Erysipelas occurs commonly around the stump of the umbilical cord in the newborn, around chicken pox and impetigo sores, on areas of eczema or psoriasis, around sores caused by scabies, and as a complication of open wounds, operative wounds such as mastoid wounds, and those caused by burns.

Erysipelas has an incubation period of two to five days, after which a sharply demarcated area of redness and swelling appears. The edge of this area is thickened and rounded, which distinctly separates it from the surrounding normal skin. The center of the patch heals as the infection spreads outward. Erysipelas of the face often spreads over the entire head, resulting in marked swelling and temporary disfigurement.

The child may have a fever of 103° to 105°, starting at the same time as the rash or a little before it. He feels chilly and may have shaking chills. He quickly becomes quite sick and toxic, and as the disease advances, he may become delirious, even comatose. The skin usually heals after a week or ten days, but it may break down into abscesses. Unless actively treated with penicillin or sulfa drugs, it is a very serious disease; without treatment it is fatal in many, especially in the very young, the very old and in people who are weak from other causes.

Erysipelas can be cured in twenty-four to forty-eight hours with the proper antibiotics or sulfa drugs given internally. After this time the patient feels well and the skin begins to lose its swelling and redness. As the swelling subsides, the involved area of skin becomes purple, wrinkled and peels. These changes last a week or two. There is no scarring unless the skin becomes abscessed.

Erysipelas may recur, especially in people with chronic skin diseases. After several recurrences, these people seem to develop resistance to the infection. There are no tests for erysipelas, and immunization with vaccine or gamma globulin is not recommended.

The patient should have a separate room until after recovery from the disease, but exposed children need not be quarantined or given preventive treatment because the disease is almost never spread directly from person to person.

QUESTIONS & ANSWERS

SCARLET FEVER

Q. *Is scarlatina a mild form of scarlet fever?*

A. No, they are the same disease.

Q. *Is scarlet fever the same everywhere—in New York, China, Rumania, Chicago and Miami?*

A. It is the same disease, but it varies when the climate and the populations do. In New York and Chicago its incidence and severity would be about the same, but in China and Rumania it would vary. In Miami, as in other areas with warm climates, it would probably be less frequent and less severe.

Q. *Do all streptococcus germs produce scarlet fever?*

A. No. There are hundreds of different germs of the streptococcus family, but only about forty are known to produce this type of disease.

Q. *Is scarlet fever spread only from person to person?*

A. Most often it is, but some large outbreaks have been started by contaminated food and milk.

Q. *How contagious is scarlet fever?*

A. Of those exposed, about 15 to 20 per cent develop the disease with a rash, but many more are infected. The percentage may be higher where many people live together, for instance, in army barracks and boarding schools.

Q. *Why is it so much less contagious than measles, whooping cough and mumps?*

A. Probably because more of our population has some resistance to the streptococcus as a result of previous contact with it. And infection with bacteria is less easily spread than infection with viruses.

Q. *Does the sore throat of scarlet fever differ from other kinds of sore throats?*

A. It is likely to be more severe, but sometimes it feels like any other sore throat. Generally it looks different to the experienced eye of the doctor—it is redder and swollen.

Q. *Is the scarlet fever rash sometimes confused with other rashes?*

A. Yes, with the rashes of German measles, roseola and rashes caused by sensitivity to some drugs.

Q. *Is it necessary to send a scarlet fever patient to a hospital?*

A. No, unless home conditions make it impossible to care for him properly. Hospitalization is always necessary for troops living in barracks or for children in boarding schools and camps.

Q. *Do sulfa drugs and antibiotics always help scarlet fever?*

A. Yes. Some strains of the streptococcus may become resistant to the sulfa drugs, but this never happens with penicillin or other antibiotics used against streptococcus infections. Penicillin is rapidly effective in eliminating the streptococcus.

Q. *Do convalescent serum and gamma globulin help scarlet fever?*

A. Yes. Penicillin is preferable.

Q. *How do you know how long to treat scarlet fever when there is no rash?*

A. We know from experience that treatment with an antibiotic for ten days will rid the patient of the streptococcus and in most cases keep it away. If there are complications, treatment has to be continued until they are cured.

Q. *May my boy return to athletics immediately after isolation is over?*

A. He might undertake the less active athletics if he was given sulfa or penicillin, since the chances of complications developing are very much reduced in patients treated with these drugs. But if he received no drug treatment, he should avoid strenuous athletics for three or four weeks. Several complications, kidney disease, rheumatic fever or swollen glands may appear in the third week or later.

Q. *Should all persons exposed to scarlet fever be given something to prevent it?*

A. Yes, they should have antibiotics if they are susceptible.

Q. *Should antibiotics be given to infants of six months?*

A. Yes, it is safer.

Q. *Since you can get scarlet fever more than once, why not give every exposed person antibiotics?*

A. Second attacks are not so common as to justify it.

Q. *Is it easy to get scarlet fever convalescent serum?*

A. No. It is becoming harder and harder to get. Very few laboratories make it.

Q. *Why is active immunization against scarlet fever not practiced generally?*

A. The toxin injections necessary to produce immunity often
cause reactions and the resulting immunity may not last
very long. It is much less troublesome and much safer to
treat the disease with sulfa drugs and/or antibiotics since
they are so effective.

Q. *Does one attack of scarlet fever make you immune for life?*

A. Yes, usually, though second attacks do occur.

Q. *If you have scarlet fever a second time, is it milder than
the first?*

A. Not necessarily.

Q. *How soon after scarlet fever do you develop immunity?*

A. After the first three to five days of the illness.

Q. *How can you tell that?*

A. By the Dick test becoming negative. A positive Dick test
indicates that you are not immune to scarlet fever and a
negative one that you are.

Q. *My child has been exposed to scarlet fever at school. May
he play with other children in his class who were exposed
at the same time?*

A. Yes, after two days of penicillin treatment.

Q. *How soon after scarlet fever should a child return to
school?*

A. He may go back to school as soon as he is released from
isolation if he is well and was treated with antibiotics. I
prefer to have the child up and about and out of doors for
a few days before he goes back. If the isolation period is
fourteen days or longer, the child may be sent to school
as soon as it is over.

Q. *How soon after scarlet fever may my child go to the
movies?*

A. The answer is the same as for returning to school.

Q. *I run a nursery school. A case of scarlet fever broke out in
my four-year-old group. Should I disband the group?*

A. The children who have had the disease could keep coming.
It might be possible to keep the class together if all the

children who had not had scarlet fever were given preventive treatment with the local health authorities' approval.

Q. *If my child has scarlet fever, must it be reported to the local board of health?*

A. Yes. Your doctor will report it.

Q. *How do you clean a room that has been occupied by a scarlet fever patient?*

A. You wash the horizontal surfaces such as floors, table tops and window sills with soap and water or a commercial antiseptic. Wash all washable objects which have been in direct contact with the patient. Leave things which cannot be washed in the open air for several hours. Wash the child's dishes separately with soap and hot water before returning them to the family cupboard.

STREPTOCOCCUS SORE THROAT

Q. *Does immunity follow a streptococcus sore throat?*

A. Yes it does, but the immunity is specific for the germ which caused it. There are many different members of the streptococcus family which produce the same infection, so it is possible to have streptococcus sore throat more than once.

Q. *Why, then, does it become less common after ten years of age?*

A. By that age children have probably been infected with several of the streptococci and the chances of being infected with streptococci to which they lack resistance are reduced.

Q. *How soon after having had streptococcus sore throat may my child return to school?*

A. A week after the onset, provided he has had no fever or other signs of illness for at least two days.

Q. *If he is treated with penicillin for seven to ten days may he return sooner?*

A. Yes. If he looks and feels well before his treatment is

finished, he could return to school and the penicillin could be continued even though he is not at home.

Q. *Is there anything different between scarlet fever and strep sore throat in treatment, prevention, quarantine, isolation, complications, etc.?*

A. None, except that the rash makes scarlet fever easier to diagnose.

ERYSIPELAS

Q. *Is erysipelas a common disease?*

A. Yes, but not as common as it was before antibiotics were used for treatment of ordinary skin diseases.

Q. *Is erysipelas contagious?*

A. It is for those who have open sores or wounds. The germs enter through broken skin.

Q. *You say that erysipelas can be cured in one or two days. I thought it took longer, even with antibiotics.*

A. I mean that the bacteria causing it can be destroyed in that time, but it would take the skin many more days to look normal again. Also, if the child had a high fever with erysipelas, his temperature would become normal in one or two days, but it might take several more days to get over the effects of the fever and the toxicity of the disease.

Q. *Will any hospital accept a patient with erysipelas?*

A. Most will not, since treatment can be given with ease.

Q. *Should a child with erysipelas be taken to a hospital?*

A. Not usually—only if the child is so ill that he requires treatment difficult to give at home, such as intravenous feeding or oxygen treatment.

Q. *How soon after erysipelas may my son return to school?*

A. He might return after the swelling is reduced, the skin is healed, and he has regained his strength. It would probably be several days after his temperature has become normal, or about a week from the onset of the disease.

Q. *I have heard that erysipelas is a dangerous disease. Is that no longer so?*

A. It is no longer dangerous because we have antibiotics for treating it, but without treatment it would still be a horrible disease.

Q. *Can I have my child immunized against erysipelas?*

A. There is no vaccine and none is needed since the disease can be cured so rapidly.

Q. *Is there really a difference in management of any of the diseases caused by the beta hemolytic streptococcus of Group A?*

A. No, they should be treated in the same way.

20: Rheumatic Fever

Rheumatic fever occurs everywhere, but more often in some parts of the world than in others. In general, rheumatic fever is more frequent in damp, cold climates, and less common in warm, dry ones. It is therefore more frequent in the area east of the Rocky Mountains and on the eastern coast of the United States. It becomes less common as we approach the southern states, Florida, Arizona, New Mexico and southern California. It is quite common in England, Ireland, Scotland and the Scandinavian countries, and along the west coast of Germany, and is also observed in the colder, damper areas of Egypt, Syria, Israel and in other Middle East and Eastern countries, such as India.

Thirty or forty years ago rheumatic fever had reached the position of being one of the leading causes of death between the ages of five and twenty. It occurs more often among people living in crowded quarters where hygiene and nutrition are poor, but I have seen rheumatic fever many times among children who live in luxurious homes and have all the food and shelter that can be obtained.

The great danger of rheumatic fever in childhood is that it usually attacks the heart. In a small percentage of cases, the effect on the heart is very rapid and very severe, and it becomes a life-saving procedure to recognize the condition and to treat it actively. Generally the heart involvement develops a little more slowly, but rheumatic fever is a disease which recurs and the heart involvement becomes more severe with each recurrence over a period of years. Because of the involvement of the heart, rheumatic fever carries with it an appreciable mortality. Approximately 80 per cent of the heart disease of young people under twenty years of age is caused by rheumatic fever. Undoubtedly some of the remaining heart cases are also due to unrecognized rheumatic fever. Between twenty and twenty-nine years old, about 65 per cent of heart patients have had rheumatic fever. About 55 per cent of the heart disease in the thirty to thirty-nine year age group is due to rheumatic fever, and so on, diminishing as the person gets older, when the chance of heart disease due to hardening of the arteries becomes greater.

Rheumatic fever occurs at all ages, but is most common between the ages of five and fifteen. It is rarely observed in the first year of life, and not often before three years, after which it increases in frequency, reaching its peak at eight to ten years. It begins as an acute illness, and there may be acute recurrences of the symptoms, but it most often remains as a chronic disease and lasts for many years, usually becoming inactive before the age of fifteen.

There had been a great deal of question as to what causes rheumatic fever. It is now clear that rheumatic fever is a reaction of the body to an infection with a hemolytic streptococcus germ of the kind that frequently causes tonsillitis, scarlet fever, and septic sore throat. Whenever there is an epidemic of scarlet fever or tonsillitis caused by a hemolytic streptococcus, it is reasonably certain that there will be an increased incidence of rheumatic fever. It is most likely to occur in the late winter and spring when throat infections are most common.

Rheumatic fever had been dropping in frequency for about twenty to thirty years until about 1950 when an increase occurred throughout the world. The sharpest rate of drop occured after sulfa drugs and antibiotics became available for the treatment and prevention of streptococcal infection. During World War II, in U.S. army installations, out of more than seven hundred soldiers who had throat infections caused by the hemolytic streptococcus and who were treated with penicillin or aureomycin, three, or less than 0.5 per cent, developed rheumatic fever. On the other hand, of a similar number who developed a similar infection and who were not treated with antibiotics or sulfa drugs, twenty-one, or about 3 per cent, developed rheumatic fever. Such figures suggest that with early recognition and treatment of streptococcal disease, rheumatic fever might be prevented or reduced to a minimum.

Yet there is no reason why we should be complacent. It is true that the incidence and severity of scarlet fever have declined spontaneously over a period of many years. It is also true that simultaneously there has been a progressive and equally striking decline in cases of rheumatic fever. But it is curious, and distressing, that within the past ten to fifteen years there have been epidemics of scarlet fever in Canada and Switzerland with a subsequent increase in the number of cases of rheumatic fever. Whenever such an outbreak of streptococcal infection occurs, we may expect an upsurge in rheumatic fever.

Contagion: Rheumatic fever is not a contagious disease. Neither is it inherited, but there may be an increased tendency toward it among children whose parents have had it. This suggests the inheritance of a predisposition to the disease, but the disease must follow infection with a hemolytic streptococcus.

Incubation Period: The term *incubation period* does not apply to rheumatic fever, but usually the onset follows the streptococcal infection by two, three or four weeks. Sometimes it is as short as a few days or as long as eight weeks.

Symptoms: If a child has frequent nose and throat infections with many episodes of tonsillitis or sore throat, and a week or two after apparent recovery he has a period during which he feels tired, has a low-grade fever, and is not his usual self, rheumatic fever should be considered. If he looks pale and gets tired easily, and has frequent nose bleeds and migratory pains in the joints, rheumatic fever is even more likely. If, in addition to that, the child has a low-grade temperature which is unexplained in other ways, and if a heart murmur is heard which was not there before, the suspicion that the child has rheumatic fever becomes very great, almost a certainty. The illness often begins in a much more abrupt fashion and may be severe right from the beginning. The child may be extremely sick, he may have a high fever of 103° to 105° and feel achy and chilly. One or several joints may be red, swollen, very painful and exquisitely tender when touched, and he may have early signs of involvement of the heart, a rapid pulse, an irregular pulse, a murmur, and signs of involvement of the pericardium (the sac surrounding the heart). Such a child is in imminent danger and requires urgent care. The slower and less extensive the heart involvement is at the beginning, the better is the outlook for the child's progress, although it sometimes becomes severe after a mild beginning.

It had been observed that between 25 and 50 per cent of all children who developed rheumatic fever developed a rash early in the illness. But in the past twenty to twenty-five years rashes, nodules and chorea have been less common in the New York area, but more common in such areas as Europe, the Middle and Far East, and South America. The rash occurs most frequently on the outer surfaces of the arms and thighs and on the buttocks, and almost never on the face. It is called erythema multiforme because of the many shapes it takes. The most common variety appears in irregularly shaped flat patches. About 10 per cent of the rashes look like hives. Another kind of rash, which may accompany the other symptoms of early rheumatic fever, is called erythema nodosum. It appears as painful reddish or purplish lumps on the shins, and occasionally on other parts of the body. Usually these nodules leave purple staining of the skin for some time after they have healed. Rheumatic nodules, or little firm lumps about the size of a pea along the spine, in the scalp, over the elbows, over the knuckles may occur in some children with rheumatic fever. These nodules are usually unmistakable evidence of acute rheumatic fever. They may come and go in a few days. Occasionally they remain as long as a week.

Diagnosis: When the diagnosis of rheumatic fever is in doubt and needs confirmation, laboratory examinations of the blood and an electrocardiogram may be helpful. An increased number of white blood corpuscles and an increased sedimentation rate of the red blood cells (the speed with which the red corpuscles settle out in a narrow glass tube) usually accompany acute rheumatic fever. Certain other laboratory tests (such as the antistreptolysin titre of the blood) may also be helpful in arriving at a correct diagnosis.

Treatment: If a child develops rheumatic fever, he should be put to bed and kept there. He must not even be permitted to get up to go to the bathroom. He should be given a wholesome, liberal, and well-balanced diet, with an adequate amount of milk and vitamins. Company should be limited. The room should be comfortably warm, about 70° F. The doctor will undoubtedly treat the child with either salicylates (aspirin) or cortisone. There is a great deal of discussion among doctors at the present time as to which of the drugs is more effective. There is also a great deal of disagreement on how long the drugs should be given. Usually there is little or no difference in the effectiveness of one drug as opposed to another if doctors are unable to decide which one is more helpful to the child. The doctor draws his own conclusions from his experience and that of other doctors, and thus arrives at a plan of treatment.

ASPIRIN: It has been my practice to treat rheumatic fever with aspirin, approximately 1 grain per pound of body weight per day divided into four doses given every four hours. For example, if a child weighs sixty pounds, 60 grains of aspirin would be given each day, 15 grains every four hours during the waking day. I prefer to let the child sleep through the night, since rest obtained during sleep seems to me very important. I continue the aspirin until the temperature becomes normal and for a period of about two weeks thereafter. This is the routine of aspirin treatment adopted at one of our better hospitals, not because it is the only form of treatment which might be recommended, but because it represents the opinions of many excellent doctors—pediatricians as well as heart specialists. But this is not the routine of every doctor. In fact, very few doctors treat rheumatic fever patients in exactly the same way. Some give more or less aspirin, some give it every four hours around the clock, some continue the aspirin for months, etc. Aspirin is usually well tolerated, but if it is continued for weeks, blood levels should be determined. Low levels may be ineffective and high levels may be toxic.

CORTISONE: Some physicians prefer substitutes for aspirin, such as amidopyrine and especially cortisone or A.C.T.H., one of the cortisone-like drugs. Some give both. The dosage of cortisone and the duration of treatment has been under study for several years. It varies considerably according to the doctor's experience and the results of studies previously made. Your doctor will know what the best plan of treatment is for your child.

It is the belief of doctors that almost all children with rheumatic fever develop some involvement of the heart. This may be, and it is quite serious in some children, but it is much less so in most. In fact, it is often so mild and there is such complete healing of the heart muscles and heart valves that the child may resume all his usual activities with no limitations.

BED REST: A child with rheumatic fever is kept in bed for at least six weeks or until such time as he has been without fever for a minimum of two weeks after drugs are discontinued, and until it becomes evident by the doctor's examination and an electrocardiogram that the progress of heart injury has stopped and the heart has begun to improve, and until the white blood count becomes essentially normal and the red blood cell sedimentation rate has become normal or become stabilized at a low level. At that point the child is allowed to start exercise, very little at first, perhaps to dangle his feet over the side of the bed, then to take a few steps, finally to walk a little farther, a city block, then two, four and so forth, until he gradually is able to go back to school. Other activities requiring more effort, such as sports, are postponed for several months and are then allowed only when the doctor finds that the child has recovered without extensive injury to the heart, and that he can safely take part in such activity.

There is great difference in doctors' opinions as to how long a child should be kept in bed with rheumatic fever. Twenty-five to thirty years ago many doctors recommended bed rest for six to eighteen months for acute severe rheumatic fever. Now we believe that six weeks or longer may suffice depending on the progress of the heart, the findings on the electrocardiograph, the red cell sedimentation rate, the disappearance of other conditions such as rash, joint pains and joint swelling, nodules and, of course, fever. Some recommend shorter periods of inactivity. And this may be suitable for the very mild cases. Keeping a patient in bed too long softens him and it tends to make him heart-conscious, possibly for life.

Psychological Aspect: During my service in the army, I saw many young men who said they were unable to undertake any physical exertion because in their childhood they had spent many months in bed with a disease called rheumatic fever. They had been told by their doctors never to undertake strenuous exercise, not play football, not to take up any competitive sports. They were told it would be dangerous for them to do much work because exertion might tax the heart to a dangerous degree. Probably some of these men never did have rheumatic fever as judged by careful examination, but having been told they did they never could believe that they could behave like other young men without danger to their welfare. To become an invalid without having the disease is almost as serious as to become one with it. In both situations the person is incapacitated. A diagnosis of rheumatic fever is serious and no person should be told he has it unless it is definitely so. And it is very important that the condition of the heart be properly evaluated so that correct advice can be given as to the child's future behavior.

St. Vitus' Dance: Chorea, or St. Vitus' Dance, is believed to be a form of rheumatic fever. It is a condition in which the child is unable to control the actions of his muscles, which results in facial grimacing, awkward motions of the arms, legs, hands and feet, a constant wiggling and moving about, and marked emotional instability, crying, hysterical laughing and moodiness. Unlike the other forms of acute rheumatic fever, chorea is rarely accompanied by joint pains, high fever or heart involvement, but it occurs in about 5 per cent of children who have acute rheumatic fever. Perhaps 10 per cent of the cases of chorea are complicated by involvement of the heart. Like the other manifestations of rheumatic fever, chorea also may occur once or several times. It is more common in girls than in boys under fifteen years and relatively rare in adults. About half of the episodes diagnosed as chorea are probably not associated with rheumatic disease but are emotional in origin. These are difficult to diagnose and even more difficult to treat.

Prevention: There is no immunization against rheumatic fever, and no serum which offers any positive advantage. A vaccine has recently been reported, but it is still in the experimental phase.

Once a child has had rheumatic fever it becomes very important to protect him from infection with the hemolytic streptococcus for many years. This is done by giving him regular doses of antibiotics over this period. We know that if such children go without a recurrence of rheumatic fever for a period of about five years, the chances of recurrence subsequently are sharply reduced. Some doctors feel that when the disease starts early, it is important to protect the child for more than five years, or until he is fifteen years old, after which there seems to be a sharp drop in the number of recurrences. If a child developed rheumatic fever at the age of twelve, antibiotics would be recommended until he was seventeen, since the exact period for penicillin prophylaxis is not known. Some recommend it indefinitely. We used to give daily doses of sulfa drugs, but lately we have found that penicillin given daily is preferable because it is more certain to be effective. The penicillin is given throughout the winter, spring and fall, and even during the early summer. This kind of penicillin is given by mouth and, of course, may be given at home. There is another kind which may be injected once every two or three weeks, and while the injections must be made by a doctor or a nurse, the cost is about the same because the doses are so much less frequent. Many children object to having injections, however. When a child is given penicillin regularly, the chances of recurrence of the acute form of rheumatic fever are reduced by about 60 per cent as compared to those rheumatic fever patients who have not been treated with antibiotics.

An additional safeguard against recurrences of rheumatic fever, if family circumstances permit, is to spend the entire fall, winter and spring in an area where the climate is warm and dry, and where streptococcus infection is less frequent. Florida, Arizona, New Mexico and southern California are such places. Since this is likely to be both inconvenient and expensive, and since antibiotics are so effective, a change of climate is recommended only for those children who get frequent colds in spite of treatment with all available drugs, and then if it does not impair family life.

If a child has tonsillitis frequently, the chance of developing rheumatic fever may be reduced by removing his tonsils, since scarlet fever and hemolytic streptococcus infection seem to occur less frequently in children whose tonsils have been

removed. But merely removing tonsils which are not infected
will not prevent rheumatic fever. Tonsillectomy is only effective when chronically infected tonsils are the cause of frequent
episodes of tonsillitis, because it is the frequency of throat infections which is important.

One very important thing to remember is that if a child
has a sore throat—and any sore throat might be due to a streptococcus—it is important that it be treated with a suitable
antibiotic. If a child has scarlet fever, the same is true. Measles
occurring in a child who has, or has once had, rheumatic fever
should also be treated with antibiotics to eliminate the hemolytic streptococci which are often present. In general, rheumatic fever is altogether too frequent and too vicious a disease
to be allowed to occur and recur. With proper medical attention, the incidence of the disease can be reduced greatly, as
can many of the relapses.

Isolation and Quarantine: Since rheumatic fever is not a
contagious disease, a child who has it need not be isolated, but
he should be in a room where he is not disturbed. A child exposed to rheumatic fever need not be quarantined.

QUESTIONS & ANSWERS

Q. *Rheumatic fever is often called a crippling disease. How
does it cripple?*

A. It usually involves the heart, particularly the valves, whose
function is to close the openings between the different
chambers of the heart. There are three groups of valves
and if they become first inflamed and swollen and then
scarred and shrunken, they cannot perform efficiently because they inevitably leak. When there is a leak, the heart
must overwork, and this causes it to become enlarged and
heavy and thickened and more easily exhausted. Rheumatic
fever is a crippling disease because many children with
serious heart damage have to be limited in their activity.
Their hearts just will not stand the excessive strain.

Q. *If one parent or both have rheumatic fever, is it more
likely that their child will have it?*

A. Yes, but it is by no means certain that he will.

Q. *Are living conditions responsible for rheumatic fever?*

A. Not directly, but rheumatic fever does occur more often among the less privileged, among those who live in crowded quarters, who have less food with little variety, fewer clothes and fewer opportunities for good hygiene. Nevertheless, I have seen rheumatic fever many times in children of parents who lived comfortably in large apartments where there was ample food, ample care, good hygiene, enough of everything. The children developed rheumatic fever, primarily because an initial infection with a streptococcus was not adequately treated.

Q. *Does rheumatic fever occur in several children in the same family?*

A. Not very often.

Q. *Can you tell that rheumatic fever is about to begin?*

A. No, usually not. A child who has had a sore throat or tonsillitis seems to be perfectly well and goes back to school, only to find that he begins to feel irritable, tired, has fever, maybe joint pains, and now has rheumatic fever. There is no way to tell in advance that this particular child is going to develop the disease rather than others who had similar sore throats and did not develop rheumatic fever.

Q. *Do repeated joint pains mean rheumatic fever?*

A. Not necessarily. Many children have pains in their muscles or joints. Sometimes they are even awakened at night with pains in their legs. These used to be called growing pains and we have learned since that many of them are really caused by rheumatic fever. But most of the children who complain of pains in their joints on and off never have swollen joints and never have rheumatic fever.

Q. *Does a fever which continues for a week or longer with no explanation mean rheumatic fever?*

A. No, although that is a very common misconception of parents. While it may be rheumatic fever in some cases, it usually indicates incomplete treatment of some infection, usually of the nose and throat or the adenoids or tonsils or sinuses.

Q. *Are the joint pains of rheumatic fever the same in children as they are in adults?*

A. Not usually. Mostly in adults the joints are swollen and red and hurt to the touch. In fact, they may be so tender that as someone approaches the bed or leans on it, there is a great deal of pain. In children, while this is sometimes true, the pain is usually of a more transient type. It might last a few hours, a day, two or three days, with some swelling in a few joints. These subside, new joints are involved, they clear up, and sometimes the inflammation recurs in a joint that was affected before.

Q. *Is there ever only one joint involved?*

A. Yes, but not often in children. Usually there are several at the same time, or one after another is inflamed.

Q. *Do you have a cough with rheumatic fever?*

A. Not unless there is still some inflammation in the back of the nose and throat, the sinuses or the bronchial tubes. But this would not be due to rheumatic fever. It would be left over from the original infection that caused it.

Q. *Should my child be treated in a hospital when he has rheumatic fever?*

A. Yes, I believe so, during the acute phase. It is usually easier to keep a child inactive in bed in a hospital than it is at home. A child is apt to take advantage of his parents' sympathy for him when he is ill and to get away with many things he cannot get away with in a hospital. When he is told to stay in bed in a hospital, he will usually do it. At home he may, but the chances are he will roam around, if he can. Also, we find that it is much easier to give medicine to children in the hospital. I have seen unpleasant-tasting drugs taken with nothing more than a grimace, whereas at home there was a struggle, followed by vomiting.

Q. *Should the child be sent home after the acute phase is over, or to a convalescent home?*

A. In general, it would be preferable to send the child to his own home. His convalescence must be restful but this is manageable at home.

Q. *Can a child recover completely from rheumatic fever?*

A. Yes. He can recover so that the doctor can find no trace of damage either by listening to his heart or making an electrocardiogram. He can do everything a normal child can do.

Q. *After my child has recovered from rheumatic fever, will she be able to go back to school and climb stairs and join in other school activities?*

A. Very likely. The American Heart Association has classified the degree of damage to the heart and the amount of activity to be permitted in school in five groups. In Group A, the heart damage is so insignificant that the children are allowed full physical activity without any restrictions. In Group B the heart injury is such that the children are allowed to take part in all ordinary activity, but are advised against unusually severe or competitive efforts. In Group C are the patients whose regular physical activity should be moderately restricted, and whose more strenuous habits should be completely discontinued. In Group D are the patients who should be restricted in all their activities. And finally, in Group E are the patients who must be at complete rest, confined to a bed or a chair.

Q. *Should children with heart disease be in separate classes at school?*

A. There is considerable difference of opinion about this. Unless a child's condition makes it absolutely necessary to put him in a class whose activity is limited, it is wiser for him to be in his regular class. When he is in a class with normal children, he will probably adjust to an average life much more easily.

Q. *You said that doctors disagree about how long a child should be kept in bed. Why is this?*

A. We all agree that a child with rheumatic fever should be kept in bed until the heart disease has stopped being active. We are not always absolutely sure when the disease has become quiescent, but we can tell by listening to the heart, by the pulse rate and by the electrocardiogram whether the heart is overacting, whether the damage has stopped progressing, whether there has been any improvement, and so forth. At this point some of us feel that the

child should start getting out of bed, a little at a time, and
should start working toward whatever kind of a life his
condition will allow. There are many doctors, however,
who feel that the child should have bed rest for a much
longer time. I feel, and so do many others, that the disad-
vantage of this prolonged rest is the psychological damage done to the child by impressing him with the idea that
he is an invalid, that he cannot make any physical effort
without endangering his life. Many children have fallen
prey to this way of thinking, and their entire attitude
toward living has been influenced by the fear of doing too
much.

Q. *Does a child recover more completely if he stays in bed
longer?*

A. There is considerable doubt about it. Many of us feel that
when it becomes clear that the heart affection is making
no more progress or has begun to improve, further inactivity will not help the heart particularly.

Q. *Can you, by giving penicillin daily to children who have
had rheumatic fever, prevent streptococcus infection and
thus prevent relapses?*

A. Yes, years of experience have proved this to be true.

Q. *Isn't there any kind of penicillin which can be given less
often?*

A. Yes, there is a kind which can be given every two or three
weeks, but it must be injected by a doctor or a nurse. The
cost, including the doctor's fee, is about the same, but most
children do not like injections, particularly every two or
three weeks for five years.

Q. *Is it still necessary to send children away to warm, dry climates?*

A. No, not since penicillin has become available as a preventive. Of course, it is much better to keep a child at home
and not uproot him from his customary environment, his
friends and his school.

Q. *You said there is no way of preventing rheumatic fever,
but you also said it follows a streptococcus infection and
that they can be prevented. Isn't this inconsistent?*

A. Not as much as it seems. We can prevent the various streptococcus infections that lead to rheumatic fever. We could inject children with scarlet fever toxin and with the streptococcus toxin for each type of streptococcus germ which causes rheumatic fever, but there are at least forty of these and we would have to keep on immunizing indefinitely since the immunity does not last very long. So the only practical preventive is to treat scarlet fever and sore throats, any of which may be caused by one of the streptococcus germs, actively with antibiotics.

Recently a new effective vaccine against the streptococcus has been developed. It is still in the experimental stage and should not be substituted for penicillin, which is now well established as an effective agent to prevent infection with the streptococcus.

21: Rickettsial Diseases: Rocky Mountain Spotted Fever, Typhus, Q Fever, Rickettsialpox

The rickettsiae which cause the diseases we are discussing in this chapter are small organisms which fall between bacteria and viruses in size. They are named in honor of a scientist named Ricketts who died of typhus while studying it. Rickettsiae live within cells of animal tissue. They can be stained and seen with an ordinary microscope. They are essentially parasites which live on arthropods such as fleas, lice, midges, ticks and mites. Rickettsiae are able to produce disease in man only where man lives near to those blood-sucking arthropods and to mice and rats, because the infection is carried by the host (the tick or the louse) to man. It is not transmitted directly by man to man.

In the case of Rocky Mountain spotted fever, a disease common in the United States, the infected dog tick or wood tick attaches itself to man and feeds on him and thus infects him. But man is not the source of infection for others. The cycle of infection is rather complicated. The infected tick, while feeding on the dog, lays eggs which fall to the ground. These infected eggs develop into baby ticks (nymphs), and they are already infected at birth. The infected nymphs attach themselves to the rat, feed on it, and thus transmit the disease to it. The rat then becomes the source of infection of other ticks which bite the dog. This cycle is repeated over and over again, and man really has nothing to do with it except that he sometimes is bitten by an infected tick.

Rocky Mountain spotted fever, which is also known as tick fever, black fever, blue fever and tick typhus is uncommon in the eastern part of the United States, but it has been found in every state except Connecticut, Maine, Rhode Island and Vermont. Infected ticks have been found on Cape Cod and Long Island. It is thought that Western cattle brought east were infected with infected ticks. We still have a few cases in the summer in eastern Long Island.

Rocky Mountain spotted fever is the same whether it is seen in the northwestern United States, where it is carried by the wood tick, in the southeastern United States and Mexico where the dog tick is responsible, or in the southwest where the lone star tick carries it. In Brazil the same, or a closely related, disease is carried by a different tick. Apparently Rocky Mountain spotted fever is the same or similar to São Paulo fever in Brazil, Colombian spotted fever in Colombia, Mediterranean fever in the Marseilles area and South African tick typhus.

In other rickettsial diseases the person is infected by the bite of an infected louse (epidemic typhus). In turn, other body lice bite the infected person and become infected by him. These lice may then spread the disease from one person to another. Typhus fever has been very important historically. In some epidemics entire populations have been decimated. During World War I, typhus was a very serious problem in many European countries and was extremely difficult to cope with. During World War II, an epidemic in southern Italy was rapidly and effectively stopped by dusting large parts of the population with DDT and injecting several hundreds of thousands of people with vaccine.

In many instances, the bite of the tick or the louse is not necessary to acquire the infection; contact with them is sufficient. In taking a tick off a dog or a child, a person may crush it and either he or the child may be infected by the contaminated blood of the tick, even on unbroken skin. In other instances, the feces of the flea are left on the child's skin. The skin itches, the child scratches, and the infected material is introduced into the skin. Wearing old contaminated clothing may also infect the skin, as in Q fever. This infection is usually acquired by persons working in stockyards and meat-packing concerns who come in contact with contaminated animal carcasses, wool, fertilizer or dust, or by consuming contaminated milk. Laboratory technicians are especially prone to infection when working with the Rickettsia burneti, the agent causing Q fever.

Incubation Period: Symptoms usually begin six to fifteen days after a person has been bitten by a flea, but in three to ten days in Rocky Mountain spotted fever and fourteen to twenty-one in Q fever.

Symptoms: There is considerable similarity in the symptoms of all rickettsial diseases. They all result in fever, chills, loss of appetite, vomiting, headache, backache, general muscular aches, and most of them are accompanied by rashes or spots which may cover the entire body. The rash usually appears between the third and the fifth day of the disease and varies from flat, pink spots to purpura, or areas of bleeding into the skin. The diseases last between seven and fourteen days and most people recover. Q fever usually starts with pneumonia, and is likely to have more rash than the other rickettsial diseases.

Epidemic typhus lasts fourteen days and is more severe. In this disease coma and delirium set in rapidly and recovery is less frequent. The mortality is between 10 and 50 pe[r] unless treated actively with the broad-spectrum [ ] especially one of the many tetracyclines. These [ ] rickettsial diseases very quickly—in two to four days.

Immunity: Rickettsial diseases leave specific [ ] which may or may not be permanent. A child who has [ ] becomes immune to the rickettsiae which caused it and [ ] to that one kind. If a child has Rocky Mountain spotted fe[ver] he becomes immune to the rickettsiae which caused it. He a[lso] acquires some immunity to the diseases which are caused b[y] related rickettsiae, for instance, the ones which are responsible for São Paulo fever and Mediterranean fever.

The tick must be attached to the skin for at least four to six hours to transmit. Miller explained that there is an incubation period of the bite, infectious agent.

During this time, high fever and chills appear. The 10 to 12 days, severe headaches, muscle aches, high fever and chills resemble influenza or gastritis. Early symptoms resemble influenza or gastritis.

About the third day, a rash appears on the palms of the hands and soles of the feet and later spreads to other parts of the body. The victim may also be delirious and have convulsions. Miller said.

Prevention is the best treatment for Rocky Mountain spotted fever, according to state epidemiologists. Miller made the following recommendations to avoid contracting the disease:

★Tuck pants legs into your socks and wear long-sleeved shirts when in the woods or high grass areas.

★Use insect repellents if desired.

★Check yourself and family members at least twice a day for ticks. Remove ticks with a piece of tissue or a pair of tweezers.

★Keep yourself tick-free. Use an insecticidal power or spray dogs with insecticide.

★Keep animals tick-free. Use insecticidal power or spray dogs with insecticide.

★Keep lawns sprayed to kill ticks.

Prevention: In areas where arthropods are numerous, insect hygiene or decontamination is necessary. In the case of Q fever, the ticks are found in tall grass. The grass should be cut and the area decontaminated with DDT before camping. Sleeping on the ground in such areas is not wise.

Vaccines are available for immunization against Rocky Mountain spotted fever, typhus fever, and against some of the other rickettsial diseases. These are recommended for people traveling to or living in areas where the diseases are always present. Usually two injections of vaccine given a week apart give immunity for a year. Booster injections should be given if there is a possibility of reinfection.

Isolation and Quarantine: It is not necessary to isolate a person who has a rickettsial disease, but in the diseases caused by lice, the patient is isolated until he is deloused, and people who live in the same household are quarantined until they are deloused.

Rickettsialpox: This disease is relatively new in the United States. It was discovered in an epidemic form in a new housing area in the Rego Park section of New York City. The history of its discovery is fascinating. When the illness was first observed, there was no name for it, but alert doctors described it as resembling typhus fever, another rickettsial disease. An exterminator in Rego Park noticed in the course of his work some dead mice near the door of an incinerator, and he also noticed that they were swarming with mites. He had heard about the new disease and he had never seen this kind of mite in the area, so he associated the two and reported his discovery to the health department. His ideas were not at first taken seriously, but he was persistent. Finally an investigation was made which proved his idea was correct—that the infected mice are bitten by the mites, the infected mites bite humans and thereby transmit the disease.

Persons who have the disease become immune to it. Since immune persons have been found in other parts of the world, it is quite certain that the disease is not new, but has up to now not been recognized as an entity. It is caused by the *Rickettsia akari*. The incubation period is ten to fourteen days.

The symptoms are fever, headache, severe malaise and a

Disease	RICKETTSIAL-POX	ROCKY MOUNTAIN SPOTTED FEVER (tick typhus) & MEDITERRANEAN FEVER	EPIDEMIC TYPHUS FEVER (louse-borne)
Cause	Rickettsia akari	Rickettsia rickettsi Rickettsia conori	Rickettsia prowazeki
Source of infection	Infected house mouse	Infected dog and rodent ticks	Infected persons
Mode of transmission	Bite of mite infected by biting infected mouse	Bite of infected tick and contact with tick material (blood, feces)	Bite of human body-lice from infected persons
Incubation period	10 to 14 days	RMSF: 3 to 10 days MF: 5 to 6 days	6 to 15 days
Communicability from man to man	None	None	None
Susceptibility	General	General	General
Resistance	Immunity duration unknown	Immunity may or may not be permanent	Immunity may or may not be permanent
Prevalence	Seen only in New York, but probably more widespread	Entire U.S.A. Along entire Mediterranean coast, Kenya, South Africa	Widespread where crowded unhygienic conditions exist; more cases in colder months
Symptoms	Fever, headache, chills, light sensitivity, muscle pain. Rash on 3d–4th day	Same as rickettsialpox	Sudden fever, chills, headache, general aches. Severely toxic. Rash on 5th–8th day
Rash	Resembles chicken pox	Pink spots, slightly raised	Flat, red spots
Methods of control	Rodent control, including proper care of and firing of incinerators. Report disease	Rodent control. Destroy ticks. Restrict dog travel. Remove ticks without handling. Isolate patient. Report disease	Vaccination of exposed population. Spray populace with DDT. Report disease
Quarantine	None	None	15 days or may be released after delousing with DDT
Epidemic measures	None	None	Yes
Treatment	Broad-spectrum antibiotics: Terramycin, Chloromycetin, Achromycin, Tetramycin		
Immunization	None	RMSF: 3 injections, good for one year, then booster MF: None	2 injections of vaccine. Booster after one year

MURINE TYPHUS (flea-borne)	Q FEVER	SCRUB TYPHUS (tsutsugamushi fever)
Rickettsia mooseri	Rickettsia coxiella burneti	Rickettsia tsutsuga-mushi
Infected rodents	Infected cows, sheep, goats, ticks, bandicoots	Infected larval mites
Flea bite. Flea is infected by biting infected rat	Occupational handling of carcasses. Drinking milk of infected cows	Bite of infected mite
6 to 15 days	2 to 3 weeks	7 to 14 days
None	None	None
General	General	General
Immunity may or may not be permanent	Immunity duration unknown	Immunity not always permanent
Widely distributed in temperate, semi-tropic, tropical areas. More cases in warmer months	Australia, Panama, U.S.A., France, Mediterranean basin	Southeast Asia
Similar to epidemic typhus, but lower mortality. Less dangerous disease. Rash on 5th–8th day	Similar to murine typhus. Rash on 5th–6th day	Similar to RMSF, but less severe. In addition, cough and signs of pneumonia. Rash on 5th–8th day
Flat, red spots	Flat, red spots	Pink spots, slightly raised
Rodent and flea control. Report disease	Pasteurize milk. Rapid recognition and reporting of disease	Cut grass low and burn camp area with oil. Avoid sleeping on ground. Spray clothes with miticide agents. Report disease
None	None	None
None	None	None
2 injections of vaccine. Booster after one year	Vaccine being studied	None

rash which resembles chicken pox. There is usually one sore larger than the rest at the place first bitten by the mite.

Treatment with the broad-spectrum antibiotics is successful.

People infected with the disease need not be isolated since it is not spread from man to man, and those exposed to it are not quarantined.

There is no vaccine for prevention, but none is needed in view of the success of the antibiotics.

QUESTIONS & ANSWERS

Q. *Are rickettsial diseases very important?*

A. Yes, especially epidemic typhus. This disease seems to follow poverty and disaster. It has erupted periodically in the past two centuries, often at the same time as the plague, another very bad epidemic disease. During World War I, epidemics of typhus in central Europe were of immense proportions, reaching a height of some ten thousand cases a day in Serbia. The epidemic was not only very large but very severe. Epidemics in Poland, Rumania and Russia were also very extensive.

Q. *Can you stop an epidemic once it gets started?*

A. Yes, now we can. During World War II, an epidemic started in southern Italy and was stopped as its spread reached a dangerously high level. About a quarter of a million people were vaccinated, a very large number were sprayed with DDT powder to destroy lice, and to avoid the spread from one community to another, only vital travel was permitted. These precautions were successful.

Q. *Is typhus common in children?*

A. Less so than in adults, and it is less dangerous in children.

Q. *Are the rickettsial diseases seasonal?*

A. Typhus, being carried by the body louse, is more frequent in the winter when more clothes are worn. Rocky Mountain spotted fever and others like it which are carried by ticks are more common in the summer when the adult ticks emerge from the larval stage. In countries where the weather is always warm, rickettsial diseases are likely to be present throughout the year.

Q. *Can an infected mouse or rat transmit rickettsial diseases by biting a human?*

A. That is not the usual manner of infection. The tick, flea or mite which gets infected by sucking blood from infected mice or rats carries the disease to man.

Q. *Can household pets carry rickettsial diseases?*

A. Yes, if they go through woods and pick up infected ticks. These ticks can then light on humans and infect them.

Q. *Do bedbugs, cockroaches and house mice transmit rickettsial diseases?*

A. Not bedbugs and cockroaches, although bedbugs have been found to harbor rickettsia. House mice transmit rickettsialpox indirectly by harboring the infected mite which transmits the disease to humans.

Q. *Does recovery from one rickettsial disease result in immunity to others?*

A. Not generally, but there may be some cross-immunity. Immunity to Rocky Mountain spotted fever, for instance, results in partial immunity to some of the diseases which are kindred to it.

Q. *Who should be immunized against Rocky Mountain spotted fever?*

A. Anyone who lives in, or is traveling to, an area where the disease is prevalent.

Q. *Does the same principle apply to other rickettsial diseases?*

A. Yes, if there is an effective vaccine. For example, all American military personnel who are sent to areas where typhus fever is endemic are vaccinated against it, as are soldiers and sailors of other countries.

Q. *If the diseases can be cured so rapidly with antibiotics, why do you give vaccine to prevent them?*

A. The reaction from the vaccine is insignificant compared with the diseases themselves, and it is always better to prevent disease than to have to cure it.

Q. *Are the vaccines always effective?*

A. There is never an *always* or *100 per cent* in medicine, but the vaccines are successful enough to justify their use.

Q. *How do you avoid Rocky Mountain spotted fever and other diseases caused by ticks?*

A. By keeping ticks off yourself. When you go through fields where there are ticks, wear boots or protective socks over your trouser legs to keep the ticks from climbing up your legs. Afterward, inspect your body and clothes, and if you find any, remove them gently without crushing them because you can be infected by the contaminated blood of the tick, even on unbroken skin.

22: Diseases Transmitted by Animals (Zoonoses)

It may be difficult to imagine that your children's favorite dog or cat or even canary could be the cause of serious diseases. But it is true, and every family should be aware of the possibility.

Zoonoses are animal diseases which can be transmitted to man or other animals. There are some eighty-two of them known all over the world. Of course, some of them are very rare and do not concern us here, but according to authorities on the subject, people in North America can contract twenty-four diseases from dogs and twelve from cats, and a number from domestic and wild animals and birds. Some of them are skin diseases. These are discussed in the chapter on that subject.

RABIES (HYDROPHOBIA)

Rabies is not by any means the most common of the zoonoses; in fact, it is rare, but it is the most feared because once the infection develops, it is invariably fatal unless promptly treated. It is a horrible disease, which was described by Claudius Galen, the great Roman physician in the third century A.D., thus: "Hydrophobia is a disease which follows the bite of a mad dog and is accompanied by an aversion to drinking of liquids (hydrophobia or water-fear), convulsions and hiccoughs. Sometimes maniacal attacks supervene."

There is no such thing as natural immunity to rabies. Everyone is susceptible. It is a virus disease of the brain and spinal cord. There would be no point in describing the symptoms and course of the disease here. The reason I have included the chapter in this book is to acquaint parents with the steps they should take if a child is bitten by a dog or some other animal which might be infected with rabies.

All mammals are susceptible to rabies, especially dogs, cats, wolves, foxes, jackals, wildcats, badgers, coyotes, mongooses, squirrels and vampire bats. They contract the disease by being bitten by rabid animals which have the virus in their saliva. Cattle, horses, sheep and swine can also have rabies and have, on occasion, been the source of human infection, but the dog bite is by far the most frequent cause of rabies in man, particularly in the United States. In South Africa the mongoose, in Iran the wolf and in South America the vampire bat have been responsible for a considerable number of cases of human rabies.

In the United States, a very large number of children and adults are bitten by dogs each year, but the number of these cases which become infected with rabies (based on all dog bites, not only bites by rabid dogs) has been estimated at .0007 per cent to .0005 per cent. When the animal is definitely rabid, 5 to 16 per cent may get rabies, except when the wounds are deep, multiple, or on the face, in which instances as many as 60 per cent may develop rabies because with multiple bites there is a heavier infection and with bites on the head or face, the infection travels a shorter route to the brain. There is less chance of the rabies virus getting from the saliva to the wound if the bite is through clothing rather than on bare skin. Although the virus of rabies is in the saliva of rabid dogs, it is rare to become infected without being bitten or scratched by the dog. If a rabid dog merely slobbers on a fresh wound not inflicted by the dog itself, the chance of infection is 0.1 per cent. If the wound is more than twenty-four hours old, there is no chance of being infected.

Incubation Period: The incubation period in humans varies widely. It is usually from ten days to six weeks, but it may be as long as six months, and in rare cases, a year. When the bite is on the head, neck or face (near the brain) or when there are many bites on any part of the body, the incubation period is considerably shortened. In animals, the incubation period is similar, but they are not capable of transmitting the rabies during all of this time. The virus is in the saliva for only three to seven days before the symptoms begin, so the disease can be transmitted only during that interval. If a dog remains well for seven days after a bite, it is most unlikely that it is rabid.

Symptoms in Animals: In animals the symptoms of rabies are any unexplained changes in behavior such as when an ordinarily timid wild animal becomes very friendly with humans, or an ordinarily friendly dog becomes snappish. This period is followed by one of excitability or paralysis, and then death within ten days of the first symptoms. It is wise to remember that all animals with rabies do not appear to be "mad" in the accepted sense that they run wildly and foam at the mouth. In the first place, they may not have reached that stage of the illness, and in the second place they may have the paralytic type of rabies in which they become quiet and seem to be strangling on a foreign body because the swallowing muscles are paralyzed.

What to Do if Bitten by a Dog or by a Wild Animal: If your child is bitten by a dog, even his own pet dog, this is what you should do:

1. Wash the bite with kitchen or laundry soap for twenty minutes, getting the soap well into the wound. Bites were formerly treated with nitric acid, but this is painful and disfiguring and the soap and water wash is now considered just as effective.
2. Consult your doctor, your health department or your police department *immediately. Do not delay. This is urgent.*
3. Do not kill the animal unless it is absolutely necessary. If you must kill it, try not to damage the head. The surest sign by which rabies can be diagnosed is the presence of certain bodies called Negri bodies in the brain. If the brain is destroyed, it may be impossible to make the diagnosis and then the child may have to be subjected to a course of injections unnecessarily.

4. Capture the biting animal, if possible, and keep it penned up so that it can be observed for ten days. Or better still, place it with the health department, police department or a veterinarian for observation.

Even if you know the biting dog has been inoculated against rabies, it should be watched. If the dog begins to show signs of illness, it should be killed, and its brain examined for signs of rabies. All dogs and cats bitten or suspected of having been bitten by a rabid animal should be killed at once. Waiting to see whether it develops rabies is too great a chance to take. If there is rabies in your community, do not examine the mouth of a sick dog or cat. Let a veterinarian do it because the saliva may be infectious.

Treatment: There is no treatment for rabies once the infection has developed. Treatment for a bite has already been discussed, but in addition to this you must consult your doctor quickly. He may want to start vaccine or give rabies antiserum (which gives a temporary immunity) or both, and delaying treatment by even a few hours may make the antiserum ineffective. It should be given within twenty-four hours and it *must* be given within seventy-two hours.

Details of the procedure followed in giving rabies antiserum and vaccine and the indications for using them are discussed in detail in the chapter on immunization.

Prevention: The first great accomplishment in the control of rabies was the discovery of a vaccine in 1885 by Louis Pasteur. He found that the rabies virus lost its virulence for dogs and for men if it was injected from one rabbit to another five times or more. He made his vaccine from the spinal cord of the rabbits which had been infected with the weakened virus and observed its effect on dogs and men, and today we still use essentially the same type of vaccine. Its efficiency is proven by data collected between 1932 and 1935. During these years, 46,000 people were bitten by dogs which were proven rabid by laboratory tests. They were treated with the Pasteur vaccine, and only 188 (0.4 per cent) contracted rabies. If they had not been treated, at least 6,900 (15 per cent) of them would have died.

Antiserum is a new development in the treatment of rabies.

It is made in horses which have been rendered immune by injections of weakened virus, but it is made of blood serum rather than from the spinal cord as the vaccine is. Like other antiserums it gives only temporary immunity and sometimes causes serum reactions. Since 1953 enough data on its use has been collected to show that it does have a beneficial effect when it is correctly used. If it is given early enough after the bite, it is able to block the development of the infection. It *must* be given within seventy-two hours; within twenty-four hours is much better.

Control of Rabies: Rabies control is entirely a public health problem. There are about 25,000,000 dogs in the United States. By law they must be licensed, and there should be a law that they must also be vaccinated against rabies. There is a vaccine for dogs, the Flury vaccine, which seems to be very effective in protecting them against rabies. One injection of vaccine makes a dog immune for at least four years or more. If all dogs were vaccinated, rabies could be eliminated, but that is a big problem, and there is always the stray dog. A control program which has been successful in several cities where rabies was a threat consists of:

1. Registration of all dogs and immunization at the time of registration.
2. Revaccination after one year. (The manufacturer of the vaccine recommends now that in communities threatened with rabies, dogs be vaccinated every year for three or four years, and then, after immunity has been established, every third year. In rabies-free communities, vaccination every three years is sufficient.)
3. Impounding and vaccination of stray dogs.
4. Education of the public as to the importance of having dogs vaccinated.

Enforced muzzling of dogs and/or quarantine of dogs when rabies is prevalent are very effective ways of controlling rabies. These measures and vaccination have practically eliminated rabies from Great Britain, Holland, Australia and the Scandinavian countries.

PSITTACOSIS (PARROT FEVER)

Psittacosis is a relatively rare disease in the United States, and yet when it does show up in a community, the fear of it creates considerable panic. Since parakeets, parrots, love birds, canaries, pheasants, pigeons, ducks, turkeys and even chickens may harbor the infection, and since many of them have become so popular as household pets, I have frequently been asked about the safety of having them at home. When the mother of one of my patients suddenly became seriously ill with pneumonia which was thought to have been due to psittacosis, almost every parent of the children in my patient's school telephoned me to ask what to do with their parakeets. Most of them got rid of their birds, even though there was no evidence that the birds were infected.

Contagion: The disease is caused by a virus which is transmitted by contact with the bird or its cage and surroundings. These can be highly infectious. Psittacosis is hardly ever passed from man to man, though it has been on rare occasions. Young children (and young birds) may be infected, but they rarely show any evidence of it as older ones do.

Incubation Period: The incubation period is seven to fourteen days.

Symptoms: Psittacosis causes pneumonia which starts with fever, headache, chilly sensations, loss of appetite and constipation. A cough develops after a while. The disease is very severe and the patient is prostrated and often delirious; but in most cases he recovers. In children the disease is almost always milder than in adults.

Treatment: Recovery is faster if the child is treated with antibiotics. The psittacosis virus is one of the few against which antibiotics are effective. The patient is best treated in a hospital because of the strict isolation that is necessary, and to avoid spreading the disease in the family. To prevent recurrence the treatment should be continued for ten days or longer.

Isolation and Quarantine: The child is isolated for the entire illness, or a minimum of seventeen days. Those exposed to the child or the sick bird need not be quarantined, but they should be watched closely and treated promptly if they show any signs of illness. The doctor will report the disease to the health department and you should report it to parents of children who have been in contact with your child or with your sick bird.

Hygiene: If the child is at home while he is ill, his dishes and laundry must be soaked in a disinfectant solution or boiled. His discharges and excreta should also be disinfected. The person who is taking care of him should be careful to wear a mask and gown in his room and to observe strict isolation technique. The room, after the illness is over, should be thoroughly cleaned and disinfected. The room the sick bird was in should be cleaned and disinfected immediately after the bird has been disposed of.

Prevention: One attack of psittacosis gives immunity, but there is no vaccine or serum for immunization, nor is the disease common enough to justify its use even if it were available.

There are public health measures which regulate the importation of birds which carry psittacosis. The birds are quarantined and laboratory examinations are made to be sure they are free of the disease. Bird-breeding places should be inspected and quarantined if psittacosis is found.

BRUCELLOSIS (MALTA FEVER, UNDULANT FEVER, BANG'S DISEASE)

Brucellosis is a widespread disease which occurs everywhere. It is called brucellosis because it was first discovered in 1887 by a British scientist, David Bruce. It is called Malta fever because Bruce first observed it in Malta, and it is called undulant fever because of its tendency to undulate—that is, it occurs in waves of several days of fever and illness separated by periods of well-being and normal temperature. It is caused by several similar bacteria, found in different areas and in different animal hosts. Bang's disease, described by B. L. F. Bang in 1932, is the name commonly attached to the same disease when it is found in cattle, goats and swine in which it causes contagious abortion. People of all ages are affected.

Contagion: In children the disease is caused primarily by drinking raw milk and by eating cheese, ice cream and other products made from raw cow's or goat's milk, and less frequently by eating inadequately cooked, infected meat of cattle, swine or goats. Adults acquire the disease in the same way, and may also contract it by handling infected animal carcasses. It is not transmitted from one person to another, but is transmitted from animal to animal and from animal to man.

Incubation Period: The incubation period varies from five to thirty days. It is usually fourteen days.

Symptoms: Many infected children remain well. In the children who become ill, the symptoms may be very light or quite severe. The child may feel tired, have a low-grade fever of 100° to 101°, poor appetite, and sometimes joint pains and vague muscle aches. Or he may have symptoms indistinguishable from those of typhoid fever with headache, sweating, nausea, loss of appetite and daily peaks of temperature of 102° or higher. This sometimes lasts for two weeks. The child may then seem to recover, only to have a recurrence of the signs and symptoms. Occasionally the infection is severe and is accompanied by chills and fever of 104° to 106°. Brucellosis can involve the bones and the nervous system, but this is relatively uncommon.

Diagnosis: The doctor suspects brucellosis when there are fever, joint and muscle pains, possibly an enlarged spleen or liver or both, and a low white blood cell count. His diagnosis can be confirmed either by finding the bacteria in the child's stool, urine or blood or by other tests such as a skin test and the demonstration of an increasing antibody concentration in the child's blood.

Treatment: The child should be kept in bed, on a soft diet. Antibiotics seem to be the most effective drugs. The choice of which one or ones should be left to the doctor. When untreated, the disease recurs fairly often, but recurrences are less frequent with antibiotic treatment.

The child may be treated either at home or in a hospital, but because the infection is not easily diagnosed, most children with active brucellosis are sent to the hospital for diagnosis, and usually the disease is treated there.

Prevention: Preventive measures consist mainly of not drinking unpasteurized or unboiled cow's or goat's milk and not eating cheese or other products made from such milk, careful inspection of animal carcasses by health departments, and avoidance of handling of cattle, swine and goat carcasses. Infected cattle can be detected by skin testing. They can be injected with a vaccine which seems to reduce the incidence of abortion in cows and the spread of disease to man. Vaccine is not used for human beings.

Isolation and Quarantine: The infected person need not be isolated nor contacts quarantined. The disease is not spread from man to man.

Hygiene: Ordinary cleanliness should be observed in the disposal of the patient's urine and stool. No other precautions are necessary.

TULAREMIA (RABBIT FEVER)

This disease is caused by a bacterium called *Pasteurella tularensis*, which seems to be able to penetrate unbroken skin. It occurs all over North America and in Europe and Japan. In Japan it is known as Ohara's Disease. Here it gets its name from Tulare County in California where it was first discovered in an epidemic among ground squirrels. Since it is transmitted mostly by wild rabbits, it is found most frequently among hunters, trappers and butchers, and there are more cases during the hunting seasons than at other times. One attack seems to give permanent immunity; at least there have been no second cases reported.

Contagion: While 90 per cent of the cases in humans are transmitted by wild rabbits and hares, the disease is occasionally acquired from tree squirrels, quail, and less frequently, skunk, woodchuck, opossum, deer, fox, coyote, muskrat, sage hen, bull snake and water rat of Europe. The disease is caught by skinning and handling infected carcasses or eating inadequately cooked meat. Occasionally it is acquired from the bite of a deer fly, dog tick or wood tick which has previously bitten an infected rabbit, and rarely by drinking water contaminated by an infected animal. It is not transmitted from man to man.

Incubation Period: The incubation period is usually three to five days, but may be as few as one or as many as ten days.

Symptoms: The disease begins with a chill, fever, sweating, malaise, headache, vomiting, body pains and, in severe cases, prostration. A rash may appear. At the place where the infection entered the body, usually on the skin, the conjunctivae or the mucous membrane of the mouth, swelling and redness develop about the same time as the fever does. This spot becomes ulcerated, the path from the ulcer to the lymph glands in the area becomes swollen and red and the lymph glands become sore and swollen. Often the lungs are involved, very much as in pneumonia. The illness lasts two or three weeks and may behave like typhoid fever in some cases or like psittacosis in others.

Treatment: The patient is usually too sick to stay at home and is taken to the hospital for diagnosis and treatment. Treatment is both general and local. The swollen lymph gland may become abscessed and have to be opened and drained. Fluids and such food as the child can take are given freely. Aspirin reduces discomfort and fever and antibiotics are effective. They have to be continued for several days after the child seems well. Relapses may occur, though this does not happen as often with antibiotics.

Isolation and Quarantine: The patient is usually not isolated and contacts are not quarantined.

Prevention: State and county health departments usually issue warnings to hunters that infected rabbits or other animals have been found in the area. If a warning is issued, it is best not to hunt that particular animal in that area.

There are no serums or vaccines to prevent tularemia or to treat it.

RAT BITE FEVERS (SODOKU, HAVERHILL FEVER)

Rat bites are not as uncommon these days as many people believe, especially in slum neighborhoods and where garbage is carelessly disposed of. In hospital clinics or out-patient departments requests for treatment for rat bites are quite frequent. The bite of a rat can introduce several diseases. Tetanus is one example, but the term *rat bite fever* refers to either of two unrelated conditions, Sodoku and Haverhill Fever.

Sodoku: Sodoku is caused by the rat's teeth introducing the *Spirillum minus* into or under the child's skin. A sore forms at the site of the bite, then heals, and one to four weeks later the child becomes sick. He has malaise, fever as high as 104° or 105° daily, chills, nausea and vomiting. The sore breaks down and forms an ulcer and the lymph glands near the ulcer become swollen and tender. A rash appears over the entire body. It consists of bluish-red, slightly raised spots, some of which are quite large. This illness lasts three to five days, then the child feels better for three to five days. After this interval he becomes sick again, and all the signs and symptoms may be repeated.

The doctor may suspect rat bite fever because he knows the child has been bitten by a rat, but in order to prove it the spirillum must be found in scrapings of the sore, or infected material must be injected into a laboratory animal.

A week's treatment with antibiotics or arsenical drugs will usually cure the disease. It is best to treat the patient in a hospital.

While the description I have given is the accepted pattern of the disease, I have seen two cases which behaved peculiarly. Both of them required years to be diagnosed because in neither case was it known that the child had been bitten by a rat. In the first case the child was walking through the woods and thought his ankle had been injured by a broken twig. In the second, the child had been in Florida during a hurricane while rats were abundant and wild. The child's bite, which occurred while he was asleep, was thought to have been made by a spider. Treatment after this length of time was very difficult, though finally successful.

In order to prevent the disease, rats must be eliminated from the home, and if a child is bitten, you should consult your doctor promptly.

Haverhill Fever: This disease is caused by a different organism, a fungus called *Streptobacillus moniliformis,* and was first described in Haverhill, Massachusetts. While it can be acquired through a rat bite, it is also transmitted by milk or food which has been contaminated by rat urine. When food or milk is the source of infection, the disease is likely to appear in epidemic form.

Usually the child becomes ill three to five days after being bitten by a rat, or ingesting contaminated food or milk. There may be fever, a milder rash than in Sodoku, and swollen, painful joints. The local infection around the bite is much milder, and there is usually no lymph gland involvement. The fever lasts three to five days, then there is improvement, followed by another period of fever and joint swelling. This condition may continue for weeks or months if it is not treated, but one injection of penicillin is usually enough to cure it. Larger doses are preferable and treatment for several days is safer and wiser.

I have seen a nine-month-old infant who had meningitis caused by this organism. Mice were seen in the kitchen of his home.

WEIL'S DISEASE (SPIROCHETAL JAUNDICE)

This is another disease transmitted by rats, though not by biting. It is caused by the organism *Leptospira icterohemorrhagiae*. The infected rat harbors the germ in its kidneys and passes it in its urine. Usually the child is infected by eating or drinking urine-contaminated food or water, or by washing in contaminated water, in which case the infection may enter through a sore on the skin.

The incubation period is four to nineteen days, usually nine to ten days, after which the child is very ill with fever, chills, headache, vomiting, congested eyes and muscle aches. In about half the cases, the child becomes jaundiced after the first week of illness. Symptoms of meningitis are sometimes present right from the beginning. If there is no jaundice, the acute part of the disease lasts about two to nine days. If there is, it lasts longer.

The only treatment is for the symptoms of the disease, though some doctors believe that penicillin is valuable if it is given in the early stages.

None of these three diseases, Sodoku, Haverhill Fever or Weil's Disease, is transmitted directly from man to man, so the patient is not isolated and contacts are not quarantined. There are no vaccines or serums for prevention or treatment. Penicillin, tetracyclines and other antibiotics are helpful and often curative.

CAT SCRATCH FEVER (BENIGN INOCULATION LYMPHORETICULOSIS)

About thirty-five years ago it was discovered that a cat's scratch may have more annoying results than the initial sting. This was first observed in France by Robert Debré in 1930, and since then several hundred cases of cat scratch fever have been reported from many parts of the world, including North America. The disease is not only transmitted by barn cats and alley cats. Apparently even the well-cared-for house pet can introduce a virus into the skin and start an infection. Occasionally a meat handler develops the disease without having been scratched and, rarely, a rabbit or a porcupine is responsible. In about a third of the cases, there is no history of contact with a cat at all. Possibly the infection can be acquired through contact with contaminated objects.

Incubation Period: The incubation period is three to seven days.

Symptoms: The scratch may seem unimportant, but any time from seven to forty-two days later the lymph glands which drain the scratched area become swollen, inflamed and tender. The child has a high fever which goes up and down in daily peaks for weeks. He feels sick, and as the glands swell, the scratch seems to become more inflamed and irritated. Occasionally, a purplish elevated skin eruption appears early in the disease, and sometimes the child has involvement of the lungs (pneumonia) similar to the infection with the psittacosis virus. In rare instances, encephalitis follows. In more than a third of the cases, the glands become abscessed and either rupture and drain to the outside, or have to be opened surgically. After this, they drain for a while and then heal and the disease is over.

Diagnosis: When a child has swollen glands in an area where he has been scratched and there is no other explanation for it, the doctor will suspect cat scratch fever. There is a skin test which is helpful in confirming the diagnosis.

Treatment: Antibiotics have been given, but it is not certain whether they actually destroy the virus, help prevent secondary infection, or whether they help at all. Other treatment is only a matter of making the child as comfortable as possible. Aspirin will relieve the painful glands and lower the temperature. When the fever is very high, lukewarm water and alcohol rubs are helpful.

Prevention: The only known preventive is avoidance of cat scratches, including those of your own pet.

Isolation and Quarantine: A child with cat scratch fever is not contagious and need not be isolated, and an exposed person need not be quarantined.

Hygiene: The eating utensils and clothes may be treated in the ordinary manner, but the person who takes care of the child should be careful not to come in contact with the pus from the abscessed glands. If he does, he should wash thoroughly with a strong antiseptic. A brush should not be used, to avoid injuring the skin.

QUESTIONS & ANSWERS

RABIES

Q. *If rabies antiserum is effective when given early enough, why should the child who has been bitten also be subjected to the Pasteur treatment, or the duck embryo vaccine?*

A. Together they seem to be more effective.

Q. *Does the Flury anti-rabies vaccine work for humans?*

A. It does if it is given before exposure. There is very little reason for giving it unless the child is sure to be exposed —or has been bitten by an animal which may be rabid.

Q. *Is the Pasteur or Flury vaccine always effective?*

A. Usually, but not always. The mortality among patients who have been bitten by rabid animals and vaccinated is 0.4 per cent as against about 15 per cent in untreated patients.

Q. *Why must the Pasteur or Flury vaccine be injected into the abdominal wall?*

A. Actually, it can be injected anywhere, but it is less painful in the abdomen.

Q. *Can't a pet which has been bitten by a rabid dog be vaccinated just as a child can?*

A. Yes, it can. It could be given antiserum and then the Flury vaccine. Even the smallest possibility of the pet developing rabies would make it necessary to have it destroyed. The animal should be impounded by the health or police department for at least fourteen days to determine if he is rabid.

PSITTACOSIS

Q. *Can one person get psittacosis from another?*

A. Yes, by contact with the secretions or excretions of the patient, particularly his sputum when he coughs. The disease is more often transmitted from bird to man, however.

Q. *Do birds which are not sick ever pass on the infection?*

A. Yes, but not as often as sick birds do.

Q. *When I buy a bird in a pet shop or a department store, how can I be sure it is not diseased?*

A. You cannot be, but buy the bird from a reputable dealer and before you buy it, ask whether the bird has been inspected by the health department.

Q. *Must I consider psittacosis if my child develops pneumonia?*

A. Not unless you have a pet bird which has become ill.

Q. *What should I do if I suspect my bird is sick?*

A. Take the bird to a veterinarian or the board of health immediately.

Q. *What will they do if the bird is found to have psittacosis?*

A. It will have to be destroyed.

Q. *Are canaries susceptible to this disease?*

A. Yes.

Q. *Do pigeons, chickens, ducks or turkeys get infected?*

A. Yes, especially wild ones. Do not worry about dressed poultry you buy for the table, however. It has been inspected and found to be free of disease.

Q. *Is there an injection which birds can be given to cure them of psittacosis after they have become infected?*

A. No, and this is one of the reasons they must be destroyed. They are too great a source of danger. But antibiotics can be given them to keep them from getting psittacosis if they are liable to be exposed to it, or if they have already been exposed, but have not yet developed symptoms.

Q. *Are antibiotics effective in psittacosis?*

A. Yes, treatment with tetracycline drugs must be continued for ten days or longer.

BRUCELLOSIS

Q. *Is there any public health measure which controls brucellosis in cattle?*

A. Yes. Cattle and meat are inspected for infection. The U.S. Bureau of Animal Husbandry and the U.S. Livestock Association recommend that calves be vaccinated against the disease.

Q. *Is this control universal?*

A. No. It is quite general in the United States, and vaccination of cattle is officially advised in Great Britain.

Q. *If I am traveling abroad, is it safe to eat raw meat or meat which is not well cooked?*

A. It may be, but it is safer to eat only well-cooked meat. Milk should be pasteurized or boiled. Eat cheeses, ice cream, etc., only if they are made of pasteurized milk.

Q. *Is it safe to drink raw milk from our own cow?*

A. Only if the cow has been tested for brucellosis and tuberculosis and found free of both. Otherwise, the milk should be pasteurized.

Q. *If you have brucellosis, do you develop immunity?*

A. Yes.

Q. *Is the immunity permanent?*

A. We do not know how long it lasts.

Q. *Is brucellosis ever confused with other conditions?*

A. Yes, with typhoid fever, salmonella infections, dysentery and occasionally with rheumatic fever.

Q. *If my son has brucellosis, may his brother go to school or the movies?*

A. Yes, if he is well.

Q. *Is antibiotic treatment always a cure?*

A. Not always. Relapses may occur after treatment is discontinued.

Q. *Should contacts be given antibiotics to prevent the infection?*

A. No. The disease is not passed from one person to another.

TULAREMIA

Q. *How common is tularemia in children?*

A. Quite infrequent. It is rare in city children.

Q. *Is it a serious disease?*

A. Yes. It can be very severe and dangerous.

Q. *Is it safe to handle rabbits or hares which are bought from local grocers or butchers?*

A. Yes.

RAT BITE FEVERS AND WEIL'S DISEASE

Q. *Are all rats infected with the germs which produce rat bite fevers and Weil's disease?*

A. No, but in one study made in several cities 10 to 30 per cent of the adult rat population was found to be infected with the organism which produces Weil's disease. One must assume that the rat is infected in case of a bite and treat the child accordingly.

Q. *What should be done for a rat bite?*

A. Wash the wound thoroughly with soap and water. Call your doctor or go to a hospital emergency room where your child will probably be given something, possibly penicillin, to prevent rat bite fever and tetanus.

Q. *Why is it necessary to give a preventive for tetanus? Does the rat cause that, too?*

A. Yes. The rat lives in dirty areas, around barns and stables where tetanus germs are found. The rat may be contaminated and introduce tetanus germs into the wound.

Q. *Can Sodoku, like the other two, be transmitted by contaminated food or milk?*

A. Apparently not. It seems to be transmitted only by a bite.

Q. *Is the rash of Sodoku or Haverhill Fever like a measles rash?*

A. Sometimes, but more often with Haverhill Fever than with Sodoku. Usually the rash of Sodoku is quite different.

Q. *Does the rash appear with each period of fever in Sodoku and Haverhill Fever?*

A. Not necessarily. It may not appear until after the second or third bout of fever. It may appear with the first and not again, or it may appear with every bout.

Q. *Is Weil's Disease the only one of the three which involves jaundice?*

A. Yes, usually.

CAT SCRATCH FEVER

Q. *Can every house cat transmit cat scratch fever?*

A. No, most of them do not, but we know no way of finding out which can and which cannot.

Q. *Would you advise against having cats as pets?*

A. No, but I would not play roughly with them, and thus avoid being scratched.

Q. *Can a cat be vaccinated against cat scratch fever?*

A. No. There is no vaccine.

Q. *Is the disease contagious?*

A. No.

Q. *Is it safe to take care of a child who has the disease?*

A. Yes, provided you are careful not to be contaminated by the pus from the broken-down glands.

Q. *Can you get cat scratch fever more than once?*

A. We do not know, but probably not.

Respiratory Diseases
& Related Conditions

23: Common Upper-Respiratory Infections

Upper respiratory diseases are a large group of infections. Of these, the common cold is the most important example because colds are more frequent in man than any other disease. Most respiratory infections—tonsillitis, sinusitis, rhinitis and laryngitis are some of them—are named after the part of the respiratory system most affected. The common cold, grippe and influenza are not.

If sneezing and running nose indicate that the infection is in the nose, the disease is called rhinitis (*rhino* in Greek means nose). Coryza is another name for this (*coryza* in Greek means catarrh, or running of the nose). If the throat is red and sore, it is called pharyngitis (after the Greek word, *pharynx,* throat). Since *nasus* is Latin for nose and *pharynx* means throat, nasopharyngitis means an infection of the nose and throat. When there is a hoarse voice and a barking cough, the disease is located in the voice box and is called laryngitis (after *larynx,* the Greek and Latin word for voice box). Sometimes, when there is a spasm of the larynx and drawing air past the vocal chords causes a crowing noise, it is called croup, which is a combination of the words *croak* and *whoop.* If the windpipe is involved and there is an irritating, hacking cough, it is tracheitis (from the Latin phrase *arteria tracheia,* meaning rough artery or windpipe). All of these may be a part of the common cold, or each may be a separate infection or a complication of the common cold.

Most of the common respiratory diseases are caused by viruses, but the complications such as tonsillitis, swollen glands in the neck, middle ear infection, bronchitis, pneumonia and sinus infection are often caused by bacteria like the streptococcus or pneumococcus. In other words, in most instances the infection by the virus seems to make the inflamed tissue fertile ground for the invasion of bacteria which then produce another infection at or near the original place. In some cases viruses may not enter the picture and the infection is caused entirely by bacteria, as in most instances of follicular tonsillitis.

Upper respiratory infections tend to run a fairly uniform course at a given time in a certain area. For example, if your child has tonsillitis, you are likely to find that there are a number of cases of tonsillitis in your area. At another time, most of the infections will involve the nose, sneezing, running nose, tearing eyes and cough. At still another time, there may be an outbreak of fever, chills, aches, headaches with rapid recovery. This similarity of symptoms is undoubtedly due to the prevailing viruses or bacteria responsible.

THE COMMON COLD

The cold is the most frequent infection of man from infancy to old age. More days are lost from school and work because of colds than because of any other single reason. Colds are caused by one of several viruses, at least some of which are known. People everywhere in the world have colds all through the year, but most often when it is cold and wet or cold and wet and windy.

Infants under a year old do not get as many colds, but this is because they are more apt to be protected from contact with people who have them, not because they are immune to them. If an infant is exposed to a cold, he catches it just as readily or more so than an older child or an adult would. When an infant is the first child in a family, he often does not catch a cold until he is well over a year old, but second babies get them earlier and third ones even earlier than that, because they are exposed to their brothers and sisters.

Colds become more frequent during early childhood when children mingle in playgrounds and at parties, and especially when a child is old enough to go to school. Usually the increase is dramatic at the time of entering nursery school, kindergarten or grade school. Often, much of the first year of school is spent at home, and this is true no matter how old the child is when he starts. Colds become rarer at about age eight or ten, but they recur all through life.

The average child living in a temperate climate has at least two or three obvious colds a year, and probably an equal number of mild colds, too slight to be noticed. Some children have colds every month except in the summer, while others rarely have any, though this last is more true of adults than of children. Children who have respiratory allergy are more susceptible to the acute respiratory infections, such as colds. They also seem to be more sensitive to the bacteria which cause the complications. If such a child develops asthma with respiratory infections, it is called infectious asthma.

Children do not develop a strong immunity to colds, and if some immunity does develop, it lasts a very short time, possibly two to four weeks.

Colds begin to be very frequent with the opening of school in September. They increase in the fall and winter, are prevalent in the spring, and least numerous in the summer in temperate climates or in the warm, dry seasons anywhere.

Contagion: Colds are highly contagious. They are spread through droplet infection from the nose and throat of an infected child to healthy susceptible children who are close to him. They can be spread by using common drinking cups and common towels. When a child coughs or sneezes without covering his nose and mouth, he can spread an infection to anyone within a radius of six to twelve feet.

On several occasions when I have been examining a child's throat, he has coughed, spraying my face with droplets of moisture. Within six to eight hours, I have begun to have a stuffy nose and a scratchy throat, and have actually caught a cold.

Incubation Period: The incubation period may be very short (several hours) or as much as two or three days.

Symptoms: Usually the common cold consists of sneezing, tearing of the eyes, a running nose, a low-grade fever and a general let-down feeling. The child may develop a sore or scratchy throat and possibly a cough. The running nose and the cough are apt to be most annoying when the child is lying down and the mucus from the nose and sinuses runs down into his throat and causes irritation.

Occasionally a cold is more severe, and the child feels very much sicker. His temperature is higher and his eyes look dull or sleepy. His head feels full, he may have a headache and feel chilly and achy and very tired.

At different ages the symptoms vary. The infant or young child usually has more fever with colds than older children or adults. When an infant is starting a cold, he is cranky and cries more than usual. He may want to be held more, and even this fails to comfort him. His mother knows it is a cold when his nose begins to run. It becomes blocked, and when his mouth is closed around a nipple, it is very difficult for him to breathe. The young child also is made miserable by the running nose. He too has difficulty eating and sleeping on his back, but since he can sit up and turn in bed and walk about, he is somewhat better off.

After the cold improves and the fever goes, the infant or child may go on having a running nose and cough for days, even for a week or two. This is also true of the older child and adult, and in all of them it probably means there is some infection of the nasal sinuses.

Treatment: A child with a cold should stay at home, and if he has a fever, he should stay in bed. In fact, he is probably better off in bed during the first day of a cold even if he has no fever. He may eat anything he wants, but not too much of it, and he should have plenty of fluids. If it is summer and the weather is fair, he may find sitting in the sun comforting.

There are many different cold "cures" and "preventives" put up commercially in pills, capsules, powders and syrups. These contain various drugs which are not well tolerated by all. Some are of questionable value. There are no truly curative drugs for colds, and those used are valuable only for the relief of uncomfortable symptoms. If medication is to be used at all, it is much better to have your doctor prescribe it. If you use these commercial products without your doctor's advice, you are overlooking the fact that while doctors may prescribe any of the drugs in them for colds, they usually prescribe special mixtures of them which they consider most suitable for the particular patient's particular cold. The dose of a drug in a commercial product, a trade-name mixture, which one child can tolerate might be too much or too little for another.

In general, I recommend aspirin for the fever and aches and in most instances watery nose drops or sprays of a drug which shrink the nasal lining and reduce the secretion for an hour or more. The nose drops should not contain oil since the child may draw the oil into his lungs and set up lipoid pneumonia.

The antihistamines often suppress the symptoms of a cold, but they neither prevent it nor cure it. If you do use them, you must use them with care. On several occasions I have been asked to see children who after five or six days of treatment with antihistamines seemed sicker than they were while taking the drugs. In each case the child had pneumonia. The fact that the drugs had suppressed the cold symptoms had made the parents feel that the child was much better and instead of keeping him in bed, they felt that he was even well enough to go to school.

Ointments and liniments containing drugs like camphor or eucalyptol are pleasant, and they do help to relieve nasal congestion. They also may relieve the cough which is due to irritation of the voice box and windpipe. But they do not prevent or cure the infection.

Children with colds are better off in comfortably warm and moist air day and night. If opening a window at night makes the room cold or drafty, keep it closed, but open the door and a window in the next room or the bathroom. If the child's nose is very stuffy, it might be helpful to have him inhale steam to thin the secretions. If this is done, the steam kettle must be out of his reach. If he wiggles and throws off the covers at night, dress him warmly enough so that it will not matter if he does.

When an infant's nose is stuffy, spoon feeding of both solids and milk will probably be more successful than bottles. Propping him on a pillow when he sleeps or turning him on his stomach are usually comforting because his nose will drain better.

Cough syrups may be helpful to thin the mucus and keep the child from coughing all the time, but of course it is not a cure. I would like to emphasize that whenever you give a child medicine for a cold, it is important to know how much to give and how often to give it and when to stop. Your doctor should tell you this. Even aspirin can be poisonous if it is not properly used.

Convalescence: A child should be allowed several days of convalescence after a cold. As he improves, the discharges from the nose thicken and the cough gets better. Most children recover rapidly, but some take a week or more. You should let your child be out-of-doors for a day before he goes back to school, although this may be difficult with older children who feel they are missing out in their school work.

Complications: If the fever caused by a cold lasts more than a few days, if the temperature rises after the first few days, or if the cough becomes more severe or more frequent, a complication probably has set in. In children the complications are apt to be ear infections, sinus infections, swollen glands, bronchitis and pneumonia. In adults, ear infections are not very common, but sinusitis and bronchitis are.

Prevention: There is no special vaccine or serum for the prevention of colds. Good hygiene, keeping away from people who have colds, keeping physically fit by getting enough rest and enough food with the necessary vitamins, and avoiding excesses of all kinds are all helpful in warding off colds. If the diet is well balanced for normal body development, additional food and vitamins are not needed to prevent or cure colds. If a child is run-down, if he is malnourished, if he has a vitamin deficiency, he is more likely to catch colds as well as other infections.

When children become cold and wet, they become less resistant to colds. Infants and little children are especially apt to catch colds on very windy days and when it is wet. One of the more dangerous times of year as far as colds are concerned, is the season when there is melting snow and high winds. The wind blows all sorts of germs (viruses) around which have accumulated in the standing snow.

The term *cold vaccines* is misleading. So is the term *catarrhal vaccine*. They are not made of the viruses which start colds, but of various bacteria which invade the nose and throat. They are usually injected, but they are also made in a form to be taken by mouth. The results of their use vary from doubtful to fair, but they seem to be more effective when given by injection to allergic children who have frequent upper respiratory infections and are apt to develop asthma.

Isolation and Quarantine: A child who has been exposed to a cold is not quarantined, but a child who has one should be isolated. He should not go to school (nor should an adult go to work) where he will infect others. He should not go to the movies, play groups, parties or on public conveyances. It is sometimes impossible to isolate a child with a cold because it can be so mild that you do not know he has it, and then he will infect other people unwittingly.

GRIPPE

Grippe is a common respiratory infection which often is grouped with colds and influenza. It is usual for a person who has body, muscle and joint aches, fever, chills or a chilly feeling and a scratchy throat to say "I feel grippy," and the name has come to mean a combination of these symptoms. Actually, grippe is another word for influenza in many parts of the world, especially in Europe. Here in the United States, too, we recognize that many cases of grippe are akin to influenza. Whenever there is an outbreak of grippe, medical and public health authorities investigating the cause find that many of the cases are caused by one of the influenza viruses. Still others are caused by the group of APC (adenoidal-pharyngeal-conjunctival) viruses, such as parainfluenza, coxsackie and respiratory syncitial viruses, and the rest have not been determined. These unidentified cases are grouped with the common cold.

Grippe attacks people of all ages, though it is less common in infancy. Immunity is short-lived, probably not more than a few weeks, but the exact time is not known. A person who has had the grippe may develop a similar infection two or three months later. Some people have the same combination of symptoms once or twice a year. Many of us living in temperate climates have had the grippe several times. This suggests that the same type of disease can be caused by many different viruses, or that we do not develop adequate immunity to some and become reinfected.

Contagion: Grippe spreads very easily and very rapidly by droplets of moisture from the mouth of an infected person to people near him.

Incubation Period: The incubation period may be less than twenty-four hours, or it may be from two to four days.

Symptoms: Unlike the mild form of the common cold, this severe form may suddenly make you feel very sick. Your throat feels scratchy or raw, you may have a headache or feel dizzy, you may feel hot or chilly, or even have a shaking chill. Children usually have a fever as high as 104° or 105°. In adults it is usually between 101° and 103°, but it is sometimes higher. You feel tired, even to the point of exhaustion. You want no food, but you may be thirsty. You take to bed and want to keep warm, go to sleep and be left alone.

Treatment: If your child has grippe, you should call the doctor. Often, what seems like a severe cold or grippe is the beginning of influenza or pneumonia, or some other serious infection. Your child may need special treatment other than bed rest, hot drinks and aspirin.

Complications: If the illness lasts longer than two or three days, you should suspect the possibility of an infection like influenza or of a complication such as bronchitis, pneumonia or sinus infection.

Prevention: The only way we know to prevent grippe is to keep away from people who have it. When there is an epidemic, it is best to avoid crowds, theaters and parties, to get plenty of rest, and not to overindulge in anything, whether it be food or exercise. There is no vaccine or serum which is effective, except the new vaccine against Group III of the APC viruses, which according to human experiments seems quite effective.

Isolation and Quarantine: People who have been exposed to grippe are not quarantined, but a person who has it should be isolated for as long as he has any fever and a day or two more.

INFLUENZA

Influenza is a disease known everywhere. It usually occurs in epidemics and, on rare occasions, in pandemic form. The pandemic of 1917–18 infected perhaps as many as half a billion people and killed hundreds of thousands of them.

Influenza attacks people of all ages, usually in the late fall, winter and spring. It can be caused by several viruses. The virus which seems to have produced the pandemic of 1918 is thought to have been the Virus A. We now recognize about fifteen different strains of influenza viruses, most of them subgroups of Virus A, B and C. This is important to remember, for, unlike the common cold or grippe, a person who is infected with Virus A, for example, develops a lasting immunity to Virus A. If he is infected with Virus B, he develops immunity to Virus B, but not to Virus A. In the case of the fifteen or more recognizable subgroups of A and B, there may be some cross-immunity. That is, there may be some immunity to both Virus A and Virus A^1 after an infection with Virus A^1, but the immunity is not of the same degree to both viruses. It may be high and protective to the virus with which the person was infected, A^1 for example, but slight to Virus A.

Contagion: Influenza is highly contagious and is spread by droplet infection from the nose and throat of a sick person to all susceptible people who are near.

Incubation Period: The incubation period varies between one and three days.

Symptoms: The child with influenza has a headache, is drowsy, tired, chilly or has real shaking chills, backache, and muscle and joint pains. He loses his appetite, sometimes is nauseated and possibly vomits, and has a sore throat. He may feel very weak and exhausted, even to the point of collapse. Although influenza sometimes produces intestinal symptoms, it is an entirely different disease from what people call "intestinal flu." The symptoms of this disease are abdominal pain or cramps, nausea, vomiting and/or diarrhea, and sometimes fever, which may be low or quite high. But this disease is not usually caused by the influenza virus. The exact cause or causes (for there may be several) are not known.

In influenza the child's temperature usually rises quickly to somewhere between 100° and 102°, but it may reach 104° or more. Coughing may start quickly and often goes with dryness and irritation of the throat and a tickling sensation in the windpipe. Running nose is not usually a part of this disease. The child looks flushed and quite sick. If he is very sick, he may be a little blue around the mouth. His joints and muscles not only ache, but the muscles are tender when you press them. His eyes hurt and are red and inflamed looking. The fever usually lasts two to four days, after which the child begins to improve unless a complication sets in.

Treatment: The child should be put to bed, given a light diet, plenty of liquids and some fresh air. Aspirin or an equivalent drug is helpful, but only to relieve the aches and reduce the fever. There are no antibiotics or sulfa drugs which are effective against the influenza virus, but since so much of the difficulty from influenza is due to secondary infection by bacteria, some doctors start giving one of these drugs right at the beginning to ward off bacterial infections before they get started. This is not necessary in the milder forms of influenza, but it may be helpful for the very sick child who is likely to develop early complications.

Convalescence: The child should be kept in bed until he is well over the disease and has convalesced for several days.

Complications: Influenza varies tremendously in its severity from a mild grippelike ailment to a very severe disease. In recent years most of the outbreaks and small epidemics have been mild, but occasionally one is reported with appreciable mortality, sometimes up to 10 per cent. When it occurs in small outbreaks, it is not nearly as serious as when there are large epidemics as in 1918 when the disease was absolutely devastating. There has been no epidemic of such proportions since, and in the more recent epidemics, complications (bronchitis and pneumonia) have not been a major concern.

Prevention: In case of an epidemic of influenza, it is important for both adults and children to keep in as good physical condition as possible. They should have adequate rest, nutritious food, and a well-balanced diet. They should not become overtired or chilled and wet. They should avoid crowds. If the epidemic is extensive, it may be safer to keep children away from schools and play groups, or wherever there are many people together, since the disease is rapidly spread from person to person. This is not recommended except when the epidemic is severe and the health authorities believe closing the schools is necessary to control the disease.

It is possible to immunize people against any one or all the viruses of influenza, but this kind of immunization is not recommended as a routine because: (a) the vaccine available may not contain the virus causing the current outbreak, and even if it does, (b) the immunity from the vaccine lasts only a few months; (c) as soon as there is an outbreak and the virus causing it is found, it may be possible to make a suitable vaccine—this vaccine confers immunity very quickly.

Newer vaccines have been prepared which render a child immune for one to two years. These vaccines are made with many of the viruses known to cause influenza. If they prove as effective as they now seem to be, our feeling about routine immunization may have to be revised.

At present the vaccine should be given to children living in child-care institutions, particularly if an outbreak has started or if the disease has occurred in the past. It should be given to children with chronic diseases, such as cystic fibrosis of the pancreas, asthma, chronic bronchitis, congenital heart disease, rheumatic heart disease, chronic kidney disease (nephrosis, nephritis, pyelonephritis), diabetes and other metabolic diseases, and all other debilitating illnesses. If such vaccine is available, be sure to ask for polyvalent vaccine, the kind made with many different strains of the influenza viruses and which results in immunity for at least a year, two years or longer.

Isolation and Quarantine: A child with influenza should be isolated until his temperature has been normal for forty-eight hours, but people who have been in contact with him are not quarantined.

QUESTIONS & ANSWERS

COLDS AND GRIPPE

Q. *Is the common cold the same all over the world?*

A. The viruses which cause colds may be of the same or different groups and the bacteria causing the secondary infection may also differ. Therefore the entire illness may vary in one part of the world or another. Also, colds usually do not make you feel as ill in warm, dry climates or in warm weather in temperate climates.

Q. *Do you catch colds more easily when exposed to bad weather?*

A. Yes. For example, many more people have colds in the winter when the weather is wet and cold. Dry weather, hot or cold, is not as conducive to colds. Children, especially, catch more colds when exposed to windy weather. This is particularly true of infants when exposed to wind accompanied by severe cold.

Q. *Why does wind make you catch cold more easily?*

A. Probably because wind makes all sorts of germs fly around in the air.

Q. *Shall I not take my infant outside when it is windy?*

A. If you cannot keep him sheltered, it may be wiser to keep him indoors.

Q. *At what temperature may my child go out?*

A. Infants should not be taken out when the temperature is

below freezing, and children one to three years old should not go out when it is much below freezing.

Q. *Can you have a cold in other parts of the body, for instance a cold in the bladder or kidneys?*

A. Infection in the bladder, the kidneys or in other parts of the body may not be caused by the viruses of the common cold. Infection of the bladder is called cystitis, and that of the kidney nephritis.

Q. *Do you feel that a cold is some form of allergy?*

A. Usually no, but people with allergic rhinitis (inflammation of the nose) may have all the signs of a cold. Also, allergic children whose allergy affects the nose and throat seem to get colds more easily and more frequently.

Q. *What is the Devil's grippe?*

A. It is the name of an infection which we now know to be caused by a specific virus, one of the Coxsackie B viruses. It differs from ordinary grippe in that it produces a sensation of burning or tingling or pain in one or another part of the body. It very commonly causes pain in the chest which is known as pleurodynia. It is this pain that originally gave it its name. The pain was said to feel like the "Devil's grip" on your chest; otherwise it may resemble ordinary grippe.

Q. *Is Devil's grippe contagious?*

A. Yes, it is. You should avoid contact with people who have it.

Q. *I was at work today with a man who came down with grippe after he got home. Will I get it?*

A. It is certainly possible. If you feel uncomfortable or sickish, you may be getting it.

Q. *When my child went to school this morning, his throat was examined by the nurse and he was fine, but now he has come home with a cold. Did he get it in school?*

A. Maybe he did, but probably he was coming down with it before he went to school and it did not show up until several hours later.

Q. *Do you mean that you cannot tell whether a child is beginning to get a cold?*

A. No, not usually. If his throat is red, his nose is running or
his eyes are tearing, it has already started.

Q. *Do you often have pains in the chest with a common cold?*

A. No. Usually that means a different type of infection.

Q. *Should I keep my child indoors when he has a cold, no
matter what the weather is like?*

A. No. In the summer when the sun is warm he may feel more
comfortable in the open air, if he has no fever.

Q. *Are the antihistamines as good for treating and preventing
colds and grippe as the advertisements say they are?*

A. They make you feel more comfortable by reducing the
amount of secretion when you have a cold and sometimes
by making you feel better, but they neither cure nor prevent infection with the cold viruses. Sometimes the feeling
of well-being is misleading. I have been called to see children suffering from pneumonia who were being treated
with antihistamines at a time when sulfa drugs or antibiotics were urgently needed. Antihistamines may be
helpful for an allergic child who develops respiratory infections, but they will not cure him.

Q. *Are the sulfa drugs and antibiotics useful for treatment of
the common cold and grippe?*

A. No, but they may be useful for curing the bacterial infections which often follow. For example, they would be
helpful for ear infections, sinus infections, bronchitis and
pneumonia which often complicate colds and grippe as
well as influenza.

Q. *Do all doctors use these drugs for treatment of colds and
grippe?*

A. No, nor do they treat all people in the same way. It is best
to ask your doctor whether they are useful for the particular infection in question. The same doctor may give
such drugs to one person and not another, depending on
the circumstances. In the same way, he may prescribe
antihistamines, but I believe you should not use these
or any other drugs without his advice.

Q. *Do the drugs which are advertised on the radio help colds?*

A. Only in that they may make you feel a little better. If you do try any of them, do not rely on them for longer than a day or two because your child may be developing complications for which they are essentially useless. Your doctor should see your child and prescribe for him if he has a cold or grippe which lasts longer than two or three days, or if he has high fever on the first day, or if he feels particularly ill. Remember that many infections begin as a common cold. For example, diphtheria, scarlet fever, chicken pox, whooping cough, measles, meningitis and many others seem very much like a cold on the first day. So it is wiser to consult your doctor when a child gets sick than to make the diagnosis yourself.

Q. *May my son go swimming in a private pool now that his cold is improving?*

A. No. He should not go swimming at all. It might make his cold worse, and he would surely infect other people.

Q. *May he swim in the ocean with a cold?*

A. No. He should not swim at all because the likelihood of a sinus infection would be very much increased and he might get chilled or be unnecessarily exposed, and lay himself open to complications.

Q. *Is it all right to wash my child's hair when she has a cold?*

A. It would be wiser to postpone it until she is well.

Q. *What about bathing my children when they have colds?*

A. Do not put them in the tub if they are very ill. If they need washing, give them a quick sponge bath without exposing them too much.

Q. *Is there any special diet for a child who has a cold?*

A. No. He may eat what he wants, but he should not overeat and he should have extra fluids.

Q. *Is it necessary to give a cathartic to a child with a cold?*

A. Not unless he is constipated. Then ask your doctor what to give him.

Q. *My daughter is supposed to graduate from high school on Thursday and she was sick with the grippe until Wednesday. Should I let her go to graduation?*

A. If she has had no fever for at least twenty-four hours and feels well, I presume that an occasion as important as a graduation should not be missed. But anything less important might be skipped.

Q. *I felt very sick with grippe yesterday, but I feel fine today. I have a date and would like to go dancing tonight. What do you think?*

A. I think you should stay home because, although you feel a great deal better, your resistance is lowered, and you will probably be very unhappy after a strenuous evening of dancing. Also, you may infect other people.

Q. *How can I prevent colds in my children?*

A. If you or anyone else in the family has a cold, try to keep away from those who have not. Do not let the children use each other's towels, drink from the same cup or use each other's toothbrushes. Try not to have children with colds sleep in the same room with children who are well. In time we may have vaccines against colds.

Q. *If I have a cold, is it all right to take care of my baby?*

A. It would be better not to if you have someone else to do it for you. But if there is no one else to help, wear a mask and wash your hands before you handle the baby. Do not breathe directly into his face. If you must cough, direct the cough away from him, preferably into a tissue, and then destroy the tissue. Do not touch the mask with your hands while you are with the baby. A mask is quickly contaminated, and if you handle any part of it except the strings, your fingers will be, too. If you do touch the face part of the mask, wash your hands before you touch the baby again.

Q. *Is air conditioning good for a cold?*

A. I don't think so, especially if the temperature outside the room is very different from the temperature inside and you go in and out a lot.

Q. *Is air conditioning dangerous for my baby?*

A. Probably not, if he is kept in that one room and properly clothed for the temperature. But he may catch colds more easily if he is taken in and out. Keep the temperature around 70° F.

Q. *Is anything being done to try to find out how to prevent the common cold?*

A. Yes. A great deal of research has been done and is constantly going on in an attempt to find out exactly which viruses cause colds and how to combat them. Until now, all we know is that colds are caused by viruses, that they are spread from person to person, that they usually run a course and that some viruses cause cold symptoms.

Q. *How can I avoid the grippe?*

A. By avoiding people who have it.

Q. *If one of my children has a cold, should the others stay home from school?*

A. No, but be careful. Watch the others closely and at the first sign of illness, keep them at home.

Q. *If my child has a little cough, can't I send him to school? If I keep him out for every cough, he will miss half the year.*

A. It is unfortunate, but keeping him out is really necessary. It is important that he avoid getting other infections while he is rundown with a cold, and it is equally important for him not to infect other children in the classroom.

Q. *If I visit a friend with the grippe, will I bring it back to my children?*

A. Yes. You may catch it and give it to them.

Q. *My friend has just recovered from the grippe. May she visit my newborn baby?*

A. No. I believe that it is unsafe for anyone who has been sick in any way in the last three or four days to visit a newborn baby.

INFLUENZA

Q. *Is influenza the same in Great Britain, in Germany, in China as it is in New York?*

A.   Yes, it is, if the virus causing it is the same.

Q.   *Is the disease ever different when the virus is the same?*

A.   Yes. It may vary in individuals according to the condition of the patient when he caught it, how much of the virus infected him, and what stage the epidemic was in when he was infected.

Q.   *How do we know there are so many different viruses which produce influenza?*

A.   There are laboratory tests by which we can tell which viruses are present. We can wash the nose of an influenza patient with salt solution and filter the washings through a porcelain filter. The fluid which goes through the filter will contain the influenza virus which has infected this particular patient. The virus can be kept alive and grown and then matched against various samples of animal serum which we know contain antibodies to certain influenza viruses. If one of these serums is particularly active in destroying this virus, we know we can identify it with this serum. So if the serum contains antibodies to Virus A, the virus we are testing must be Virus A. If only the serum containing antibodies to Virus B is effective, the virus is Virus B. Recently a third group—Group C—has been isolated. It has occurred sporadically, not in epidemics. There are other tests, too, which can be done on the blood of an influenza patient, but these are too involved to warrant describing them here.

Q.   *Should a person with influenza be treated at home or in a hospital?*

A.   If the house is large enough so that the patient can be separated from the rest of the household, he is just as well off at home as anywhere else. If there are several people living in crowded quarters, it is much wiser to take the patient to the hospital. In that way you will lessen the risk to the rest of the family.

Q.   *I have been invited to dinner at my friend's house. One of her children has flu. Would it be safe for me to go?*

A.   Not if it is really influenza. If it is a cold or the grippe, however, and you will not come in contact with the child, then I believe it would be all right.

Q. *My child recovered from influenza two days ago and now wants to go to the movies. Is that safe?*

A. No. I think at least a week should elapse after such an illness before the child is exposed to large groups of people. This is important not only for his sake, but for the people he comes in contact with.

Q. *Does the influenza germ live in the patient so long after the illness is over?*

A. Probably not, but there is no use in taking chances for the sake of a few days.

Q. *Is it safe for a well child to use the room of a child who has just recovered from flu?*

A. Yes. If the room is thoroughly aired and cleaned and different bedclothes are used, the chances of infection are remote.

Q. *Is there any special soap needed to destroy the virus?*

A. No. Almost any soap or detergent will do it.

Q. *May letters be sent by a person who has influenza?*

A. Preferably not, unless they are aired for an hour or so in the sun first.

Q. *What should I do with my child's dishes and eating utensils when he has influenza?*

A. They should be thoroughly washed with soap and water.

Q. *Should they be kept apart from the family dishes?*

A. Not if they are well washed. Also, it would be easier if disposable plates and utensils were used.

24: Croup (Acute Obstructive Laryngitis)

Croup is the name for various kinds of laryngitis. It causes swelling of the larynx (the voice box) or swelling of the tissues above or below it. This swelling narrows the air passages and makes it difficult for the child to draw enough air into his lungs. Forcing the air through this narrowed passage results in the noisy breathing which is typical of croup. It is a disease of late infancy and early childhood. Though it can occur at any age, the usual age is between one and five or six years. This is because the passage to the larynx in small children is so short that infection settles there more easily than in older children and adults. Also, germ-carrying mucus which drips down the throat is not coughed up as easily by small children.

Much of the croup we see is caused by viruses—the parainfluenza viruses 1 and 2, respiratory syncitial, adenoviruses, rhinoviruses and probably others, many of which also are associated with colds. Often croup is a secondary infection—the invasion of bacteria after the child's resistance has been lowered by virus infection or another bacterial infection. The influenza bacillus (which causes many types of pneumonia and is not the influenza *virus* which causes influenza), the staphylococcus, the streptococcus and the pneumonia germ all may play such a secondary role, and any one of them alone may be the sole cause of the disease. Croup also may be the result of a combination of infection and allergic reaction to that infection. Swelling and inflammation of the epiglottis is almost always associated with the bacteria of H. Influenzae.

Croup is often caused by diphtheria, and although diphtheria has become relatively rare in this part of the world, it still must be considered in every case of croup. At one time we had to distinguish between "croup," meaning diphtheria of the larynx, and "simple croup," which is caused by other germs and is the one we are discussing here. This is still so in parts of the world where diphtheria is a common disease.

Contagion: Simple croup is as contagious as any other cold. Croup caused by diphtheria is the same as diphtheria. It is transmitted from the child who has it to susceptible children by droplets of moisture from the throat and is contagious until the secretions of the throat are free of the diphtheria bacillus, which is usually about two weeks, occasionally up to four.

Incubation Period: The incubation period of croup varies according to the infection which causes it. It may be as short as eight to twelve hours, if it is part of a cold, or two to five days if it is part of diphtheria.

Symptoms: Croup is very frightening when experienced for the first time. It is equally frightening to the child, to his parents and often even to the doctor. Fortunately, most of the cases are mild and pass off rather quickly, but since some are very serious and it is impossible to tell at the beginning which ones may become urgent, it is safer to have a doctor see the child as soon as possible.

Your child may have seemed perfectly well during the day, or he may have had a mild cold with or without hoarseness and have gone to bed feeling only slightly uncomfortable. He may wake up late in the evening with a loud, shrill, barking cough and with noisy and difficult breathing. He has croup. In a mild attack, the temperature is about 100° or 101°. The child does not look very sick, but the cough is shrill and the breathing noisy. He sounds worse than he is. He is apt to be frightened by not being able to breathe easily, but his color remains good. By the next morning he will probably feel much better, his voice will be softer and his cough looser. This type of croup passes off as a cold does, but at the beginning you must treat the child as if it were more severe.

In the more serious type, the temperature may rise to 102°

to 105°. The breathing difficulty is more apparent, the child's color becomes poor, and you can see that the lower part of his neck and the lower part of his chest are sucked in with the struggle for every breath. The child looks quite sick and is quickly exhausted. His pulse is very rapid. In such a case, the doctor should see the child immediately. If you cannot reach him right away, get another doctor, or failing that, take the child to the nearest hospital, preferably in an ambulance that has oxygen and the facilities for performing a tracheotomy (making an artificial opening in the windpipe below the swelling of the larynx). This is not often necessary in croup, but when it is, the situation is urgent.

Treatment: In every case of croup it is necessary to find out whether the child has been immunized against diphtheria, and whether a Schick test has been made recently. If there is any doubt about the child's immunity, and if a membrane has formed in his throat, he should be treated with diphtheria antitoxin. This will do no harm if it turns out that he does not have diphtheria, and it is a necessity if he does.

Antitoxin is not usually necessary since most cases of croup are not due to diphtheria, but antibiotics are very helpful and should be given. The doctor will probably prescribe antibiotics which will protect the child against all of the bacteria usually associated with croup—probably penicillin, plus one other which works against the influenza bacillus (not virus).

If your child wakes in the middle of the night with croup, the emergency treatment which you can carry out at home is to have him breathe steam for an hour or two. The quickest way to do this is to take him into the bathroom and run the shower hot, if your water runs hot at night. It will quickly fill the room with steam. It can also be done by running hot water in the bathtub and basin with the drains closed if there is no shower. While you are doing this, you should have a steam kettle of some kind running in the child's room, so that when you put him back to bed the air in the room will be moist.

Another method, which will steam up the bedroom while relieving the child, is to make a steam tent out of the crib or the bed. Put a sheet or blanket over the rails of the crib, or over an open umbrella over the child's head in the bed, and leave one side of it open. Direct through this side the steam from a tea kettle on an electric plate, an electric percolator or a regular croup kettle.

You can also, if your kitchen is small, put several pots of water on the stove and let them boil uncovered. Hold the child on your lap with an umbrella over him, you and the steam.

If the child does not show signs of satisfactory improvement after thirty minutes—easier breathing, a softer cough and less anxiety, or if any of these signs or symptoms are getting worse—it may mean that he needs oxygen. He may even need a tracheotomy, and while doctors can do this at home in an emergency, it is best done in a hospital.

If the child does show definite signs of improvement, he may be put back to bed in a warm, moist room. A responsible member of the family should stay in the room with him to make sure that he does not burn himself on the croup kettle. Cold vapor may be as helpful as hot steam and oxygen is undoubtedly best of all.

Sometimes making the child vomit will relax the spasm. The easiest way to do this is to give him a teaspoonful of syrup of ipecac. If one teaspoonful is not successful in a few minutes, a second one is almost sure to work. But do not give more than two.

It is very frightening to a child to have trouble breathing. If his parents seem frightened, too, he will be even more anxious and his breathing will get worse. On the other hand, if he can be reassured, his breathing usually becomes less difficult and his general condition will be improved. If a child with croup improves enough to fall into a restful sleep, it is usually a good sign because it means he is getting enough oxygen into his lungs. If the croup begins to show improvement after an hour or so, the improvement is usually progressive. The child may remain hoarse, but his breathing is less labored, less noisy, his cough is less frequent and less harsh, his temperature drops, and he looks better generally and is happier. There may be a slight recurrence of the symptoms on the second and third nights, but they are less severe and the child is well on the way to recovery.

If the child seems to improve for a while, and then his condition remains the same or gets worse, this should suggest a more severe infection than ordinary simple croup. A child with the more serious infection, in addition to the high fever and difficulty in breathing, may be very restless and unable to fall asleep. *Do not give him sedatives without a doctor's advice.* What he needs is oxygen. It is the lack of it that makes him restless.

During the whole course of the illness, you should keep the windows closed in the child's room, and the room should be warmer than usual, 72° to 75°. The room should be kept moist and warm for two or three nights to try to avoid the recurrence of the symptoms. You should encourage the child to take light foods and liquids, and as he gets better, he may eat anything he wants. He may get out of bed to go to the bathroom as soon as the acute phase is over.

If a child has once had croup, especially simple or allergic croup, the chances are that he will have it again. Therefore it would be wise to keep a croup kettle and syrup of ipecac handy for later use.

Convalescence: After an attack of croup, the child should be kept indoors away from cold air for several days, until all signs of the illness have disappeared. In the summer or in a warm climate he need not be kept indoors so long.

Isolation and Quarantine: Children who have been exposed to croup are not quarantined, but the patient is isolated as he would be with a simple cold. Of course, if the doctor suspects diphtheria, isolation and quarantine are carried out just as in the case of diphtheria.

Hygiene: No special precautions are taken with bedding, clothes and dishes unless diphtheria or some other contagious disease is suspected. In that case, the precautions are the same as for that disease.

QUESTIONS & ANSWERS

Q.   *Is croup known everywhere?*

A.   Yes.

Q.   *Does it occur only in certain months of the year?*

A. No, but it is more frequent in winter and spring when there are more acute upper respiratory infections like colds and grippe.

Q. *After an attack of croup, does the child become immune?*

A. No. On the contrary, a child who has a tendency to have croup may get it again and again.

Q. *Does a child get croup by crying a lot or shrieking?*

A. No. Abusing his voice may make him hoarse, but this swelling of the vocal cords is not caused by infection.

Q. *Does croup accompany other infections besides colds and diphtheria?*

A. Yes, it frequently occurs on the third or fourth day of measles.

Q. *Does croup ever occur in epidemics?*

A. No, but in some areas during certain periods most of the cases of croup may be caused by the same germ.

Q. *Is the child who gets croup repeatedly allergic?*

A. He is more likely to be than the child who does not.

Q. *Under what conditions does croup become an emergency?*

A. When, in addition to the high fever and difficulty in breathing, *the child becomes very restless and pale,* seems unable to get enough air and is unable to fall asleep. This restlessness indicates lack of oxygen and if you wait until the later phase in which his lips and fingertips get blue, it may be too late.

Q. *Are drugs to quiet the child helpful in croup?*

A. They sometimes are, but they should never be given without the doctor's advice because occasionally extreme restlessness is a sign of beginning asphyxiation and sedatives will slow down the child's efforts to breathe, and may mask the restlessness which is so important as a sign for the need for oxygen.

Q. *Is fresh air good for croup?*

A. Yes. After the acute symptoms are over, the necessary moisture does not have to be steam. If the weather is warm, the amount of moisture you get in the room by opening the window is enough. If, however, it is cold enough to make it necessary to close the windows and keep a radiator going, the air in the room becomes too dry and you must make artificial moisture by running a steam kettle or putting pans of water on the radiator.

Q. *Are both steam and cool air ever helpful during the acute phase of croup?*

A. Yes, they may be. If the child has a high fever, cool moist air may be preferable to hot steam.

Q. *How do you go about making cool moist air?*

A. By forcing compressed air or oxygen through a container of water.

Q. *Is oxygen preferable to steam?*

A. Sometimes, especially if it is given along with cool water vapor. At times, however, steam is more useful and possibly more effective.

Q. *Does cortisone help croup?*

A. It has often been tried in the hope that it would quickly reduce the swelling of the larynx, but the results are not definite. Some doctors are quite enthusiastic about it, and others think it has no value. I think it may be tried in severe croup but it is generally not needed.

Q. *Should a child with croup be fed as usual?*

A. Usually he does not want solid foods, but he should be encouraged to drink fluids of all kinds. An infant with croup should be spoon-fed, because closing his mouth around a nipple may interfere with his breathing and he will fight the nipple. If a child is unable to take enough fluid, he should be treated in a hospital.

Q. *How can I tell whether my child is getting enough fluid?*

A. An infant should take about 2½ ounces of fluid a day for each pound of body weight. If he weighs 16 pounds, he should be given 40 ounces of fluid a day. In both infants and children, if the eyes are not sunken, if the skin, when pressed between the thumb and forefinger, springs back quickly after the pressure is released, if he is urinating as usual, he is probably getting enough fluid.

Q. *Is there any way of preventing croup?*

A. Only by keeping your child away from people who have colds.

Q. *Should a child with croup be isolated?*

A. He should until the doctor finds out what is causing it. Also a child with croup needs special care which might disturb another child in the same room, and a well child might disturb the sick one.

Q. *How soon after my child recovers from croup may he return to school and to his play group?*

A. He may return to school when all signs of the infection have disappeared, but he should not join in hard play or athletics or join a play group for two or three days after that.

25: Acute Cervical Adenitis (Swollen Glands in the Neck)

Lymph is a slightly cloudy, almost colorless fluid which bathes most of the tissues of the body. It is like a dilute form of blood, minus the red blood cells. This fluid is picked up by lymph vessels which are similar to but thinner than veins. The lymph travels through them into the bloodstream. It enters the bloodstream by way of the largest vein in the body (the vena cava) which is attached to the heart. Lymph nodes, or glands, are small bean-shaped structures which are strategically distributed at various segments of the lymph vessels. The lymph has to pass through the lymph glands in its course into the bloodstream. These lymph glands are like filter stations and are the first line of defense against bacteria which enter the body through the mouth, throat, stomach, wounds and so forth.

The lymph glands in the neck are called cervical nodes. Others are also named according to their locations, for instance, axillary nodes are in the axillae or armpits. In the abdomen the glands are called abdominal lymph nodes. The cervical lymph vessels collect much of the tissue fluid in the neck and it passes through the cervical lymph glands, which are placed so as to intercept any bacteria that may get into the lymph by way of the throat, nose and skin, as in cases of tonsillitis, scarlet fever and diphtheria.

The lymph glands consist largely of lymphocytes, a form of white blood corpuscle. As bacteria reach the glands, they may be destroyed by the white corpuscles. If, however, more bacteria get into a gland than can be destroyed by the cells, the gland becomes infected, swells, becomes painful and tender to the touch. If the cells finally succeed in destroying the bacteria, the gland heals, becomes smaller and is no longer painful and tender. If the bacteria get the best of the cells, an abscess may develop.

If the source of the bacteria is infected tonsils and the infection becomes low-grade and long-lasting, the lymph glands in the neck become slightly enlarged and remain so as long as the infection lasts. Swelling and inflammation of the glands in the neck is known as cervical adenitis.

Acute cervical adenitis is usually a secondary disease, that is, it is a complication of tonsillitis or a throat infection. Swollen cervical glands may also follow scalp or neck infections due to eczema, head lice, superficial pus pimples or boils. In most cases they are caused by the streptococcus or staphylococcus. They are most often seen in young children, in the late fall, spring and winter. Cervical adenitis is not contagious.

One attack of cervical adenitis does not give the child any immunity to subsequent ones. They may recur repeatedly with sore throat or tonsillitis or skin infections. When this happens, it implies that there is a general body infection.

Another form of swollen glands in the neck is caused by the scratch of a cat. Cat scratch fever causes enlargement of the glands near the scratch, and it is not uncommon for the scratch to be on the neck and for the cervical glands to become enlarged and, in this case, often abscessed.

A child may have swollen and inflamed glands in places other than the neck. For example, if he is vaccinated or has an infection on the leg or the thigh, the lymph gland in the groin may become swollen and tender. It is common for the lymph glands in the armpits to become swollen and inflamed after vaccination on the arm, or when there is a boil or eczema in this area. Some general diseases like infectious mononucleosis cause swollen glands all over the body.

Incubation Period: There is no known incubation period for cervical adenitis. It may start anytime after tonsillitis or a sore throat begins. It may become severe even after recovery from a sore throat, scarlet fever, measles, diphtheria and other diseases.

Symptoms: If the lymph glands in the neck become infected, they become enlarged, painful and tender to the touch. The temperature usually climbs to a high level, 101° to 105°. It may drop as quickly as it rises and go up again in the same day. More than one peak of temperature within twenty-four hours is not at all unusual. Any one of them may be accompanied by a chill, and in young children, sometimes by a convulsion.

Acutely swollen glands in the neck may be so painful that the child is unable to move his head from side to side without considerable pain over the glands, in the neck and even in the head. As a result, he prefers to keep his neck stiff. If he must move his head sideways, he usually does it by moving his entire body. The stiff neck and headache sometimes frighten the child's parents into thinking he is really suffering from some other disease, like polio or meningitis.

The pain, the fever and the chills may last for several weeks unless the child is treated actively and adequately with antibiotics.

Treatment: Unless the glands are abscessed, it is not certain which bacterium is responsible, but it is usually the same type of germ that causes boils, the streptococcus or the staphylococcus. These can be destroyed quickly with a number of different antibiotics. It is important that swollen glands be treated promptly. The treatment must be continued not only until the swelling and the tenderness disappear and the temperature is normal, but for several days more so that the inflammation will not start up again.

When the glands are very painful, the child may be comforted by having wet compresses on them. They should usually be cold, but sometimes warm ones seem to feel better. Whichever is most comfortable is best. Salves are of little or no value. X-ray treatment is occasionally used, but rarely needed. Abscessed glands caused by tuberculosis are sometimes removed surgically, otherwise they are treated in the way that is recommended for tuberculosis.

Complications: If cervical adenitis is left untreated for some time and an abscess forms, the abscess may point toward the outside and break through the skin, in which case it is obvious. Or it may point toward the inside of the throat. In that case, the child finds it difficult and painful to swallow and his voice and speech change. He sounds as if he were talking through his nose or as if he had something in his throat. This kind of abscess usually has to be opened surgically. When this is done and the pus is released, relief is dramatic. The improvement in speech and swallowing is striking and pain almost completely disappears. The abscess drains for a few days and then heals.

Many adults have scars on the neck which are the result of the draining of abscessed lymph glands. Most of these have been caused by tuberculosis, but some are the result of an infection which started as tonsillitis or sore throat. If abscessed cervical glands drain for months or years, the infection is almost always caused by tuberculosis. The acutely abscessed glands act more like a boil and drain for only a short time. Draining abscessed glands of the neck due to tuberculosis have become less common in parts of the world where tuberculosis is better controlled. The acutely abscessed variety is also much less frequent because the kind of inflammation that causes them is easily cured with antibiotics.

Prevention: The only way to prevent cervical adenitis is to avoid the diseases which lead to it. If it is due to tonsillitis and recurs often, removing the tonsils may help. It can also be avoided if the diseases which cause it are cured quickly with suitable antibiotics or other medicines. The skin and scalp should be kept clean and cat scratches avoided.

Isolation and Quarantine: A child with cervical adenitis need not be isolated unless the disease which caused the adenitis is still active and requires it. An exposed child need not be quarantined.

QUESTIONS & ANSWERS

Q. *My child had cervical adenitis several months ago, and still has enlarged glands in the neck. Why is this?*

A. The glands may be somewhat scarred from the infection, or there may still be a low-grade infection in the throat or tonsils. Slight enlargement of the glands may continue for months, but this is not cause for concern.

Q. *Does cervical adenitis accompany other specific diseases besides tonsillitis and sore throat?*

A. Yes, it is particularly common in diphtheria in which the glands become very large and cause what is known as bull neck. This is usually a very serious sign of a severe diphtheria. In scarlet fever the lymph glands also swell, but this is the same swelling as in tonsillitis. Cervical adenitis may be caused by impetigo and by infected chicken pox on the neck.

Q. *Is cervical adenitis ever caused by a virus?*

A. Yes. In infectious mononucleosis the glands in the neck often become quite large and this disease is believed to be caused by a virus; similarly the A.P.C. or adeno-pharyngeal-conjunctival viruses produce swollen cervical lymph nodes.

Q. *Are there any other causes of swollen glands in the neck?*

A. Yes. They may be caused by such diseases as leukemia, Hodgkin's disease, German measles and occasionally a tumor in the neck. These differ from the acute inflammation which goes with sore throat in that they are usually neither painful nor tender. There are usually many swollen glands and the swelling may be quite striking, entirely out of proportion to the child's symptoms. There may be swollen glands elsewhere in the body at the same time. It is usually not difficult for a doctor to distinguish between swollen glands due to a sore throat and those due to other diseases like leukemia.

Q. *Should I worry about these serious diseases when my child develops cervical adenitis?*

A. No, not at all. These diseases are quite rare and cervical adenitis is quite common. The best way to tell that the swollen glands are not due to one of the more serious diseases is by giving antibiotics. The glands become smaller, the temperature becomes normal and the child gets well in a few days in the case of a throat infection. This is not true in leukemia, Hodgkin's disease or other such diseases. Antibiotics have no effect on them, but they may be influenced by special drugs which are used for these diseases.

Q. *Is it always possible for the doctor to tell the difference between swollen glands due to infectious mononucleosis and leukemia and those due to acute infection?*

A. Yes, but not necessarily by just looking at and feeling them. If the swelling in the neck is warm, possibly red, and hurts a great deal when pressed, the chances are it is due to an infection of the throat and tonsils. When the glands are swollen, but not tender or only slightly so, and not painful, the swelling is more likely to be due to some other condition such as infectious mononucleosis.

Q. *Why aren't swollen glands due to infectious mononucleosis and leukemia painful like acutely infected glands?*

A. The difference probably has something to do with the speed with which the gland capsule becomes distended. In the case of infection, the gland tissue is inflamed and is swollen with extra fluid and pus cells and bacteria, and the tissue around the gland is also swollen and tender.

Q. *Is it helpful to treat cervical adenitis with ultraviolet light?*

A. If the infection is caused by tuberculosis, it may be. But it does very little good for swollen glands caused by streptococcus or staphylococcus germs, and is not used widely in the United States.

Q. *Do you recommend X-ray treatment for cervical adenitis?*

A. No. X-ray specialists may, but in my experience it is not necessary. Antibiotics and the sulfa drugs do a good

job, and they are much simpler to give, more dramatic
in their results, cost less and can be given at home.

Q. *Is tying a warm piece of flannel around my child's neck
helpful when he has swollen glands?*

A. It may be comforting, but it has no particular effect in
curing the infection.

Q. *Are any of the salves good to rub on his neck?*

A. Salves are not helpful against the infection, but irritants
like camphor cause a coolness of the skin which may re-
leave some of the pain. They do not cure the disease nor
do they keep the glands from becoming abscessed, so they
are not ordinarily used.

Q. *Is quinsy the same as an abscessed gland?*

A. No. Quinsy usually means an abscess within a tonsil.

Q. *Can you prevent cervical adenitis from recurring?*

A. The only way is to prevent the conditions which cause it.
For example, if a child has repeated attacks of cervical
adenitis following tonsillitis, removing the tonsils will
prevent recurrence from that cause. This does not mean
that tonsillectomy will eliminate swollen glands in the
neck altogether. Children have sore throats even after
their tonsils have been removed, and the glands in the
neck may swell then.

Q. *Can you be immunized against cervical adenitis?*

A. No, only against some of the diseases which might lead to
it. For example, you can be immunized against scarlet
fever and diphtheria and thus swollen glands due to them
would be eliminated. But at present we cannot prevent
colds and the secondary infections which go with them,
so cervical adenitis is still likely to occur.

Q. *Is cervical adenitis contagious?*

A. Not in itself. It is always part of another infection which
may or may not be contagious. It is not necessary to isolate the patient, nor to quarantine anyone exposed to him.

26: *Bronchitis and*
Bronchiectasis

Bronchitis is an inflammation of the bronchial tubes. It occurs throughout the year, but is especially common in the winter and spring because it is likely to follow colds and grippe which are more numerous then. Bronchitis may be acute or chronic. When it is acute, it is usually the result of a cold, sinus infection, tonsillitis or adenoiditis. It is always a part of measles and whooping cough and is usually a part of influenza. The bacteria or viruses which cause these diseases get into the bronchial tubes and cause inflammation of the linings. The cells of the linings secrete more fluid to fight the infection. When the doctor listens to the chest with his stethoscope, he hears sounds of air bubbling through this fluid (rales) as the child breathes.

Bronchitis may be complicated by an allergic reaction to the bacteria causing it. When this happens, the bronchial muscles tighten in response to the reaction and the bronchial tubes become narrowed. The narrowing of the tubes causes wheezing. This kind of bronchitis is often called asthmatic bronchitis, but most allergists believe, and I agree, that the wheezing actually indicates the presence of asthma, not only bronchitis, and that the condition is due to bacterial allergy. This may seem to be hair-splitting, but it is important to differentiate between them because the treatment would vary depending on whether the condition is due to allergy or infection.

ACUTE BRONCHITIS

If your child has a cold and after a day or two begins to cough, and if the cough is loose and occurs frequently in spells, he may have acute bronchitis. With each cough he may bring up some mucus which he spits out if he is old enough or swallows if he is not. If the child has no fever, the bronchitis may be mild and will pass off in a day or two. If, on the other hand, he seems quite sick, has fever, has the kind of cough I have described and the illness lasts longer than three or four days, the bronchitis may have been complicated by pneumonia.

It is frequently necessary to distinguish between acute bronchitis and pneumonia, or between bronchitis and asthma. Since this is impossible for the average parent to do, and since the bronchitis should be treated promptly to avoid pneumonia, it is important to get the advice of the child's doctor.

Treatment: A child with acute bronchitis should be kept in bed, but if he is not too sick you may let him go to the bathroom. He might watch television in another room if he can be kept off the floor, on a couch. You should keep him warm and keep the air in his room moist. This is done by putting several containers of water on the radiators or by running a steam kettle. Steam inhalations under a tent, as I have suggested for croup, are not usually necessary because, while moist air helps to thin the bronchial secretions, no such concentration of moisture is needed. You may give the child whatever he wants to eat and he should have plenty of fluids. Warm drinks are comforting and may help to loosen the mucus, so that it can be coughed up more easily. As for medication, you should follow the doctor's directions carefully.

Do not let the child out-of-doors until his temperature has been normal for at least twenty-four hours after all medication has been stopped. Keep him out of school until the cough has stopped.

CHRONIC BRONCHITIS

If a child has bronchitis which does not clear up for weeks or months even though he feels reasonably well and his temperature has become normal or low-grade, the doctor may find that the continuing cough is due to chronic bronchitis. A chronic sinus infection is one of the most common causes of this because it results in a constant dripping of mucus into the throat which spreads the infection into the bronchial tubes. Other frequent causes of chronic bronchitis in children are measles, whooping cough and influenza. After the acute phase of these diseases has subsided, the bronchial tubes may remain infected or irritated for a long time.

Treatment: Chronic bronchitis is very difficult to cure unless the infection which caused it in the first place is cured. If the cause is a sinus infection, the sinuses must be treated until they are well with steam inhalations, drugs which shrink the lining membranes of the nose and with antibiotics. Occasionally they have to be drained and irrigated, or even operated on by a nose specialist. If the cause is chronically infected tonsils or adenoids which cannot be cured otherwise, removing them may be helpful. If chronic bronchitis is the aftermath of measles, whooping cough or influenza, the doctor will want to find out which bacteria are causing the infection and give the child the most suitable antibiotic. If it is due to an allergy, it is often possible to find out what the child is allergic to, and remove it. If these measures fail to help, a change in climate will sometimes do the trick, especially a change to a warm, dry climate where respiratory infections are less frequent. If you can avoid repeated infections, chronic bronchitis will heal.

Prevention: The prevention of bronchitis is the same as the prevention of an ordinary cold. It consists mainly of keeping away from people with colds and coughs and observing good hygiene in general. There is no injection or vaccine to prevent bronchitis except in the case of an allergic child. As in the treatment of any allergy, these vaccine treatments do not always work, but they can be expected to help some of the children who receive them.

The kind of bronchitis caused by inhaling powder (especially zinc stearate), kerosene, peanuts and other nuts, and other foreign objects can be prevented by keeping these things away from infants and little children. If you do not give babies who have not yet cut their molar teeth candy, cake, cookies and ice cream with whole pieces of nuts in them, they will not choke over them and draw them into their lungs. If you do not let your infant play with the powder can he will not spray powder into his face and inhale it.

Isolation and Quarantine: A child with acute bronchitis is only as infectious as the disease which caused it and is or is not isolated accordingly. A child with chronic bronchitis is not isolated, and, in fact, may go to school. If the bronchitis is part of a cold and the sick child infects another child, the second child will probably have a cold, but he will not necessarily have bronchitis.

Hygiene: It is not necessary to take any special precautions with the patient's clothes or dishes or utensils.

BRONCHIECTASIS

If chronic bronchitis is allowed to go on for months or years, the inflamed walls of the bronchial tubes may become scarred. As the scarred tissue shrinks, the result is a shortening and a change in the shape of the tubes. Little localized bulges are created which act as traps for mucus and for infection. This condition is known as bronchiectasis and is very serious. It is difficult to cure.

QUESTIONS & ANSWERS

BRONCHITIS

Q. *Are there other types of bronchitis besides those caused by germs?*

A. Yes, foreign-body bronchitis for instance. A child may inhale some solid object into a bronchial tube, which acts as an irritant to the lining. The oil which is set free when nuts or seeds deteriorate in a bronchial tube is particularly irritating. A child may inhale kerosene, powder (especially zinc stearate) or fumes and gases. All of these are irritating and cause bronchitis.

Q. *Can you develop immunity to bronchitis?*

A. Not to bronchitis itself. If you have become immune to a disease which is often complicated by bronchitis, you probably will not get bronchitis from that disease, but you could still get it from any disease to which you are not immune. Once we have effective vaccines made from the viruses which cause bronchitis we may be able to prevent it.

Q. *Can you tell whether a child has bronchitis by X-rays?*

A. Not usually, if it is acute bronchitis, but if it is chronic or long-standing or very severe, there is usually a thickening of the bronchial tubes which will show up on an X-ray picture.

Q. *Is there any laboratory test like a blood count to diagnose bronchitis?*

A. No. A blood count will only indicate that there is an infection, but it will not say where the infection is.

Q. *When a child has bronchitis and coughs up a lot of mucus, does it all come from the bronchial tubes?*

A. Yes. Inflammation in any part of the body results in secretion of fluid. In the case of bronchitis, the bronchial tubes are inflamed and give off a considerable amount, which is coughed up.

Q.   *If a child has bronchitis over and over again or chronic bronchitis, does it mean that there is a nose or throat infection?*

A.   Yes, usually the sinuses or the adenoids. When these are cured, bronchitis is less likely to occur.

Q.   *Is it good to try to stop the cough in bronchitis?*

A.   It is usually impossible to stop it entirely. Also it is undesirable because you want to get the mucus out of the lungs. If, however, the child coughs night and day and cannot sleep, it is helpful to give him a cough medicine to loosen the mucus and make the cough less frequent.

Q.   *Should my child be kept in bed very long after the bronchitis is finished?*

A.   No. As the bronchitis improves, if his temperature has been normal for at least twenty-four hours and he is not acting sick, you might let him out of bed. You should not treat him as a well child, but he could be up and around the house. But I would not let him go back and forth between a warm room and a cold one for another day or two, depending on how ill he has been.

Q.   *What can you do about chronic bronchitis?*

A.   Chronic bronchitis requires expert medical care. The infection that is causing it can be cured with antibiotics, and perhaps the child can be immunized against some of the common diseases. If these measures do not help, a change to a warm, dry climate may.

Q.   *Is convalescence from bronchitis apt to be long?*

A.   Not if the illness has lasted only a few days. I like to wait until the chest is completely clear, the temperature normal for at least two days and the cough has practically stopped before I let the child go out-of-doors or back to school. Of course, in the summer months when it is warm, I might let the child be in the open air even while the disease is acute.

Q.   *Is there a vaccination against bronchitis?*

A.   No, not an effective one.

Q.   *Is there any other way to prevent it?*

A. Only by treating nose and throat infections carefully so that the child will not develop it.

BRONCHIECTASIS

Q. *You say that bronchiectasis is a serious disease. How do you know when a child has it?*

A. When a child has had bronchitis for a long time, when he has cough and fever over and over again for months, when the doctor hears bubbling sounds in his chest, he suspects bronchiectasis. He can confirm his diagnosis by a special X-ray technique called a bronchogram. In this, a substance called lipiodol or a substitute is injected into the child's lungs to make the bronchial tubes opaque in the X-ray picture. The lipiodol will fill the little sacs which are formed in bronchiectasis so that they will show in the picture.

Q. *What is the treatment for bronchiectasis?*

A. We treat it with antibiotics taken internally and inhaled. Fine antibiotic particles are sprayed into the lungs several times a day for several weeks. Sometimes this will cure the infection and the bronchiectasis will heal. Unfortunately, this takes a long time and does not always work. A change of climate has helped some children, but in many cases the only thing to do is to operate and remove the part of the lung which has been made useless. This usually results in a cure.

27: Sinusitis

Sinusitis is one of the most frequent complications of colds, respiratory infections and virus diseases, such as measles and allergies affecting the nose. Although it is usually not a serious illness, sinusitis can be very acute and very annoying to the child and his family. It probably occurs much more often than it is diagnosed and, in most instances, clears up without specific treatment. Some sinus infections are difficult to detect and difficult to cure.

Sinusitis occurs everywhere, but most often in damp, cold climates and in the seasons when colds are most prevalent. In temperate climates this is during the late fall, winter and spring.

Actually, a sinus is merely a cavity or a pocket, and there are sinuses of various kinds all over the body, but the ones we are discussing here are the nasal sinuses. They are air pockets in the bones of the face and the skull which are lined with mucous membrane and drain into the nose through small openings. Most people have four pairs of nasal sinuses: the frontal, in the bone of the forehead above the eyes; the maxillary (antra), in the upper jawbone below the eyes; the ethmoids which lie behind the bridge of the nose; and the sphenoids which are back of the ethmoids, deeper in the skull. At birth the frontal sinuses are not developed at all, and the others are very small. As a child's head grows, the sinuses gradually enlarge. The sphenoids are well developed after three years, and the frontal sinuses are fairly well developed by the time the child is six or eight.

Because the sinuses are so near the nose, they are particularly susceptible to infection. The openings from the sinuses into the nose are small and anything that causes swelling of the lining membrane of the nose, such as a cold or an allergy, reduces the size of these openings or closes them off altogether. This makes it difficult, and at times impossible, for the fluid normally formed in the sinuses to drain out. Since bacteria are always present in the nose, this collection of stagnant secretion makes an ideal environment for the multiplication of bacteria. The blocking of the passages is basically what causes sinusitis. It may be acute or chronic, and the symptoms vary somewhat according to age.

Contagion: As with other bacterial infections of the nose and throat, the bacteria causing the sinusitis can be transmitted from one child to another, but they do not necessarily cause the same disease. The bacteria that produce sinusitis in one child may cause tonsillitis or middle ear infection or sinusitis in another who is exposed to him. Therefore, a child with acute sinusitis should not be close to other children since the infection is spread by droplets of moisture from the nose and throat.

Symptoms: Acute sinusitis has been observed in infants a few days old, but it is not common until after the first year. In infants and very young children, it usually is an acute infection of the ethmoid sinuses, since they are the ones which are most fully developed at this age. The baby is usually quite ill, with fever from 101° to 104°. In most cases, only one side is involved. There may be no discharge from that side at first, but at some point there will be a profuse discharge which often is thick and yellow or greenish and consists of mucus and pus. If the eye socket is involved, the eye becomes red, swollen and bulges forward. This condition is serious. It should serve as an urgent signal to call the doctor immediately. Until he comes, the baby should be given steam inhalations to thin the secretions and allow them to drain more easily, and a nasal spray or nose drops to shrink the membrane in the nose.

The older child with acute sinusitis may have involvement of the frontal, ethmoid, maxillary or any combination of these sinuses. He is acutely ill with a fever of 101° to 104° which may be accompanied by a chill. He usually complains of headache and pain over the affected sinuses. If the maxillary sinus is involved, he may feel as if he had a toothache, or he may have a pain over the cheek and it may be swollen, red and tender. His nose may be stuffed or there may be a thick nasal discharge and an irritating cough. This kind of infection usually clears up within a week, but it may last longer and need active treatment.

Some children are inclined to have a fever of 99.5° to 100.5° for three or four weeks, or to cough for weeks after a cold. This is usually due to a sinus infection. Sinusitis has a tendency to recur with each cold in children who have once had it. In others, especially older children and adults, the original infection may continue in a chronic form. The characteristic symptoms of chronic sinusitis are a stuffed or running nose, headaches, eyestrain or fatigue, sometimes chronic conjunctivitis, pain or pressure over the maxillary or frontal sinuses, a general let-down feeling and a persistent cough which is usually at its worst when the child gets up in the morning. The cough is caused by irritation of the larynx and windpipe from secretions which drain down the child's throat while he sleeps. When he gets up, the change of position releases the secretions which have accumulated while he was lying flat, and the cough increases. The temperature in chronic sinusitis is often normal, and when there is a fever, it rarely goes higher than 101°.

Sometimes, however, symptoms are almost entirely absent and diagnosis is very difficult. Sometimes the only indication that something is wrong with the child is that he has a low-grade fever, up to 101°, that persists for weeks or even months after an infection of the respiratory tract or one of the virus diseases like measles. Or the child may continue to cough or have a stuffy nose long after he should have been over his cold. In these cases, a general physical examination, a blood count and other tests may be completely normal and the diagnosis can be made only after a thorough examination, including the finding of certain bacteria in the nose and X-ray pictures of the sinuses, or a careful examination by a nose and throat specialist.

Treatment: Treatment of sinusitis has two purposes: first, to kill the bacteria and second, to relieve the obstruction of the passages to the nose and establish drainage. This treatment depends on the disease or condition which caused the sinusitis and on whether it is acute or chronic.

Acute sinusitis usually responds to steam inhalations and nasal sprays or drops of one of the many drugs like ephedrine or Neo-Synephrine. In some instances the doctor will add a local anesthetic like cocaine which helps to shrink the swollen lining of the nose and sinuses. The steam inhalations may have to be given for twenty to thirty minutes out of every three hours during the day, and in very severe cases this may have to be kept up until the sinuses open and begin to drain. External heat of various kinds has been used, but the results are not consistent. The type of antibiotic which is used is determined to some extent by the illness which the sinusitis is complicating. The doctor may prescribe only one or it may be a combination of antibiotics, but they must be selected with the idea that they will be helpful against not only the sinusitis, but the primary illness as well. For example, in the case of scarlet fever, penicillin would work for both diseases. If the infection were due to a staphylococcus, which is often resistant to penicillin, the drug of choice might be erythromycin or one of the newer antibiotics which are effective against penicillin-resistant staphylococci.

Chronic sinusitis may require irrigation of the sinuses plus antibiotics, and in some cases, especially where polyps (little growths in the lining membrane of the nose and sinuses) have formed, it may require surgery. Short-wave treatment may be comforting and it may help sinusitis, but it rarely cures it and is rarely used.

In children, the chronic form of sinusitis is relatively uncommon and the need for surgery of the sinuses themselves is quite unusual. Removing the adenoids may help, but it is not a cure and should only be done after careful consideration. Change of climate is helpful only if it prevents colds or other respiratory infections which are responsible for the sinusitis.

Complications: Sinusitis sometimes leads to asthma in allergic children. I have had patients who have had repeated asthmatic attacks for years until a sinus infection was cured. A long-standing sinus infection might cause bronchitis, and if it is allowed to go on for years, it may cause chronic bronchitis or bronchiectasis, or polyps may develop within the sinuses. In an acute form, sinusitis can cause symptoms suggestive of meningitis and, on rare occasions, it actually causes meningitis or brain abscess. Arthritis, kidney disease and a breaking down of the bones around the sinuses (osteomyelitis) are also sometimes the result of sinus infection.

Prevention: Primarily, the prevention of sinusitis depends on reducing the number of colds and other respiratory infections. There are no serums or vaccines which are valuable as preventives. Anything which prevents colds, grippe, influenza, measles and so forth will also prevent sinusitis. In allergic children, whatever helps hay fever and other allergies involving the nose will also be helpful in preventing sinusitis.

Hygiene: A child with acute sinusitis should be in a room by himself, or in one large enough to avoid intimate contact with a sibling. It is not necessary to sterilize his dishes and utensils. The room should be aired for twelve hours after he has recovered before it is used for anyone else.

QUESTIONS & ANSWERS

Q. *Is sinusitis more prevalent in damp areas than in areas which are dry and cold?*

A. Yes.

Q. *Is the tendency to get sinusitis inherited?*

A. No, but it is conceivable that the structure of a child's nose and sinuses may be similar to his parent's, so that if the parent is liable to infection, the child might be, too.

Q. *Why do some people get sinusitis with every cold while some people never get it at all?*

A. I am not sure there is anyone who never gets it at all with colds, or anyone who always does. It is true, though, that once a person has had his sinuses infected, they are more liable to be reinfected, possibly because the first infection leaves him with a chronic one which merely gets worse at the time of a cold.

Q. *Is it possible to develop immunity to sinusitis?*

A. No.

Q. *Is allergy a factor in producing sinus infections?*

A. Yes. It first produces swelling and redness of the lining of the nose and sinuses, after which infection may set in.

Q. *If a child gets asthma attacks from a sinus infection and the sinus infection is cured, will the asthma attacks stop?*

A. The ones which are associated with sinus infection will, but other infections of the nose and throat can still cause them.

Q. *Are infection of the nose and allergy the only causes of sinusitis?*

A. Anything that blocks off the openings from the sinuses into the nose may cause it. For instance, a child may push a bean or some other foreign body into his nose and block one or more of the openings. Then the bacteria which are always present in the sinuses multiply in the secretions which become stagnant because they are unable to drain out.

Q. *My doctor says I have many sinus infections because I have a deviated septum. What is this?*

A. The nasal septum is the dividing wall between the two halves of the nose. If it is crooked or off-center because of a break or an injury or a deformity at birth, it is said to be deviate and it may block off or reduce the size of the sinus openings and obstruct drainage. This would result in infection.

Q. *Will moving to a warm, dry climate permanently cure sinusitis?*

A. No. By preventing or eliminating the chances of getting colds and other infections of the nose and throat, a warm, dry climate may help the sinuses to improve, but the improvement may last only as long as the child stays in a place where he gets fewer colds.

Q. *Are nose drops good for sinusitis?*

A. Yes, if they are the kind which shrink the lining membrane of the nose and sinuses and keep the sinus openings from closing off.

Q. *Are nose drops or nasal sprays which contain cortisone good in sinusitis?*

A. Yes, particularly when it is caused by allergic rhinitis.

Q. *Are nose drops or sprays better in the treatment of sinusitis?*

A. Nasal sprays are probably better because of the more even distribution of the fine droplets, but some children do not like them and for these children nose drops are helpful.

Q. *How long should I keep on giving nose drops to my child?*

A. It is important not to give nose drops for more than a few days unless your doctor advises it. Some of them, when they are used for a longer time, will cause irritation of the nasal membranes so that the swelling and discomfort are greater than before the nose drops were used.

Q. *Instead of making a steam tent when my baby has sinusitis, can I get the same results by keeping a steam kettle going in the room all night?*

A. No. They are not quite the same. The steam in the room will be comforting and helpful, but it will not be concentrated enough to relieve a severely congested nose and sinuses.

Q. *Is washing out the sinuses helpful?*

A. Very, when it is properly done. It sometimes results in dramatic relief of pain and headache as well as the cough which sinus infection often causes.

Q. *What is the youngest age at which a child can have his sinuses washed out?*

A. There is no such age. As long as the sinuses can be reached, they can be washed out. Generally, we are reluctant to do this in children less than five or six years old. If it is very important for a very young child, it may have to be done under an anesthetic.

Q. *Is there any operation which will permanently cure sinusitis and prevent further attacks?*

A. In some cases, operation will cure the infection, make further attacks less likely and make the sinuses more available for medical treatment. In some cases it is necessary to operate to establish proper drainage because the sinus infection has become chronic, polyps may have developed and these do not respond to simple measures.

Q. *Is there any way of preventing sinuses from becoming infected when you have a cold?*

A. It can sometimes be done by keeping the nasal passages clean right from the beginning of the cold with steam inhalations or one of the drugs which shrink the membranes of the nose and sinuses. When the sinuses can drain, they are much less likely to become infected.

Q. *If allergy is a factor in producing sinus infections, will antihistamines prevent them?*

A. They may, if they are effective against the allergy which causes the swelling of the membranes of the nose and sinuses.

Q. *Will removing my child's tonsils and adenoids make a difference in the number of sinus infections he has?*

A. Removing the tonsils probably will not make much difference, but removing the adenoids may help the sinuses drain and thereby reduce the number of infections.

28: *Tonsillitis*

Tonsillitis (inflammation of the tonsils) is a widespread disease. It is particularly common in the late fall, the winter, and in early spring, but it occurs in the summer, too. There is much more of it and it is much more severe in temperate climates than in warm ones, and in the tropics it is far less common. Children of two to eight get it more often than older children or adults, but it is by no means unusual in the older groups. Tonsillitis is caused by many different bacteria and possibly by some viruses. About half of the cases are produced by the bacteria called the hemolytic streptococcus which also produces scarlet fever. The word *streptococcus* has come to mean a dangerous germ to many, but such fear is unwarranted these days because it is rapidly destroyed by penicillin and other drugs. Most of the other germs which cause tonsillitis are readily eliminated by antibiotics, too.

Scarlet fever is more common in children who have tonsils, and the tonsils are always involved in the infection. Often in a home where a child has scarlet fever, another person may develop either scarlet fever or tonsillitis without a rash. Or the order may be reversed: a person, usually an adult, has follicular tonsillitis and others in the house will come down with either the tonsillitis or scarlet fever. Under these circumstances the disease is the same except for the rash.

In the case of tonsillitis caused by the hemolytic streptococcus, the child develops an immunity to the particular streptococcus which caused the disease, but since there are more than forty of them, he is still susceptible to infection with the others. In the case of scarlet fever, the child becomes permanently immune to the toxin which causes the rash, but his immunity to the streptococcus which caused the disease is the same as for tonsillitis.

Contagion: No matter which bacteria cause the tonsillitis, it is highly contagious, particularly when the child coughs and germs from his throat come into contact with people near him.

Incubation Period: The incubation period for tonsillitis caused by the hemolytic streptococcus is two to five days, and for the other types it is even shorter.

Symptoms: Many people speak of tonsillitis as if it were the same as any sore throat. This is not quite true, even though the tonsils are involved whenever there is an inflammation at the back of the throat. Tonsillitis is a specific disease, and a child does not have it every time he has a cold. Tonsillitis causes definite symptoms. The child feels very sick, the throat is very sore, the temperature may be quite high, he may feel chilly, have a chill or ache all over. If the tonsils are very swollen, swallowing may be difficult and painful. The disease lasts about a week, with fever for three or four days. If complications arise, the fever may last longer or come back after the temperature has been normal.

When the tonsils are inflamed, the throat is also involved, and almost always the adenoids are, too. The adenoids are behind the nose in the back of the throat. Like the tonsils, they can become inflamed and swollen and cause a dripping of pus or mucus. We often group the tonsils and adenoids together although the symptoms resulting from tonsillitis are quite different from those we see with inflamed adenoids.

Diagnosis: Doctors reserve the name *tonsillitis* for the condition in which the tonsils themselves are particularly inflamed, swollen and often covered with white or gray spots. When there are spots on the tonsils it is referred to as follicular tonsillitis. This is really the only kind that is easy to detect unless the tonsils are so swollen and red that it is obvious they are more infected than the rest of the throat. Sometimes the spots run together and form a membrane on the tonsils that is hard to distinguish from the membrane of diphtheria. If there is any doubt in the doctor's mind about this, he will have a laboratory test made to make sure.

Treatment: The doctor should see the child and start treatment as soon as possible. Tonsillitis can be treated very successfully with penicillin and other antibiotics. If treatment is started early, complications are very much reduced. The choice of drugs, the amount to be given and the method of giving them depend on several things and can best be decided by your doctor. The child should be kept in bed until a few days after the fever is gone, and aspirin will make him feel better as long as there is fever and his throat hurts. Do not try to treat tonsillitis yourself with aspirin alone or with gargles or by swabbing your child's tonsils with an antiseptic. At best, these are inadequate and sometimes swabbing is injurious. Call your doctor and be guided by his advice.

Complications: The most common complications of tonsillitis are swollen glands in the neck, ear infection, sinus infection and abscess of a tonsil (quinsy). Usually quinsy occurs only in one tonsil, but it may occur in both at once. If the tonsillitis is produced by the hemolytic streptococcus, it can lead to more serious complications, such as inflammation of the kidneys (nephritis) or rheumatic fever.

Isolation and Quarantine: If a child has tonsillitis, I think it is wise to isolate him just as if he had scarlet fever. The board of health does not insist on this as it does with scarlet fever unless it is known to be caused by the hemolytic streptococcus, in which case the disease is considered the same as scarlet fever. But since you do not always know which bacteria caused the disease, it seems to me safer not to take any chances. All infections with the hemolytic streptococcus are essentially the same from the standpoint of isolation and treatment. They are now called the streptococcuses, and include scarlet fever, tonsillitis and streptococcal sore throat, erysipelas (a skin disease) and childbed fever. There are many others, but these are the most important.

Reasons for Removing Tonsils and Adenoids: If a child has tonsillitis very often, two or three times in one year or once or twice a year for several years; if tonsillitis has often been the cause of swollen lymph glands in the neck; if, along with tonsillitis, there has been frequent adenoid infection, and frequent ear infection; if the tonsils are so large that they cause difficulty in swallowing or in speech; if the adenoids have become so large as to cause breathing difficulty, snoring at night, or chronic running nose or loss of hearing—if all of these signs occur or any one of them occurs in severe form, many doctors recommend removal of the tonsils or the adenoids or both. Mostly both are removed at the same operation, although the adenoids alone are often responsible for the child's difficulties. The operation is postponed, however, by most doctors if the child is very young or otherwise sick, and during and just before the polio season.

Tonsillectomy should be recommended when definitely indicated. It should not be done lightly or because "it will have to be done sooner or later." One in four thousand dies from a general anesthetic. Complication of tonsillectomy, hemorrhage, aspiration pneumonia and lung abscess are serious enough to avoid tonsillectomy unless it is a must.

QUESTIONS & ANSWERS

Q. *Is tonsillitis the same all over the world?*

A. No, not entirely. It is more prevalent in some parts of the world and it is more prevalent in certain seasons in the same community. The bacteria may be different in different parts of the world. In Europe people talk of tonsillitis as being less frequent than in the United States. We have noticed that Europeans who come to the United States rapidly become exposed to the prevailing bacteria and develop the same kind of tonsillitis we have.

Q. *Are tonsillitis and scarlet fever the same disease?*

A. Only when the tonsillitis is caused by the same germ, the beta hemolytic streptococcus.

Q. *Can you have tonsillitis in the summer?*

A. Yes. It is less common in the warm months, but it does occur.

Q. *Should I swab my child's throat when he gets tonsillitis?*

A. I believe that swabbing is very little help. In fact, it may be irritating and actually spread the infection to other parts of the throat.

Q. *Is gargling good?*

A. If it is done correctly, it is comforting, but the average child does not get the fluid near the tonsils when he gargles.

Q. *Is it better to treat tonsillitis with lozenges, medicine to swallow, or medicine by injection?*

A. Medicine is much more effective either swallowed or injected because it affects the infected layers of tissues which are under the surface by way of the bloodstream. Lozenges and gargles only reach the surface tissue. Some medicines applied locally are absorbed, but not enough to be valuable.

Q. *If my child has tonsillitis, should I isolate him just as if he had scarlet fever?*

A. I think so, because it is often caused by a streptococcus which is easily spread to contacts.

Q. *At what age should I have my child's tonsils removed?*

A. There is no special age for this or any other operation. It is done when it is necessary. The exception is that doctors don't like to operate on very young children, on children who are otherwise ill, and in seasons just before or during epidemics of polio, unless they have been adequately immunized with vaccination.

Q. *What connection has a tonsil operation with polio?*

A. It is claimed that children who have recently had their tonsils removed are more likely to get polio, and if they do get it, they are more likely to get the serious bulbar form which paralyzes the breathing muscles.

Q. *My child has a chronic cough. The doctor says his tonsils should be taken out. Will that help?*

A. Possibly, although there are usually other reasons for a chronic cough. A low-grade infection anywhere in the nose and throat may cause a drip which will irritate the bronchial tubes and induce coughing.

Q. *My son is a very poor eater. Will taking out his tonsils help his appetite?*

A. Possibly, if the tonsils and adenoids are very large or

chronically infected so that swallowing or breathing is difficult. Otherwise, no.

Q. *My child is very thin. Will removing his tonsils and adenoids help him?*

A. If the tonsils and adenoids need to be removed, he will undoubtedly improve after surgery and may begin to put on weight. But if they don't need to be removed there is probably no connection between his weight and his tonsils and adenoids.

Q. *Do doctors ever take out tonsils and adenoids in babies?*

A. Yes. Sometimes they are so large that they make sleeping, eating and breathing very difficult.

Q. *Is there any other way to remove tonsils and adenoids besides surgery?*

A. Yes, they can be shrunk by X-ray, but it is not the treatment most doctors employ because it is possible to do a more complete job by surgery, and excessive exposure to X-rays may be harmful.

Q. *Do enlarged tonsils cause deafness?*

A. Usually not. But enlarged adenoids may cut off the passage of air through the Eustachian tube to the ear. The Eustachian tube is a narrow passage from the throat to the middle ear and the opening is very small. When the adenoids block this opening and the circulation of air is interfered with, the chances of ear infection are increased. Frequent ear infections are apt to cause a thickening of the ear drum and hearing difficulties.

Q. *Do the adenoids have to be removed to correct this?*

A. Yes, if they are large.

Q. *If the adenoids have been removed and my child still has the same hearing difficulty, what can I do?*

A. Have the child examined by an ear, nose and throat doctor. If he finds that adenoid tissue has regrown and blocked the opening of the Eustachian tubes, surgery or X-ray or radium might be used to correct it. If surgery is not possible, X-ray or radium is usually quite effective.

Q. *Will my child have fewer colds if his tonsils and adenoids are taken out?*

A. I doubt very much that the number of colds will be changed, but the nature of them may be.

Q. *In what way will they change?*

A. When there are no tonsils and adenoids, colds behave differently. The tonsils no longer make swallowing difficult and the adenoids no longer obstruct the breathing. Also the glands in the neck are less likely to swell. With no adenoids there is less snoring, less severe running nose, and less likelihood of infection of the ears and sinuses. On the other hand, cough and bronchitis are more likely to result from the cold.

Q. *Our ten-year-old has had an abscess on a tonsil on two different occasions. What should be done about it?*

A. I believe most doctors would recommend removing the tonsils.

Q. *Does tonsil infection ever produce arthritis?*

A. Yes, but it is certainly not the only cause, and the situation should be carefully evaluated before anything is done about removing the tonsils.

Q. *Can chronically infected tonsils produce other diseases?*

A. Yes, sinus infection, chronically swollen glands, recurrent eye inflammation and others.

Q. *Can you remove tonsils or adenoids alone, or must they always be taken out together?*

A. They can be taken out separately and often are. Usually it is the adenoids which are removed alone because of obstruction at the back of the nose, or repeated ear infections or sinus infections. Often though, when only one has been removed, it is only a few years before the other must be, too. But it is sometimes preferable to remove only the one which really causes trouble. Some doctors feel that removing the tonsils makes the child more susceptible to chest infections and therefore they do not like to remove them unless it is absolutely necessary.

Q. *Should a child's tonsils be taken out while they are infected?*

A. Whenever it is possible the infection should be cleared up before the operation. It is a common practice to treat the child with penicillin or some other drug before and for a few days after the operation to avoid the spread of infection, and to avoid new infection after the operation.

Q. *How often does tonsillitis result in rheumatic fever and/or nephritis or kidney trouble?*

A. Between 0.5 and 3 per cent of those having tonsillitis caused by the beta hemolytic streptococci will develop rheumatic fever, and about the same number will get nephritis. The nephritis is known to follow infection with only certain strains of the streptococcus.

29: Pneumonia

Pneumonia means inflammation of the lung. It was formerly a dreaded and often fatal disease. While it is still very severe, and often dangerous, many forms can be cured rapidly. The mortality from pneumonia has dropped strikingly since the sulfa drugs and antibiotics were discovered. Nowadays pneumonia is rarely fatal in children other than the newborn except when it is a complication of some other serious disease and when it is caused by agents which do not respond to available drugs. It is usually an acute disease, but occasionally it is chronic.

Pneumonia occurs everywhere, at all ages and in all seasons. It is more common and more severe in infants and elderly people or debilitated people of any age. In temperate climates it is most frequent in winter and in spring, less frequent in late fall, and much less common in summer. It is often a complication of a cold and frequently follows measles, whooping cough and influenza. Pneumonia can be caused by bacteria, most commonly by the pneumococcus, streptococcus and staphylococcus, especially in infants, and by the influenza bacillus. Tuberculosis often produces pneumonia in persons recently infected. Pneumonia can be caused by viruses of many varieties (more especially by the influenza virus), by the mycoplasma pneumoniae (also known as PPLO), the Eaton Agent, an organism in-between a virus and a bacterium, and by rickettsiae. Pneumonia can be caused by fungi, protozoa, oil and powder.

While the influenza viruses, of which there are at least fifteen varieties, the Eaton Agent and mycoplasma pneumoniae are common causes of pneumonia, many other viruses produce the disease.

Atypical pneumonia is caused by the Eaton Agent.

An attack of pneumonia due to bacteria results in only passing immunity. Pneumonia due to one of the influenza viruses may result in lasting immunity to that particular virus, but we know of many different viruses which cause influenza.

Contagion: Pneumonia is not as contagious as measles, whooping cough or chicken pox, but it can be contagious, especially the virus type which is much more likely to spread to contacts. I have seen the virus type of pneumonia spread from one to another member of a family until all eight persons had it within a period of two weeks. Similarly, bacterial pneumonia can be spread to contacts, particularly those in intimate association for many days.

Incubation Period: The incubation period for virus pneumonia is from seven to fourteen days. It is not well established for bacterial pneumonia, but it may be two or three days.

Symptoms: Ordinarily we can tell that a child has developed pneumonia by the following: he usually has fever, ranging from 101° to 104°, but occasionally as low as 100°; he has a hacking type of cough and he may have pain in the chest. The pain in the chest is due to pleurisy (inflammation of the pleura, the membrane covering the lung and lining the chest wall). Pleurisy is always part of pneumonia. It may be very mild, or become severe enough to dominate the illness. The child may have difficulty in breathing, his face may be flushed, and if enough of the lung is involved, his lips and fingertips may become bluish from lack of oxygen in the blood. When the temperature is very high at the onset of pneumonia, the infant or young child may develop muscular twitching, and sometimes a generalized convulsion. This is more likely to happen if the child is prone to have convulsions with fever. A high white blood cell count may be helpful in suggesting the presence of infection, and in the presence of obvious pneumonia, a low white blood cell count suggests pneumonia of virus origin. Pneumonia occurs in two forms, lobar pneumonia and bronchopneumonia. Their symptoms vary considerably or resemble each other so much that it is impossible to distinguish one from the other.

LOBAR PNEUMONIA

In lobar pneumonia the bacteria causing the infection, usually a pneumococcus, get into the blood by way of the throat and then into the lungs. In this case, the disease has a sudden onset with a chill, sometimes with a convulsion in young children, pain in the chest and a high fever. The child may vomit and complain of abdominal pain, sometimes severe enough to be mistaken for acute appendicitis. The child looks very sick, and breathing is rapid and may be labored. He often becomes flushed or develops a dusky or bluish color around the mouth and fingernails. This type of pneumonia lasts for six or seven days if treatment is not started promptly, and usually ends with a crisis, or a sudden and rapid drop of the temperature and a marked general improvement. The crisis is generally a favorable, not a dangerous, event because it heralds the beginning of recovery. Fortunately, lobar pneumonia, due to a pneumococcus, is the type which responds very quickly to treatment with antibiotics. A child who has lobar pneumonia and is given penicillin or another drug may be desperately ill one day, and if promptly treated he may improve so rapidly that by the next day he may sit up and demand to be permitted out of bed, even though he might have X-ray evidence of pneumonia for several days thereafter.

BRONCHOPNEUMONIA

There are many different forms of bronchopneumonia. They usually come about somewhat differently from the lobar type. A plug of mucus from the throat or large upper bronchial tubes drops down and closes off one or more of the smaller bronchial tubes, or an infection and swelling of the larger bronchial tubes (bronchitis) spread downward, finally reaching the very small bronchioles and closing them off. This makes it impossible for air to enter the segments of the lung which are connected to these closed-off bronchioles. Because no fresh air can get into the involved part of the lung, bacteria are trapped there and start an infection. The body's fight against the infection results in an accumulation of pus cells, bacteria and fluid (serum) which oozes from the tiny blood vessels. These substances fill the air sacs and produce pneumonia. There may be few or many little areas involved at the same time in different segments of the lung, or one segment after another becomes involved. This patchy type of involvement of the lung is characteristic of bronchopneumonia.

Bronchopneumonia may be initiated in other ways—for example, by the aspiration (drawing into the lung) of a foreign body, vomitus, or blood, through injury, or through stagnation of blood because of inactivity.

Bronchopneumonia is not quite as abrupt in its onset as is the lobar type of pneumonia and ends gradually, or by lysis. The temperature becomes lower over a period of a few days, in contrast to lobar pneumonia in which the temperature drops abruptly in twelve to twenty-four hours, or by crisis. If untreated, bronchopneumonia may last eight to fourteen days. While not quite as dramatic as lobar pneumonia, bronchopneumonia is just as serious. Like lobar pneumonia, it responds to the antibiotics which are best suited for the particular germ that produces the disease, except when the causative agent is a virus.

Aspiration Pneumonia: Aspiration pneumonia occurs quite frequently in premature infants, and in very old and debilitated persons who are so weak that they cannot swallow the mucus in the throat. When mucus accumulates in the throat it may be pulled down (aspirated) into the lungs by a sudden forced breath. There it keeps the air from getting into the segments of the lung it has blocked off and sets up pneumonia. The same is true for patients who have paralysis of the throat, for example, in bulbar polio, or in paralysis of the throat following diphtheria. In the patient with polio who is in an iron lung, this condition is quite common.

Foreign-Body Pneumonia: A foreign body in the lung or in a bronchial tube also produces bronchopneumonia. An infant may vomit and then take a deep breath and inhale some of the vomitus. During a tonsil operation a child may aspirate a loose tooth, or he may pull down a great deal of blood which may set up aspiration pneumonia.

A child may aspirate a small toy. A nut, especially a peanut, is a common foreign body in the bronchial tube of a child and it not only closes off a segment of the lung, but also as the nut degenerates it liberates an oil which is very irritating and sets up an inflammation in the lung.

A foreign body in the lung may produce symptoms which are similar to those of severe bronchitis or bronchopneumonia. The fact that there is a foreign body involved is usually detected by the history of having choked over something, and the findings on X-ray of the lungs. A foreign body usually requires bronchoscopy (viewing the inside of the bronchial tubes through a long illuminated metal tube). If a foreign body is found, an attempt is made to remove it by suction through the bronchoscope or by grasping the object with a long forceps.

Lipoid Pneumonia: Lipoid pneumonia is another type of foreign-body pneumonia, or aspiration pneumonia, which was quite common years ago, but is now seen infrequently since most nose drops do not contain oil as they used to. If infants are repeatedly given nose drops containing oil, if they are given mineral oil for constipation or cod-liver oil and they vomit it and aspirate some of the oil, it remains in the lung and causes irritation and pneumonic reaction around the oil droplets. Lipoid pneumonia is a rather stubborn type of pneumonia which lasts a long time.

Kerosene swallowed by accident is often vomited and aspirated, causing pneumonia. Kerosene fumes are also very irritating.

Traumatic Pneumonia: This means pneumonia caused by injury and is another kind of bronchopneumonia. For example, if a child is in an automobile accident and receives a blow to the chest, the lung or the ribs may be injured. Small blood vessels are ruptured and bacteria drawn in with breathing lodge at the injured site and produce inflammation. If this happens the child might have pneumonia close to the part of the chest which was injured. This usually comes within a day or two and behaves like ordinary pneumonia.

Hypostatic Pneumonia: Hypostatic pneumonia is another form of bronchopneumonia which occurs in the very feeble, in the premature and collapsed infant who does not move about and in the child who is forced to remain on his back for a long time because of illness or injury. This inactivity usually results in puddling of blood in the lowest part of the lung. The blood which accumulates there is relatively stagnant; this is conducive to infection, and inflammation will set in. This is particularly true in older people who are ill or who have been operated upon, and is one of the reasons why patients nowadays are not permitted to stay in bed any longer than is absolutely necessary. If they must be in bed, their positions are changed as frequently as possible.

Virus Pneumonia, Including Primary Atypical Pneumonia: There is a form of bronchopneumonia caused by viruses rather than by bacteria. While several different viruses can cause pnuemonia, the influenza virus and those organisms, such as the Eaton Agent, producing primary atypical pneumonia are the most frequently encountered. Virus pneumonia may be severe, in which case the child feels and looks sick, coughs a great deal, has a temperature between 101° and 104° daily, and when the chest is examined by the doctor the presence of pneumonia may be easily detected. In rare instances it may be so extreme (especially some forms of influenza pneumonia) as to be rapidly fatal. On the other hand, the disease may be, and often is, so mild as to be difficult to detect.

Primary atypical pneumonia, one of the most common of the "virus" pneumonias, varies greatly in its pattern. When it is mild a child may have a low-grade temperature, 100° to 101° every day, feel tired and ill at ease, irritable and cranky, and cough occasionally. The child may act as if he has a cold, yet on examination of the chest the doctor may hear the signs of pneumonia. In some cases the doctor may hear nothing of importance for as long as seven or eight days, yet on X-ray examination of the chest, pneumonia may be quite evident. Virus pneumonia varies considerably in its duration. The primary atypical disease may last as little as three days or as long as three weeks, the average duration being about ten to fourteen days. Virus pneumonia differs from bacterial pneumonia in that it is usually less dramatic in its onset, and less dramatic in its termination. If it is determined that the pneumonia is caused by the mycoplasma pneumoniae, antibiotics of the tetracycline group are rapidly helpful. If the disease is caused by other viruses, we have no specific drugs. In such a case I prefer to withhold treatment with antibiotics. If in doubt whether the pneumonia is viral or bacterial in origin, it may be wiser to treat it as if the infection is bacterial.

Virus pneumonia is occasionally followed by bronchopneumonia due to bacteria. While this does not occur frequently, some doctors give antibiotics to patients who are known to have virus pneumonia, hoping thus to avoid this complication. Personally, I prefer to withhold antibiotic treatment if the pneumonia is known to be caused by a virus and to reserve it in case complications develop.

TREATMENT

All children with acute pneumonia of any type should remain in bed. The room should be well aired, and the temperature kept near 68° or 70° F. The patient's fever can be kept down with aspirin and tepid-water sponges or alcohol rubs. Oxygen is a great help and is urgently needed if the child is breathing very rapidly with grunting and flaring of the nostrils, or if the child is dusky or bluish around the mouth and under the fingernails, and particularly if he is restless.

The diet should be mostly liquid during the very acute phase because of air hunger, but the child may eat solid food as soon as he feels well enough. The only restriction is that the meals should not be heavy.

The child is kept in bed for about three days after the temperature is normal and after the lungs are clear of signs of pneumonia. During this period bathroom privileges may be allowed.

Antibiotics cure most types of bacterial pneumonia, and the kind caused by the psittacosis virus (parrot fever) and the type caused by the Eaton Agent, but they do not cure other virus pneumonias. The pneumonia caused by the pneumococcus responds most rapidly. Antibiotics must be prescribed by the doctor according to which he thinks most suitable in view of his diagnosis. The treatment should be started quickly and continued for two or three days after the temperature has returned to normal and chest signs of pneumonia have disappeared. I have observed a dramatic drop in temperature in twenty-four hours after beginning treatment of pneumonia with a sulfa drug or with penicillin, but daily X-ray examination of the lungs showed that it took three to thirteen days for them to become normal again. During that entire time the child was anxious to get out of bed and play, and the parents found it hard to believe that such a lively child could still have pneumonia. Do not be fooled by the child's behavior after antibiotics have made the fever disappear. It is still important to keep him from overexerting himself and to treat him for as long as the doctor thinks necessary.

Occasionally pneumonia does not clear up rapidly, but lasts for weeks and months. It becomes chronic. This, however, is rather uncommon. If the pneumonia is chronic, antibiotics should be employed, as indicated by the type of infection. Continued bed rest and house confinement may be unnecessary.

Convalescence: Convalescence depends a great deal on the severity and duration of the disease, and on the age of the child. Although some children recover very rapidly, others tire easily for several weeks. Head sweats are common for a month or longer.

After recovery from pneumonia, a child should convalesce for at least a week between getting out of bed and going back to school. Some need two weeks. Exercise should be started gradually. A short walk out of doors equal to about two city blocks may suffice at first. This is increased progressively, and the child may usually resume all activities, including sports, within two to four weeks.

Isolation and Quarantine: A child with pnuemonia ought to be isolated for the duration of the illness. It would not be safe to have other children sleep in the same room during the

acute phase of the infection, nor should other children visit
during that period. Those exposed to the disease need not be
quarantined. They may attend school just as they would if
one of their siblings had bronchitis, a cold or sinusitis.

Hygiene: If a child has lobar pneumonia or bronchopneumonia the dishes and laundry need not be treated in a special
way. The dishes should be thoroughly washed, and the
laundry washed with that of the rest of the family. It is not
necessary to sterilize the excreta.

QUESTIONS & ANSWERS

Q. *Are there other causes of pneumonia besides the ones you
have mentioned?*

A. Yes. Pneumonia can be caused by psittacosis (parrot
fever), typhus fever, tularemia (an infection that is usually transmitted by animals like deer and rabbits) and
many other diseases. In these conditions the pneumonia
is caused by the bacteria or the viruses which cause the
specific diseases and is treated accordingly.

Q. *Does the age of a child have anything to do with the kind
of pneumonia he gets?*

A. Yes. In the first year of life pneumonia is usually due to a
staphylococcus. This germ has a particular tendency to
cause abscesses in the lungs.

Q. *Is the immunity you get from pneumonia long-lasting?*

A. That depends on the cause. In virus pneumonia, it may be
for years, though we do not know the exact duration. If it
is caused by one of the pneumococcus germs, the immunity lasts about a month, perhaps longer. Again we do
not know exactly how long. Some children get repeated
attacks of pneumonia, but each one may be caused by a
different germ.

Q. *Does chilling make you more likely to get pneumonia?*

A. Under certain conditions. For instance, if a child has a
cold, sore throat or bronchitis, it may. But when he is in

good physical condition and the environment is not rich with the bacteria which cause pneumonia, chilling seems to have no effect. Children who go on overnight camping trips and get wet and chilled rarely get pneumonia.

Q. *How can you tell the difference between virus and bacterial pneumonia?*

A. The white blood cell count is usually high in bacterial pneumonia and is relatively low in virus pneumonia. In about 83 per cent of cases of bacterial pneumonia the bacteria can be found in the throat. There are other tests which indicate the presence of virus pneumonia.

Q. *How can you tell when pneumonia is finished?*

A. Pneumonia causes certain signs which the doctor can detect when he listens to a child's chest with a stethoscope. After the child has recovered, the doctor can no longer hear them. It is often necessary, however, to X-ray the patient before you can be sure that the pneumonia is completely cured. I make it a rule either to fluoroscope or X-ray every one of my pneumonia patients before I let him return to school or to full activity.

Q. *If pneumonia is contagious, should the child be treated at home or does he have to be taken to a hospital?*

A. He can usually be cared for at home. If he is desperately ill and needs oxygen treatment, or if it is not possible to keep him in a separate room, or if he cannot be attended around the clock, he should be taken to a hospital.

Q. *Is it safe to wash my child's hair while she has pneumonia?*

A. No. Wait until she is well.

Q. *May I give my child a bath while he has pneumonia?*

A. A tub bath would be unwarranted. The child is much too sick and a tub bath may present a problem. If he is uncomfortable because of sweating or because he has been ill for several days, a bed bath might be given, provided only one small part of his body is exposed at one time.

Q. *Does the treatment of pneumonia vary with the cause?*

A. The treatment is essentially the same except that the choice of an antibiotic may vary. In the case of foreign-body pneumonia, especially if it is caused by a solid object like a peanut or a toy, the object must be removed, otherwise there is great likelihood that an abscess of the lung will form.

Q. *Are all antibiotics effective against pneumonia?*

A. No, not all but many are. The choice must depend on the bacteria causing it. It is generally safe and correct to start with penicillin or a penicillin-like antibiotic. Sulfa drugs may be quite effective. If the infection is caused by a staphylococcus, some of these drugs are better than others.

Q. *Is whiskey good for pneumonia?*

A. It serves as a stimulant, but it is rarely given to children now, as it used to be.

Q. *Should a child with pneumonia be kept in cold air?*

A. Fresh air and oxygen are helpful, but cold air is not necessary.

Q. *Is pneumonia likely to spread to the rest of the household if the child is kept in a separate room?*

A. No.

Q. *Can you be immunized against pneumonia?*

A. It is difficult to do, but it is possible for some types caused by viruses.

Q. *How can you avoid pneumonia?*

A. Primarily by avoiding the diseases which cause it, and by treating colds, sore throats and sinus infections actively so that pneumonia does not set in.

Q. *Is it necessary to do anything special with a child's room after he has been sick with pneumonia?*

A. Give it a thorough cleaning, let it air for several hours and, of course, change the bedclothes. Then it will be safe for healthy children.

30: Earache

___

MIDDLE EAR INFECTION
(OTITIS MEDIA)

Infection of the middle ear is a very common disease everywhere. Almost every child has an earache sometime during
his early years. Some children have repeated infections of the
ears, often as many as two, three or four times in a winter.
They usually outgrow this tendency as they get older.

The ear consists of three parts: the auricle or external ear
(the part you can see and the canal that leads to the eardrum);
the middle ear, the space containing the little bones which
conduct sound waves to the inner ear, covered on the outside
by the tympanic membrane or eardrum; and the inner ear
which contains the nerves of hearing and the mechanism
which controls balance. When your child complains of an
earache, it is usually the middle ear which is infected.

Ear infections are usually caused by one of the bacteria
like the streptococcus, staphylococcus, pneumococcus, the influenza bacterium and sometimes some of the less common
ones. They are almost always the result of an infection of the
nose or throat or one of the acute diseases like the common
cold, the sore throat, measles, chicken pox, mumps, tonsillitis
or adenoiditis. They may also result from swimming and diving
because water is forced into the nose and into the Eustachian
tubes, the pathways between the back of the throat and the
ears.

Repeated ear infections sometimes cause permanent hearing
difficulty because the eardrum becomes thickened and misshapen when it is inflamed over and over again. In the past,

ear infections accounted for a large number of the children in institutions for the hard of hearing, and chronic discharging ears were numerous. This is less true now that we have the sulfa drugs and antibiotics which are so effective in curing them.

Symptoms: Otitis media usually starts with severe pain in the ear and fever. The child cries inconsolably. The pain may be excruciating and may continue for a variable period, six to eight hours, or even for several days. It is caused by the inflammation of the eardrum and by pressure against the eardrum from serum or pus in the middle ear. If no treatment is given, the pain may continue until the infection quiets down, or until an abscess forms, causing the eardrum to break. When this happens, the pus in the middle ear is suddenly released, and the child is temporarily relieved of pain. In some types of otitis, blisters form on the eardrum. There is pain for four to twelve hours, and then the child may hear a swishing or bubbling sound made by the motion of the fluid in the blisters.

The ear infection may be accompanied by fever of any degree, ranging from almost no fever to temperatures of between 101° and 106°. It is not unusual for infants to develop extraordinarily high fevers with a simple ear infection. Babies who are too young to speak indicate pain by crying a great deal, by refusing a bottle or food and by being restless. They may pull at or rub the ear that hurts, or turn their heads from side to side. They may react in other ways, too. For example, if the temperature is very high, the baby may be jittery, even to the point of a convulsion. He may vomit and develop diarrhea. Sometimes there is no evidence of pain at all, or even fever. In very young infants vomiting and diarrhea may be the only obvious symptoms. It is the careful physician who, in such cases, will discover that the illness is due to ear inflammation.

Diagnosis: When a doctor sees a child because he has a high fever and is crying without letup, he always examines his ears and often finds the explanation there. He may see a red, thickened and misshapen eardrum instead of a normally smooth gray one. He may find blisters on the eardrum, and if the eardrum is ruptured, he will probably find pus or blood or both.

Treatment: If an ear infection is left untreated, about 75 to 90 per cent get well by themselves, but only after a period of several days to two weeks during which the child suffers considerably. Before treatment with sulfonamides and antibiotics was available, 10 per cent or more of ear infections resulted in rupture of the eardrum with draining of pus from the middle ear. About 2 or 3 per cent developed mastoid infection (breaking down of the bone behind the ear) for which an operation was necessary.

Some time ago, when a child had a middle ear infection and it progressed, it was customary for the doctor to make an opening in the eardrum to release the pus. Often the pain would stop dramatically and the child's condition would improve. Nowadays, opening the ear is rarely necessary if treatment with suitable antibiotics and sulfa drugs is started early and continued until the child is completely recovered. Among my own patients in the past twenty years, it has not been necessary to have an eardrum opened or a mastoid operation done, except in a child whom I did not see until after the infection had advanced to the point of serious complications. Obviously, I do not encourage opening an ear except when it is absolutely necessary, but it must be said that there are many able ear specialists who feel otherwise. They continue to open (lance) the eardrum because, in their opinion, the patient fares better after that has been done.

Do not depend on your own treatment for ear infections. Call a doctor and let him look at the ear and tell you what treatment is best. When the child's temperature drops and the earache is gone, you may be tempted to stop the treatment. This would be a serious mistake since it is not unusual for an ear infection which is not completely cured to become active again. It usually takes a week or more for an infected ear to recover completely after it first appears to be normal. Therefore it is necessary to keep up the drugs for at least three, four or five, or even seven days after that time. Do not decide yourself when to stop the treatment. Let this be your doctor's decision.

Complications: Since we have had the sulfa drugs and antibiotics, it is usually the untreated or insufficiently treated child who develops a mastoid infection or other complications. If a child with an acute ear infection is left untreated, or if the treatment is haphazard, either not long enough or not intensive enough, the infection may seem cured temporarily, but it may linger and reappear. This might cause breaking down of the mastoid bone, or go on to produce one of the more serious complications, infections which might lead to meningitis. Meningitis used to be a dreaded complication of ear infections, but it is relatively rare these days. Occasionally an ear infection results in a chronic discharge. This is a very difficult thing to correct, and in some cases it may require surgical operation of the mastoid.

Adenoids and Hearing: Children with very large adenoids who have frequent colds are more likely than others to have ear infections. Sometimes it is necessary to take out the adenoids to reduce the number of ear infections. The adenoids are next to the opening of the Eustachian tubes, which are narrow canals between the ears and the back of the throat. In adults they are fairly long and winding, but in infants they are short and straight, which makes it easier for infected material to travel into the ear from the throat. When the throat end of this tube is blocked by enlarged adenoids, the passage of air from the throat to the middle ear is interfered with and infection is more likely to set in. Children whose adenoids have been removed have fewer ear infections than they did before. If, after the adenoids have been removed, the child goes on having ear infections or is having trouble with hearing, it may be due to the regrowth of adenoid tissue (lymph tissue) at the opening of the Eustachian tubes or into them. This can cause hearing difficulties as well as infection. The lymph tissue can be shrunk with either X-ray or radium, or sometimes another operation is necessary to remove it.

Isolation and Quarantine: If a child has an ear infection, he need not be isolated unless it is necessary because of the disease which caused the ear infection. A child exposed to an ear infection is not quarantined unless it is part of measles, scarlet fever, diphtheria or some disease of that sort for which there are quarantine and isolation regulations. In nurseries, or where several babies occupy the same room or ward, it is safer to isolate a child with a running ear because infants are more susceptible to infection and it is more easily spread in nurseries.

EXTERNAL EAR INFECTION
(OTITIS EXTERNA)

So far, I have discussed only middle ear infection. Occasionally the external part of the ear (the part you can see and the canal into the middle ear) is infected. This is essentially the same as a skin irritation anywhere else and is usually caused by bacteria, as in the case of a boil. It is painful, especially when the ear is pressed or moved about and when the child moves his jaw, but there is little or no fever. This is not as serious as middle ear infection, but it requires treatment. Since the infection can be quite variable, it should be seen by a doctor so that he can make the correct diagnosis and prescribe the proper treatment.

Occasionally, an infection of the external ear is caused by a fungus. This is usually painful, lasts longer than the bacterial infection, and may not respond to antibiotic treatment. It is treated with medication applied locally.

Tuberculosis of the ear is another kind of infection, but the tuberculosis is practically never limited to the ear. It accompanies tuberculosis of some other part of the body. It causes long-standing discharge with little or no pain. Other less frequent diseases may also cause ear infections, but we need not concern ourselves with these rare ones here.

QUESTIONS & ANSWERS

Q. *Can you have an earache at any age?*
A. Yes.

Q.   *I used to have earaches when I was a child, and now my little girl does. Is it inherited?*

A.   No, but possibly you are both constructed in such a way that infection gets into your ears easily.

Q.   *Does an earache always mean that you have a cold or some other infection?*

A.   Yes, except when you have forced some water into the back of your nose and into your Eustachian tube as you might while swimming or diving.

Q.   *Is a swimming ear like all other ear infections?*

A.   Yes, if it becomes infected.

Q.   *It is helpful to wear ear plugs to prevent ear infections?*

A.   No, because the infection does not begin from the outside of the ear.

Q.   *Is an ear infection contagious?*

A.   No, but the infection of the nose and throat or the cold which caused the ear infection may be contagious. In nurseries or at home, if more than one baby occupies the same room, a baby with a running ear should be isolated.

Q.   *Is it possible to have a running ear without having had pain or fever?*

A.   Yes. Children suffer pain in different degrees. In a child who has great tolerance for pain, an ear may be infected and the eardrum rupture without the child's knowing it until someone notices that fluid or pus is coming from the ear. This type of child who doesn't suffer pain acutely must be watched very carefully because he may develop complications without showing many signs of them.

Q.   *My child has had an earache for a few days. At first he didn't want to eat, but now he is ravenous. Is it all right to feed him all he wants?*

A.   Yes. The fact that he wants food usually means he is getting well.

Q.   *Must the food be liquids only?*

A.   No, it may be any kind.

Q.   *Should a child be kept in bed when he has an infected ear?*

A. He will probably be more comfortable in bed, but if he has no fever and no pain, it is usually quite all right for him to get up and be about the house. If the weather is warm, he may go outdoors.

Q. *When I was a child, I had my ear lanced several times. Should that be done when my child gets an ear infection?*

A. It is usually not necessary if treatment with sulfa drugs or antibiotics is started early and the child shows signs of steady improvement.

Q. *Do you mean that an eardrum should never be lanced?*

A. There is no "never" in medicine. It may be necessary to lance the eardrum under certain conditions, but it is quite uncommon today as compared with the frequency with which it had to be done before we had antibiotics and sulfa drugs.

Q. *My doctor advises me to have my child's tonsils taken out to avoid frequent ear infections. Is that your opinion, too?*

A. If you mean also removing the adenoids, yes. It is the adenoids, not the tonsils, which interfere with the Eustachian tubes and the middle ear, and it is the removal of the adenoids which helps to reduce the number of ear infections.

Q. *My child's tonsils and adenoids have been removed, but he gets as many ear infections as ever. What shall I do?*

A. Have the ear doctor check to see whether the adenoid tissue has grown back near the Eustachian tube. This may explain the repeated infections and it may need further treatment. Another reason for repeated infections is that some people are constructed differently from others so that infections get into their ears more easily. There is nothing you can do about such people except to treat the infection as soon as it starts.

Q. *My child has had several ear infections and now seems to hear badly. He asks "what?" whenever I speak to him. What do you think I should do?*

A. I think you should take him to an ear doctor right away. The doctor can find out whether the child's hearing is really affected and whether it is caused by blocking of the Eustachian tubes by adenoid tissue.

Q. *My doctor told me that my child's kidneys were injured by an ear infection. Is that possible?*

A. Yes. The kidneys can be injured by an infection of any part of the body. Infection of the tonsils or the throat are more likely to cause nephritis (inflammation of the kidneys), but ear infection can certainly do it, too, since it often goes with tonsil and throat infection. It must be a streptococcal infection to cause nephritis.

PART FOUR

Diseases of the Nervous System

31: Poliomyelitis (Infantile Paralysis)

Infantile paralysis is an inaccurate and frightening name for a disease which is relatively infrequent among infants in many parts of the world and which, in most cases, does not paralyze. I prefer the name *poliomyelitis*, but in the interest of brevity I shall refer to the disease in this book as polio.

It was first described some sixty years ago by Heine and Medin, but we know from paintings and writings that the paralysis which occurs with polio was appreciated long before. It occurs throughout the world.

It would be sufficient for most readers of this book if I stressed the dramatic results of the widespread use of polio vaccine. Paralytic polio in the United States is no longer a serious problem and is not likely to be, so long as all of our infants and children are vaccinated with the attenuated live-polio-virus vaccine.

I include a description of the disease and suggest treatment since it is still a dreadful disease which is altogether too common in some parts of the world. Perhaps the description will also alert the readers in countries where the disease is less common to be diligent about vaccinating their children. People in countries which do not have the live polio vaccine should urge their governments to make it available to all who need it.

Paralytic poliomyelitis was formerly a most frightening disease in the United States. During an epidemic there was real panic. People tried, often unsuccessfully, to run away from epidemic areas. They avoided crowds, carried packets of camphor and to protect themselves from the disease adopted any recommendation offered them. No one living in a community made safe by immunization of most children will ever know or appreciate the fear, the panic, that prevailed when the disease was common.

In New York we had major epidemics in 1916, 1931, 1935, 1941 and 1949. In 1949 we treated about seven hundred and fifty cases at the Willard Parker Hospital and nearly five hundred the next year. The epidemics occurred from June through November. Summer and early fall or the equivalent seasons in South America and other areas are the periods of greatest incidence of the disease in temperate climates. In tropical climates it may occur throughout the year. It is very rare in a cold season. Thanks to the polio vaccine, in 1966 and 1967 we had no cases of polio in New York City.

There are three different polio viruses, each of which is capable of producing the disease, but Type II is less likely to produce serious disease. Type I was responsible for most epidemics, and Type III to a lesser degree. The immunity which results from each type is specific—immunity from one type, e.g., Type I, does not protect against infection with Types II or III. Yet, second attacks of polio are rare, probably because repeated exposure to the various types of polio virus results in widespread immunity to all three types, just as if regular booster doses of vaccine were given.

In the United States, polio was most common in children from the ages of five to nine. A few cases have been observed already started in newborn infants, proving that it is possible for the virus to enter the mother and pass across the placenta (afterbirth) to infect the newborn infant.

Infants born to mothers who are immune to polio acquire protection from those viruses to which the mother is immune. This immunity lasts a few months in the infant, but this should not suggest delay in vaccination. Pregnant women seem to be especially susceptible.

Contagion: If you judge by the relatively small number of obvious cases of polio, you would assume that it is not highly contagious, but for each case diagnosed as polio, probably fifty to a hundred more people are infected without developing signs or symptoms. They have what is called abortive polio which gives them immunity. If they live in an area where polio is always present, the chances are that they are repeatedly exposed to it and thus sustain this high level of immunity.

The manner of spread of polio has not been definitely established. The virus is often passed on by patients who have the disease. The patient with polio harbors the virus in his throat for the first few days before he shows any recognizable symptoms and probably is a greater source of danger to other people a day or two *before* the illness than *after* symptoms appear. The virus may remain in his bowels for as long as two to eight weeks, and in rare cases, a few months.

The virus has been found on flies caught in the rooms of polio patients, and outside of their homes, but it has not been proved that flies actually cause the disease. It is possible that the infection is spread through contaminated milk and other food, but we do not know how often this happens. The virus has been found in city sewage and it is possible that children playing near it could be infected. Our knowledge of these facts is rather uncertain, but what we do know helps us in deciding on the hygienic measures to be taken to prevent the spread of the disease.

Nurses and doctors who take care of polio patients in hospitals and in epidemic areas are more likely to get polio than other adults of the same age group. One reason for this may be that doctors and nurses are apt to be exposed early in the disease when the patients still have the polio virus in their throats. Another reason may be that nurses and doctors come into intimate contact with the patients, their bedclothes and their bodies, which may be contaminated with stool containing the living polio virus.

Incubation Period: The incubation period of polio is seven to fourteen days, occasionally as much as twenty-one days, and rarely as long as thirty days.

Symptoms: The polio virus attacks the nervous system especially, but we now know that it gets into the blood and is distributed to other parts of the body, for instance, the heart. The heart is sometimes seriously involved in polio, but if the patient survives, the heart always seems to recover. It is the nervous-system involvement which makes polio so serious, because when the nerves controlling a muscle are destroyed, the muscle withers. There are several different types of polio, depending on which part of the nervous system is involved.

ABORTIVE TYPE

Abortive polio is by far the most common. It occurs without any signs or symptoms, or sometimes it is so mild as to be mistaken for a cold or a stomach upset.

NONPARALYTIC TYPE

The illness may start with a fever of 100° to 101°, headache, pain and stiffness in the back of the neck and the lower back, vomiting, sore throat, a suggestion of a head cold or a stomach or intestinal upset, or with any combination of any of these symptoms. At this time, an examination of the spinal fluid (obtained by inserting a hollow needle in the lower spine) will show an increase in the cells which are characteristic of the disease. The fever lasts about five days, the headache and nausea usually not so long, the stiffness of the neck becomes progressively better and usually disappears in three to five days, sometimes longer. The stiffness of the back may only last a day or two or it may persist long after the other signs of the illness are gone.

If the illness passes without noticeable signs of muscular weakness, it is known as the nonparalytic type. About 50 per cent of cases with recognizable symptoms fall into this class, although some observers who have examined the patients in meticulous detail with the object of discovering muscular weakness have found some minor evidence of it in as many as 90 per cent of nonparalytic cases. These weaknesses were so small, however, that usually the patients themselves were unaware of them.

SPINAL PARALYTIC TYPE

This form of polio occurs in about 30 per cent of the cases. It may start quite like the nonparalytic type except that the weakness (paresis) develops in one or both arms, shoulders or legs, or first in a part of one side and then in a part of the other. Weakness or paralysis usually sets in one to seven days after the onset of the symptoms—in some cases as long as ten or twelve days later. The spinal paralytic type may be accompanied by pain in the muscles of the arms, legs, thighs and back. In some cases of this form, the weakness or paralysis subsides. The reflexes in the affected parts may disappear early in the disease, then return. This return is a good sign, for it indicates improvement in the nerves and weakened muscles. If the recovery is going to be complete, this improvement usually takes place rapidly over a period of a few weeks. In other cases the weakness or paralysis, instead of subsiding, spreads, and if recovery is slow, some weakness or paralysis may remain permanently.

BULBAR TYPE

Another type of polio is called bulbar polio because it involves the region (the medulla or bulb of the brain) which separates the spinal cord from the brain. This part of the brain controls breathing, swallowing, body temperature and heart action. About 15 to 18 per cent of polio cases are the bulbar type. It begins as the nonparalytic type does, but after one, two or three days the child's speech becomes nasal and when he swallows liquid some of it may come up through his nose. He may complain of being unable to swallow. The situation may become urgent because of breathing difficulty. It is this bulbar type which so often requires the use of an iron lung for artificial respiration. Occasionally, especially when the child has lost the ability to swallow, an opening in the windpipe must be made (tracheotomy) through which to suction the saliva and mucus out of the throat so that it will not be pulled down into the lungs when he breathes. The bulbar type is often combined with the spinal paralytic form. Most of the very bad results of polio occur in the bulbar group and in the bulbospinal group.

ENCEPHALITIC TYPE

When polio involves the brain itself more extensively, it is called the encephalitic type. This type is also serious. The child is very drowsy and may lapse into a sleep (coma) from which he cannot be aroused. Artificial respiration may be needed, and here again a tracheotomy may have to be done so that he can get air more easily and without pulling the mucus from his throat into his lungs.

Polio is not necessarily of one type or another. It may develop as a combination of the types I have described. Bulbar polio, for instance, may begin as the spinal paralytic type, but the involvement of the spinal cord spreads upward until it involves the midbrain and causes difficulty in regulation of swallowing, breathing, blood pressure and temperature. The patient may have very high blood pressure, and may maintain temperatures as high as 104° to 106°.

If I have worried you by my descriptions of the various kinds of polio, remember, as I said before, that for each case of polio with symptoms, about fifty to a hundred people become infected and develop immunity without ever being aware of having been ill. Or they may have the disease in such a mild form that they believe it to be a cold. They do not become paralyzed or develop any muscle weakness. Also, remember that fully half of those who do develop paralysis recover their muscle power, and many more improve a great deal.

DIAGNOSIS

Polio varies so strikingly in the patterns it assumes that diagnosis is often difficult. We know that it can be so mild as to go unrecognized because we have been able to find people who are immune, yet who have no recollection of having been ill. It can be extremely severe and acute, and be fatal in a day or two. The pains in the arms and legs sometimes make it seem like rheumatic fever or osteomyelitis, an infection of the bone, and it can be mistaken for other diseases of the brain and spinal cord. On the other hand, other diseases are sometimes mistaken for polio. About 20 per cent of cases tentatively diagnosed as polio later prove to be other infections, especially mumps, choriomeningitis and other central nervous system infections, including those caused by some ECHO viruses. Fortunately, almost all of these cases recover.

If a child, especially one of the age group which most frequently gets polio in the area in which you live, develops the signs and symptoms I have described, they are probably due to polio. It is even more likely if it occurs during the polio season, or during an outbreak or an epidemic. Polio should be suspected and the child treated accordingly, even though it may turn out to be some other infection. Coarse tremors of the hands and face and stiffness of the neck and back are suggestive of polio, as is a temporary rise in blood pressure. The findings in the spinal fluid are helpful in making the diagnosis and in ruling out many other infections of the brain and spinal cord.

TREATMENT

Since polio can be so serious, it must be treated by a doctor who has had experience with it. A person diagnosed as having acute paralytic poliomyelitis should be in a hospital where the needed personnel and facilities are available. The patient may be kept at home if the disease is mild, if the isolation of the child in a separate room with bathroom facilities is possible, if one adult can be with the child around the clock and if the doctor will visit the child not less than twice a day, more often if necessary.

Changes in the condition of the child may occur rapidly, sometimes requiring emergency treatment with equipment not available at home, or in every hospital. The decision to leave the child at home or take him to a hospital must be made by the physician. The family may not, and should not, influence the doctor to keep the patient at home if the physician feels otherwise.

The child with polio should be kept in bed. If his neck or back is stiff, he will be more comfortable without a pillow. If there is any weakness of the feet or legs, the weight of the blankets should be kept off them with a foot board. He should be moved from side to side so that he is not always in the same position. He should be given sponge baths, and his skin should be freshened with alcohol rubs and powder once or twice daily. His diet should be light, but no foods are prohibited if he can swallow. Vitamins should be continued.

Hot wet packs are most comforting for painful or stiff muscles—much more effective than drugs and braces. If hot wet packs are too difficult to apply, an electric heating pad may be helpful, though not as much as the packs.

Aspirin is often given for high fever; a cooling mattress is useful for temperatures of 104° or higher. Sleeping drugs and painkillers of the narcotic type should not be given without the doctor's specific order. If the child is at home and begins to have difficulty swallowing or spitting out the accumulated mucus and saliva in his throat, he must be taken to a hospital immediately for necessary care.

After the child's temperature becomes normal, or earlier if there is muscle stiffness, weakness or paralysis, massage and passive exercise (in which the muscles are moved by someone besides the patient) may be started, in addition to the hot packs. These will help to relieve the pain of the stiff muscles, keep them from becoming stiffer, and may spare some weak muscles which are being stretched by the pull of the remaining strong ones.

PSYCHOLOGICAL REACTIONS

Polio is very frightening to the patient, even to very young children. They are usually even more frightened than their parents are. The fear of being paralyzed, of being helpless, or even of death itself, causes a child great anxiety. Some develop severe neuroses. This psychic upset is a serious complication and requires sympathetic handling and intelligent guidance right from the beginning of the illness and as long as the child remains handicapped. A parent who is incapable of concealing from her child the fact that she, too, is afraid, who hovers and worries over him, can do irreparable damage. This is the kind of parent whom I mentioned earlier as being "unable to cope with the situation." It is difficult for a worried mother to appear cheerful and hopeful, and if she cannot do it, it is better to have a professional hospital staff, which has been trained in the art of child care. If the child is not helped to conquer his own fears, they often show up in poor cooperation while he is being treated. He may not eat or rest enough; his breathing may be disturbed. All of these factors may make his condition worse or slow up his recovery.

There is no reason for a polio patient to go without the treatment he needs. Local and state health departments are most helpful, and are ready at all times to offer advice, facilities and aid of any kind you need, in whole or in part, for as long as care and treatment are recommended by your doctor.

PHYSICAL THERAPY

If the child is left with weakness or paralysis after convalescence sets in, trained physiotherapists take over. They teach the child how to use individual muscles. If some muscles have become weakened, they can show him how to use others to perform the functions of the weakened ones. They actually reeducate the child to make use of muscles he might otherwise forget to use or "alienate," as Sister Kenny used to say. Of course, it is impossible by any known means, including those I have mentioned, to get muscles to act if the nerves controlling their activity have been destroyed.

Weakened muscles continue to recover their functions over a long period of time, sometimes as long as two years, if the patient is well treated and the muscles are not further injured. Numerous drugs are available to help make this process less painful and more effective, but these are little if at all better than the passive exercise, massage and hot packs. Sister

Kenny stressed the need for earlier use of physical therapy, especially moist heat, passive exercise and muscle reeducation.

Orthopedic devices, such as braces, supports and special shoes, may be necessary. And other forms of physiotherapy such as swimming pools, whirlpool baths and so forth may be recommended.

OCCUPATIONAL THERAPY

When a child has polio, it is important for him to be occupied and to learn to use his muscles effectively, and it is most important to keep his morale high. Occupational therapy should be started as soon as possible. You should stress every return of function of a weakened muscle as evidence of progress toward recovery. It is much easier to encourage a child and to get cooperation from him if he feels he is getting well than if he has given up hope.

If paralysis has set in and it does not seem likely that the muscles will recover, you must teach the child to compensate for his handicaps. If he cannot go to school, he should have instruction at home or in the hospital. If a right-handed child has a weak right hand, you may have to teach him to use his left hand more effectively. If his legs are weakened, he may have to develop greater power in his arms to compensate. The child must be helped to make the best of a difficult situation by making the most of the powers he has left. If you can make this rehabilitation program a challenge to him, if you can keep him from feeling too sorry for himself, your job will be infinitely easier.

In my class at college the boy with the most powerful shoulders had used crutches for years because of polio in childhood. We know so much more about rehabilitation now that if he had had polio recently he probably would have been walking with a cane instead of crutches. One of my teachers had to be lifted and placed in his chair because both legs had been paralyzed in his youth. He, too, might have been helped to do more for himself physically, though he did not allow his disability to stop his progress. There are any number of examples of people handicapped by polio who have done

superb jobs. Franklin D. Roosevelt gave us the most dramatic
example of what can be done by such a person.

COMPLICATIONS

The complications of polio are mostly associated with difficulty in swallowing and inability to breathe. If a child is
unable to swallow or cough up the secretions which accu-
mulate in his throat, a tracheotomy (making an opening in the
windpipe) has to be done. If he is given solids or liquids and
cannot swallow them, he may choke or he may pull some of
the food down into his lungs when he breathes. This causes
blocking of the bronchial tubes so that air cannot get into
that part of the lung. The airless part collapses, and pneumonia
usually sets in. This is particularly hazardous after an infant or
child has vomited.

Patients lying flat in bed for long periods may develop
kidney stones. The chances of this can be lessened by using
tilt boards or tables on which they can be brought gradually
to an erect position every day.

Some muscles cause motion in one direction and some in
another. For instance, the flexor muscles of the fingers, elbows
and knees cause them to bend, and the extensor muscles cause
them to straighten out. If the muscles which are partly weakened are not protected, they may be injured further by being
stretched by the strong muscles pulling in opposition. This is
prevented by passive exercise and by supports.

PREVENTION

The preventive measures commonly employed against polio
are cleanliness, wholesome living, large doses of gamma
globulin and vaccine. It is important to teach your children
to wash their hands before eating and after toilet. During a
polio outbreak they should not exercise to the point of fatigue
or get chilled. They should not swim in polluted waters or
play in sewage drainage areas. They should not mingle in

strange crowds or travel unnecessarily. You should eliminate
flies, especially from the kitchen and dining room. All of these
precautions may help to reduce the chances of infection. The
only way of being sure to prevent polio is to immunize the
child when young with vaccine of the Sabin or live type. The
U.S. Surgeon General's Special Advisory Committee has
recommended that *oral polio vaccine* is the choice for immunization against polio. It is easier to administer, better accepted by children and stimulates better and longer-lasting
immunity. It is quite safe. Only one of 6.25 million who received Type I, one in 50 million who had Type II and one
per 2.5 million who took Type III O.P.V. developed a condition which was considered comparable with paralytic polio.
Persons over eighteen years of age may be at greater risk; it
is therefore advised that O.P.V. be used for adults if the risk
of exposure is greater, as in an epidemic, in military service
and travel to a foreign country.

TONSILLECTOMY AND MOUTH SURGERY: If your child has not
been immunized against polio, you should avoid having him
undergo unnecessary surgery, particularly the removal of
tonsils and adenoids and tooth extractions, for about three
months before the height of the polio season, and until the
polio season is over. For about three or four months after this
kind of surgery, a child will be slightly more susceptible to
polio than a nonoperated child, presumably because the open
wound allows the virus to enter more easily. Also, if his tonsils
have been removed within one month before he catches polio,
he is more likely to have the bulbar type because the virus
can more easily enter the brain through the exposed nerves
in his throat. As a matter of fact, recent investigations indicate
that a child who has had his tonsils removed at any time is
more likely to catch polio than one who has not—a good
argument against unnecessary removal of tonsils.

OTHER IMMUNIZATIONS: Infants or children who have had
injections of vaccine for whooping cough, diphtheria and
tetanus or vaccination against smallpox within a month before
catching polio are more liable to weakness or paralysis in the
injected arm or leg if they develop the paralytic type. But
there is little or no evidence that the injection makes them
more liable to have the paralytic type, or more likely to have
polio at all.

It is, however, wiser to give the polio vaccine promptly and the diphtheria or tetanus toxoid, etc., separately, as the need arises with the prevalence of diphtheria or pertussis. The tetanus toxoid may be delayed until the infant is immunized against polio.

EFFECT OF VACCINATION AGAINST POLIO ON INCIDENCE OF POLIO

The table and chart below indicate the striking reduction in the incidence of paralytic poliomyelitis in the United States which has resulted from the widespread immunization with polio vaccine. It is a tribute to medical research and its application to the health and welfare of mankind; it is monumental proof that medical scientists, with private and public support and encouragement, can and do ultimately succeed in the discovery of means by which disease can be eradicated. In this day and age when political pressure is exerted to control the types of research, the successful development of polio vaccines is striking evidence of the benefits gained by giving scientists freedom of action.

A strong and persistent educational campaign for the use of vaccine is necessary and must be continued indefinitely. As you can see, such an effort has proved to be successful in eliminating a dreadful scourge from our communities.

ISOLATION AND QUARANTINE

Patients with polio are isolated for seven days or the duration of the fever, whichever is longer. Because the virus is present in the stools for a longer time, some doctors isolate the patient for fourteen days. Since our experience in hospitals has shown that it is rare for the disease to be spread after the acute phase is over, this plan of isolation seems adequate, and the possibility of the virus in the stool spreading the infection can be controlled by careful stool hygiene.

If not immunized, children who have been exposed to polio

should be given the vaccine promptly; they are quarantined for fourteen days, as far as going to school is concerned. But since so many of the adult population are immune to polio, no attempt is made to enforce quarantine of the adults in the family. They may go to work unless they are food handlers. In that case, they should stay away from their work for fourteen days.

HYGIENE

Anything soiled with nose and throat discharges of a polio patient should be carefully disposed of or boiled since these discharges are infective during the acute phase. Bedding and clothing should be aired in the sun for a few hours if they are not washed immediately; otherwise soap is enough to kill the viruses. The person who takes care of the patient should wash carefully with soap after handling a bedpan or anything else that might be contaminated by the patient's

REPORTED POLIOMYELITIS,
UNITED STATES, 1950-64

Year	Number of Cases	% Decline from 1950-54
1950-54 Average	38,727	—
1955	28,985	25.2
1956	15,140	60.9
1957	5,485	85.8
1958	5,787	85.1
1959	8,425	78.2
1960	3,190	91.8
1961	1,312	96.6
1962	910	.97.7
1963	449	98.8
1964*	121	99.7

Provisional

Source: U.S. Public Health Service

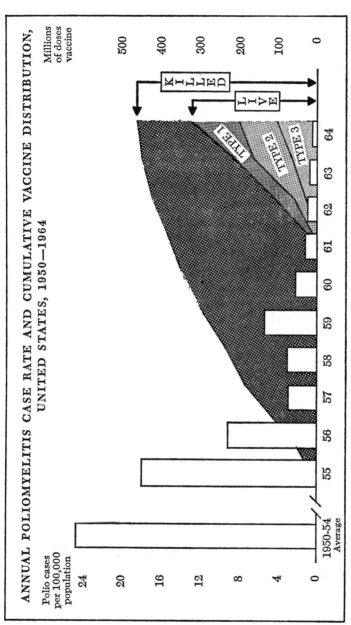

ANNUAL POLIOMYELITIS CASE RATE AND CUMULATIVE VACCINE DISTRIBUTION, UNITED STATES, 1950—1964

Polio cases per 100,000 population

Millions of doses vaccine

KILLED

LIVE

TYPE 1

TYPE 2

TYPE 3

Source: The National Foundation—March of Dimes

stool. This includes bedclothes and bedding. The bedpan should be disinfected after each use.

After the acute phase is over, if the patient has bathroom privileges, he should wash extremely carefully after toilet for several weeks. The sickroom is made safe for other people after the illness is over by a thorough cleaning with soap and water and a good airing for half a day.

QUESTIONS & ANSWERS

Q. *Why is polio called infantile paralysis?*

A. Because the early epidemics in the United States involved mostly very young children and most of the recognized cases involved paralysis. The infection still occurs in infants in some parts of the world—in South America, in Africa, and wherever hygiene is primitive, the social economic level is low and where vaccination against polio is not yet practiced.

Q. *Is polio a seasonal disease?*

A. In the United States it occurred more often in summer and early fall. Elsewhere it is a warm-weather disease.

Q. *Is polio a racial disease?*

A. It does not seem to be.

Q. *Do more boys or girls get polio?*

A. It occurs in about the same number of boys and girls.

Q. *Is polio more common in children than in adults?*

A. Yes. Only 20 per cent of the reported cases in this country were in people over sixteen years old.

Q. *Are babies ever born with polio?*

A. Yes, but rarely.

Q. *Are babies less likely to catch polio than older children?*

A. Yes, because newborn babies whose mothers are immune to polio have the same degree of immunity the mother has. Since about 80 to 85 per cent of adults are immune, an appreciable percentage of newborn babies is also, though we do not know exactly how long this immunity lasts. It is probably less than 6 months. In addition, infants are more sheltered and less likely to be exposed. In countries with primitive hygiene where infants are not as protected, many babies between one and two years of age get polio, but it is usually mild.

Q. *Can children get more than one attack of polio?*

A. Theoretically they can, because an attack caused by one virus does not give immunity to the others, but actually second attacks are very rare.

Q. *Are there variations in the frequency of the different types of polio?*

A. Yes. In one year the bulbar type, for instance, might be more prevalent than it is in another year. In nonepidemic years we are likely to see more severe cases. The death rate varies slightly from year to year, often as the percentage of bulbar cases varies, since most deaths occur from the bulbar type.

Q. *Do many people die from polio?*

A. The death rate varies from 4 to 7 per cent in different epidemics, and most of these deaths occur from the bulbar type.

Q. *What percentage of patients recover completely from polio?*

A. Counting only the recognizable cases, about 50 per cent recover with little or no weakness. Twenty-five to 30 per cent recover with some muscle weakness which does not seriously interfere with normal living. About 14 to 17 per cent are more seriously affected.

Q. *Does each of the strains of virus cause a distinct form of the disease?*

A. No. Any strain can produce any form.

Q. *Can you tell whether a person is immune to polio?*

A. Yes, but it must be done in special laboratories.

Q. *Is it true that pregnant women are more susceptible to polio?*

A. Yes, but we do not know exactly why. It has been sug-

gested that the hormone changes of pregnancy make a
woman more susceptible.

Q. *Do flies or rats and mice carry polio?*

A. Rats and mice probably do not carry polio, but flies have
been found carrying the viruses. There is no evidence that
flies themselves transmit the disease, but it has been shown
that food contaminated by flies in an epidemic was capable
of infecting chimpanzees which ate it. If polio is prevalent,
it is advisable to eliminate flies, especially in the kitchen
and the sickroom.

Q. *If a child gets polio, will the other members of his family
necessarily catch it?*

A. They may, but not necessarily. Only a small percentage
will develop any signs or symptoms of the disease. It is
possible that this exposure will make the other members
of the family immune to that particular strain of the polio
virus. Polio occurs in more than one member of a family in
only about 2 or 3 per cent of families. Sometimes several
members come down with it at the same time, usually because they have all been exposed to the same source of
infection, not because they have caught it from each
other.

Q. *Then is it useless to try to isolate a child with polio from
the rest of his family?*

A. Not at all. Intimate and long contact with any infection
makes the chance of catching the disease greater, so this
attitude would be foolhardy. The child with polio should
be isolated even from those who have already been exposed to him, particularly other children.

Q. *Is there some way I can detect polio at its very beginning?*

A. No. Polio may start like a cold or with a low-grade fever,
with abdominal pain, or with any number of symptoms
which might be typical of many other diseases. Soon after
the beginning, however, headache, stiff neck and backache
and coarse tremors of the hands are very suggestive of
polio. At this stage the suspected diagnosis may be confirmed by an examination of the spinal fluid. A doctor

should be called early for any child who is sick, especially during an epidemic of polio.

Q. *Is there any special test used to diagnose polio?*

A. The examination of the spinal fluid shows certain signs which are very suggestive of polio. The virus may be found in the patient's stool. The finding of an increasing immunity is diagnostic.

Q. *Is there a skin test for polio?*

A. No.

Q. *Can polio be cured?*

A. There is as yet no vaccine, serum or drug which cures polio. Nothing can be done to bring the dead nerves back to life, but it may be possible to prevent extra damage to muscles by proper care, and to save the lives of many patients who have difficulty breathing because of paralysis of the muscles of respiration.

Q. *Do all hospitals accept polio patients?*

A. No. Many do not because they do not have the facilities for adequate care.

Q. *For how long after paralysis sets in can you expect improvement?*

A. Under proper care, natural recovery is usually as complete as it is going to be in about eighteen months, although occasionally it goes on for two years. Of course, surgery, muscle transplants, joint fixation and so forth may help to improve function long after that time.

Q. *What do you mean by rehabilitation?*

A. In the case of polio, it means preparing a child with paralysis for a useful life, psychologically and physically. It means teaching him to get about and to make the most efficient possible use of his remaining muscle power so that he can function as normally as possible.

Q. *If a polio epidemic breaks out in the city where we live, should I take my children to the country?*

A. No. It is probably safer for everyone to stay where you are. The children may have become immune to the polio viruses in your neighborhood, and if you take them to the country, they may encounter others to which they have no immunity. Also, they may take their own viruses into communities where they did not exist before and endanger other people.

Q. *If my children have been immunized against polio, may I take them to a foreign country where polio is still a problem?*

A. If they have had the live-polio-virus vaccine within the last six months. If not, give them another dose of the live triple vaccine at least two to four weeks before traveling.

Q. *Why is fatigue bad?*

A. We have evidence that a tired person who becomes infected with polio may have a more severe attack and possibly a more serious outcome. This may explain why there was a high incidence of serious polio among athletes.

Q. *Why are crowds dangerous?*

A. A crowd is likely to consist of many people from many places. They may carry different types of polio viruses from their various neighborhoods. If a child has been exposed to one of the viruses, he may be immune to that one, but not to others. The chances of being exposed to infections of any kind are therefore greater.

Q. *Should I keep my child out of school during a polio epidemic?*

A. This is rarely a problem in the United States. Health authorities have tried closing day schools or delaying their openings, but have given it up because it does not seem to alter the course of a polio epidemic in a community. Boarding schools or schools which require bus transportation for long distances might be closed because they bring children together from many different communities.

Q. *May my child go swimming during a polio epidemic?*

A. Swimming itself is not dangerous unless the water is polluted, but swimming where there are many people from distant places is, and becoming tired or chilled is, since it lowers resistance to infection.

Q. *Should my child go to the movies during a polio epidemic?*

A. It is wiser not to let him because he will be exposed to many strangers.

Q. *Have you any suggestions for trying to protect children from polio?*

A. Yes, be sure that they are immunized in infancy.

Q. *Why have you written so much about a disease which has been almost completely eliminated in the United States?*

A. I have done so because I want persons in countries where polio is still common to become informed about the disease, and also to know how this dreaded disease can be eliminated. Also it is necessary to remind ourselves that the disease can and does reappear if vaccination is not carried out regularly for all of our infants and preschool children.

Q. *Are both the Salk and Sabin types of vaccine safe?*

A. Yes, the chances of coming down with polio because of the vaccines are extremely slight.

Q. *Is it safe for my child to get polio vaccine in the summer when polio is prevalent?*

A. Yes.

Q. *Is it safe to have the second or third injection of vaccine or a booster dose when polio is prevalent?*

A. Yes. When the child already has antibodies to the polio virus, another injection of vaccine will stimulate greater antibody formation instead of making him more susceptible. Therefore, he would be better protected than if he did not receive the second or third shot.

Q. *Does one injection of vaccine protect a child against polio?*

A. One injection of Salk vaccine may, for a short time. More injections are necessary to protect most children. One dose of live vaccine will protect some, but three doses will protect more than 90 per cent.

Q. *My child had the first injection of polio vaccine, but was unable to have the second on schedule. It is now six months since the first shot. Will he have to start the series over again?*

A. No. If the first injection was of trivalent vaccine, the next two doses may be given twenty-one to eight weeks apart.

If the first injection was of Type I, the child should now get Type III, and a month or so later Type II.

Q. *Will three doses of vaccine suffice for life, or will boosters be necessary?*

A. Boosters will have to be given every two years in the case of Salk vaccine. The live vaccine may not have to be repeated after the school age.

Q. *Is it safe to give the Salk vaccine while a child has a cold, or if he has just recovered from measles or chicken pox?*

A. Yes, but it is probably wiser to give the first dose of vaccine when the child is free of any infection and after he has convalesced from measles or chicken pox.

Q. *Does the Salk vaccine immunize you against all types of polio?*

A. Yes. So does the triple live-virus vaccine.

Q. *If a child has already had polio, should he get the vaccine?*

A. Yes. He was probably infected with only one type of virus and needs to be immunized against the other types. The vaccine would also act as a booster against the virus that caused the original infection.

Q. *Should the vaccine be given to children of all ages?*

A. Yes.

Q. *Should it be given to newborn infants?*

A. I believe it should be used much like the injections against diphtheria and tetanus, beginning at two to three months.

Q. *Are not 80 to 85 per cent of women immune and therefore their babies are immune for six months to a year?*

A. Yes, but since we do not know which are the susceptible babies or how long the immunity lasts, it would be safer to vaccinate them all.

Q. *Are children of certain ages more susceptible to polio than others?*

A. Prior to the widespread use of vaccine, they were. The National Foundation for Infantile Paralysis reported that in the United States the percentage of polio cases in different age groups was as follows:

Year	% Incidence
Birth to 4 years	24.8
5 to 9 years	27.3
10 to 14 years	15.0
15 to 19 years	8.4
20 to 24 years	6.5
25 to 29 years	7.9
30 to 34 years	5.2
35 years and over	4.9

This is why in 1955 the United States Public Health Service recommended that the five-to-nine group have top priority for vaccination.

Q. *Should adults be vaccinated?*

A. Yes, if the disease is prevalent.

Q. *Should a child receive Salk vaccine soon after a tonsillectomy?*

A. He may, but preferably before the operation, and preferably the live vaccine.

Q. *If my child has been made immune by vaccine, would it be safe to have his tonsils out during the polio season?*

A. Yes, if he has had the three doses of the live-virus vaccine, or if he has had at least three doses of the Salk vaccine, and a booster dose a month before.

Q. *Do the vaccines cause severe reactions?*

A. The live vaccine is given by mouth and causes no reactions. The Salk vaccine may cause mild reactions: stinging and slight swelling at the site of the injection. Slight fever and malaise may occur, but often there is no reaction at all.

Q. *Are some children allergic to the vaccine?*

A. In a few children allergy causes local pain and swelling, but this is usually due to the penicillin in the vaccine, not the vaccine itself. If a child is allergic to penicillin, he should be tested before receiving the vaccine.

Q. *Does the vaccine cause Rh sensitivity?*

A. If so, it has not been reported.

Q. *If a child gets live vaccine can he become a carrier of polio viruses without getting the disease himself?*

A. No, not for long.

Q. *Do you advise the Salk or Sabin vaccine for your patients?*

A. I advise the live vaccine, the Sabin type.

Q. *Have you any figures on the risk of unvaccinated children getting polio as compared with vaccinated children?*

A. See the chart on page 367.

Q. *Is it true that an injection of vaccine for the prevention of whooping cough, diphtheria, tetanus or typhoid, or a vaccination against smallpox makes a child more susceptible to polio?*

A. It may be so, but not necessarily.

Q. *Is that true of any injection?*

A. No. If gamma globulin is injected, it may prevent polio rather than increase the chances of weakness in that particular arm or leg. Penicillin and other drugs which must be injected to be effective may be given without concern.

Q. *Should I postpone my baby's whooping cough, diphtheria and tetanus injections and his smallpox vaccination until after the polio season?*

A. Not if he has had the live vaccine or if there are epidemics of whooping cough, diphtheria or smallpox in your community. Routine booster shots which can be postponed for a few months should not be given during the polio season.

Q. *Is there any health department regulation governing what should or should not be injected during the polio season?*

A. No. The health department merely makes recommendations. It is usually wise to adopt its recommendations.

Q. *What is the danger of mouth surgery during a polio epidemic?*

A. It opens up a wound through which the polio virus can enter more easily. This is particularly true of tonsillectomy. There is evidence that the virus can more easily reach the brain through the open wound in the throat which might result in the bulbar type of polio unless the child has been immunized with vaccine. Tonsils should not be removed during the three-month period before the height of the polio season. The same recommendation is made for the extraction of teeth. This does not apply to ordinary cleaning and filling of teeth, however.

Q. *How long should a child with polio be isolated?*

A. In some parts of the United States the isolation period is seven days or as long as the fever lasts, whichever is longer. Some doctors feel that the isolation period should be at least fourteen days since the virus is in the patient's stool for at least that long and is still a source of spread of the infection.

Q. *Should a person who has been exposed to polio be quarantined?*

A. Not if he has had live-virus vaccine. A booster dose of vaccine would be useful.

Q. *What about those who did not have the live vaccine?*

A. For those who have not been vaccinated the U.S. Public Health Service and most city and state health departments recommend quarantine for fourteen days after the last exposure, but in many places this is not enforced except that children must not go to school. With adults it is only enforced when they are food handlers, because immunity in adults is so general. Quarantine is unnecessary for those immunized.

Q. *If my child gets polio and is sent to a hospital, may I visit him there?*

A. Hospital regulations vary. Most hospitals will, or should, permit the parents to visit the child since the parents have already been infected. After the isolation period, others may be allowed to visit, too.

Q. *A case of polio has been reported at my child's school. Should I bring him home?*

A. I do not think so, because it is likely that your child has already been exposed. Probably the safest thing is to give him the live vaccine, if he has not yet had it. The children who have been in contact with the patient at the school should be quarantined if they have not had the live vaccine.

Q.   *Is it necessary to fumigate the room of a polio patient who has recovered or gone to the hospital?*

A.   No. A thorough cleaning with soap and water and plenty of fresh air and sunlight will clean the room in half a day.

32: Bacterial Meningitis

Meningitis means inflammation of the meninges, the outer covering which surrounds the brain and spinal cord. It occurs everywhere. In the days when ear infections were rampant and the treatment of them was inadequate, meningitis was one of the most dreaded complications. Meningitis occurs in all age groups, more frequently in the very young than in the old. Meningitis caused by some bacteria is more common at one age, while other forms are more likely at other ages. It is not always caused by bacteria; it may be due to an infection by a virus. But bacterial meningitis is what we are discussing here.

The bacteria most often responsible for meningitis in children are the meningococcus, the influenza bacillus (not the influenza *virus* which causes influenza), the pneumococcus (which frequently causes pneumonia), the tubercle bacillus and the streptococcus (which causes scarlet fever and tonsillitis). Other forms of baterial meningitis are caused by the staphylococcus, the germ that causes boils. An occasional case is caused by the germ responsible for typhoid or dysentery, or by some other bacteria which do not ordinarily cause meningitis. In very young infants the colon bacillus often is the cause of meningitis. Tuberculosis is one of the most common causes of meningitis. Before the newer drugs were available, approximately 40 per cent of infants and children up to three years old who died of tuberculosis did so after they developed meningitis.

Contagion: While bacterial meningitis is communicable, it is very much less so than measles, chicken pox or mumps. One

form (spinal meningitis) often occurs in epidemics. When
that happens, many people come in contact with the meningococcus germ which is responsible, but fortunately only a few
of those who become infected develop meningitis. They may,
instead, harbor the germ in their noses and throats with no
evidence of the disease. During the last world war as many
as 80 per cent of the soldiers in some army barracks had the
germ in their throats. Fortunately, these germs could be eliminated from the throats of these soldiers within two or three
days by the use of one of the sulfa drugs.

Symptoms: You should suspect meningitis if a child suddenly complains of headache or pain and stiffness in the back
of the neck, so that it is difficult for him to touch his chest
with his chin; if, in addition, he vomits and has a high temperature and possibly a chill; or if along with some of these symptoms he has a convulsion or, the opposite, if he becomes very
drowsy and almost stuporous; and if he has a fine rash consisting of minute hemorrhages into the skin. Such symptoms call
for immediate medical aid, and if a doctor is not available,
the child should be taken to the nearest hospital. Each hour
that elapses before treatment is started makes the outcome
progressively worse.

Bacterial meningitis is not always a very sudden infection.
It is sometimes more subtle, especially in infancy. The baby's
neck may be slightly resistant to bending, but not actually
stiff. The soft spot, the fontanel, on top of the head may bulge
because of the increased fluid content of the brain cavities, but
it may be just tense and flat. The baby may have fever, cry
a great deal, eat poorly and sometimes vomit. The cry may
become shrill or piercing. A child may only act tired, not want
to eat and may complain of a headache. He may be restless,
unhappy or irritable. He may misbehave. He may vomit if
you press food on him. At different ages such behavior will
vary, but alert parents will know that their infant or young
child is acting quite unlike himself. This does not mean that
every time your infant or child acts as I have described, he has
meningitis. It is a relatively uncommon disease.

Diagnosis: If a doctor suspects meningitis, he will probably
do a lumbar puncture. That is, he will insert a needle in the

lower part of the back and withdraw some of the fluid which bathes the spinal cord and the brain. If the patient has meningitis, this fluid is usually altered. Instead of being crystalclear it may have become cloudy. It will contain many cells and possibly bacteria, which can be seen under the microscope by the doctor and which might be identified by special staining. The fluid will be cultured. It will be placed on some specially prepared material which will enable the bacteria to multiply so that they can be accurately identified after a day or two. This is important because the proper antibiotic must be used according to the cause of the infection.

Treatment: Meningitis, at one time almost always fatal, is now curable in most cases by the timely and judicious use of the proper antibiotics. In general, the treatment consists mainly of antibiotics which work against the specific bacterium responsible for the infection. These have to be given in large doses and must be supplied by any and all routes possible. The choice of the drug, the amount to be given, the manner in which it is to be given and how long it should be continued are decisions which must be left to the doctor.

When the doctor first sees a child with meningitis, the child may be dazed or unconscious. His fever is usually high, his breathing may be irregular and he may not be able to swallow. Whatever antibiotic drug is decided upon should be injected into the child's bloodstream if possible, otherwise into a muscle. In this way, the required amount of the drug is introduced much more rapidly than if it is taken by mouth, and it is able to combat the disease more effectively. The child may have to be given glucose and salt solution for nourishment and fluid into the vein for one, two or more days, and be given medicine by the same route. When the child is lucid enough and able to swallow and does not vomit, the food, fluid and medication, except for the antibiotics, may be given by mouth. Antibiotics work best if they are injected.

Usually treatment with antibiotics is continued for about ten days or until the temperature has been normal for at least a week and until all evidence of active infection has disappeared.

Tepid water sponges, aspirin and other drugs which lower temperature are used to control high fever. Sedatives may be necessary for the child who is very restless and violent or who has convulsions.

Hospitalization: A child who has meningitis is dangerously sick and should be isolated. He needs the kind of attention which can best be had in a hospital, because the nature of the treatment and the laboratory investigations of the cause and the course of the illness are so important as guides to correct treatment. These examinations can be made more quickly and more accurately when the patient is in the hospital.

Convalescence: A child who has successfully recovered from meningitis must convalesce for several weeks. He should not return to school or join in active play until the doctor says he is able to.

Complications: Although most children recover from meningitis, the disease does injure a considerable number of those who survive. Recent surveys indicate that behavior disturbances, some muscle weakness and even alterations in vision, hearing and mental capacity are not rare.

Prevention: In case of an epidemic or a large outbreak it is best not to go to theaters or the movies and to avoid crowds. The usual type of hygiene, such as washing before eating and after toilet must be observed carefully. Preventive measures, except for the epidemic form of spinal meningitis, need only be good hygiene and prevention of the common infections—colds, ear infections, sore throats, pneumonia, etc.—and the early treatment of these infections.

Isolation and Quarantine: If a child has been in contact with a patient with meningitis, especially spinal meningitis or influenzal meningitis, he ought to be examined by a doctor, and a culture should be made of the bacteria in his throat to find out whether he is carrying the same germ. If laboratory facilities for this are not available, antibiotics or sulfa drugs are given on the chance that he may have become infected.

Hygiene: If a child with meningitis is in the hospital, the problem of caring for the bedding, clothing, dishes and utensils is solved. If the child is cared for at home, he must be isolated. His dishes must be boiled or a separate set reserved for him; his bedding and all other laundry must be boiled. The excreta, except in the case of typhoid or dysentery meningitis which are very rare, can be disposed of in the usual way. In typhoid or dysentery meningitis, the excreta are disposed of as in those diseases.

QUESTIONS & ANSWERS

Q. *Are all forms of meningitis found everywhere, or do some types occur more frequently in some parts of the world than in others?*

A. All forms may occur anywhere at any time, but they are most common when nose and throat infections are rampant. This means that in the temperate zone or where tuberculosis is prevalent in children the disease would be more common in the late fall, winter and spring and less frequent in the summer, except for tuberculous meningitis. This occurs at any time, but is more frequent at the end of February and March.

Q. *Does anything other than bacteria cause meningitis?*

A. Yes. Sometimes a head injury sets up an irritation of the brain which may produce symptoms similar to those of ordinary meningitis. Metal poisoning, such as lead poisoning, sometimes irritates the meninges of the brain. Children may get lead poisoning by eating paint, or by being exposed to the burning of lead batteries or by drinking water from old lead pipes. Painters' children have got lead poisoning by handling their fathers' paint-stained clothes and tools. This form of meningitis is very serious, but it has nothing to do with infection. The viruses of mumps, polio, choriomeningitis and many others cause irritation of the meninges, but their danger is that they cause damage of the brain tissue itself, while the irritation of the meninges is incidental. In bacterial meningitis, the brain is only secondarily disturbed because of the irritation of the meninges; however, abscesses of the brain may and do occur.

Q. *Is meningitis a frequent complication of pneumonia?*

A. Not on a percentage basis, but it does occasionally occur.

Q. *How frequently is meningitis a complication of ear infections?*

A. Relatively infrequent when the ear infection is treated early with sulfa drugs or antibiotics. When ear, nose, throat and sinus infections are treated promptly and completely, the chances of meningitis are very remote.

Q. *Is the meningitis caused by viruses just the same as bacterial meningitis?*

A. No, because it is rarely, if ever, limited to the covering of the brain. It is usually meningoencephalitis, since it also involves the brain itself. At the beginning of the disease, virus infections may be indistinguishable from bacterial infections, but the subsequent course is quite different. A spinal fluid examination usually helps to clarify the diagnosis.

Q. *Is meningoencephalitis dangerous?*

A. The aftereffects vary with the cause of the infection. When it is caused by mumps virus, for instance, most patients recover. Others are more damaging, but few of them are quite as destructive as *the untreated types* of bacterial meningitis.

Q. *Is the treatment for meningoencephalitis caused by a virus the same as the treatment for bacterial meningitis?*

A. No, because most viruses are not affected by sulfa drugs and antibiotics, and bacteria are.

Q. *Is meningitis caused by tuberculosis curable?*

A. Yes, if you mean survival. Since the development of certain antibiotics over 50 per cent of the patients recover after intensive treatment. If treated early, 80 per cent or more survive.

Q. *Is there always a rash with meningitis?*

A. No, but it occurs in about 25 per cent of cases of spinal (meningococcus) meningitis.

Q. *You said that prompt treatment is vital and that the antibiotic used must be the proper one for the type of infec-*

tion. Yet you also said that it takes a day or two to make a culture and identify the bacteria. In this case, how can you start treatment quickly?

A. It is always necessary to make a culture to identify the bacteria and to confirm the diagnosis. Sometimes the bacteria can be seen under the microscope in a smear of the spinal fluid before it is cultured. When no bacteria are seen, the doctor may suspect or decide by other means that it is bacterial, viral or some other form of meningitis. When there is any doubt about the type of bacteria causing the infection, the doctor will give two or even three different antibiotics to take care of all the possibilities until he is able to identify the specific bacterium by culture.

Q. *How soon after meningitis is over may my child go to school?*

A. Technically he would not be barred from school the day after it has been cured since he is no longer infectious, but he will probably be too weak for outside activity for several weeks. During this time he will need a great deal of rest. It will take even longer for him to become equal to a full school schedule. The convalescent period varies with each child. When he has regained his strength, is active and seems able and anxious to undertake school-work, he may return.

Q. *What about going to the theater or to beaches while he is convalescing?*

A. I believe it is wiser for any child who is recovering from meningitis to have a quiet convalescent period, and not be disturbed by going into crowds of any kind and be exposed to many possible infections.

Q. *If a child is treated for meningitis early, is the result always a complete cure?*

A. Not always, but most of the patients do recover. Some of them are left with some aftermath of the injury to the nervous system. This may take the form of a weakness of one or another part of the body, or a behavior disturbance or a disturbance of vision or hearing.

Q. *How can I keep my child from getting meningitis?*

A. It is not always possible, but many cases can be avoided if every infection is treated quickly as it is detected, whether it is of the nose and throat, ears, skin or any part of the body.

33: Encephalitis

Encephalitis, or inflammation of the brain, varies tremendously in its severity and in the pattern of illness it produces. One child may have nothing more than a mild headache and dizziness lasting a day or two, as is often the case in mumps encephalitis, or it may be so severe that within a day or two a child who looked well has lapsed into a deep coma from which he cannot be aroused.

Different types of encephalitis vary with the virus which causes them, some being more serious than others. At present there are at least thirty-five or forty different viruses that are known to cause encephalitis; it is possible that the actual number is two or three times greater. Some of the viruses are named for the places where they were first recognized, as for example, the St. Louis encephalitis virus, the Japanese encephalitis virus, the Russian encephalitis virus, and the Newcastle virus. Other viruses are named for the person who first discovered them, as Von Economo's encephalitis, or by one or another characteristic of the disease they produce. Von Economo's encephalitis is the type also called sleeping sickness. It was quite common in the early twenties but is less so now. Eastern and Western equine encephalomyelitis are so called because the viruses were commonly found in infected horses and later in human beings in the eastern or western parts of the United States. A person who has had encephalitis usually becomes immune to the particular virus which caused the disease.

Means of Infection: Some viruses are brought to humans by infected mosquitoes who carry them from birds, both wild and domestic; others are spread from person to person.

Incubation Period: The incubation periods vary from five to fifteen days.

Types of Encephalitis: Most types of encephalitis are caused by viruses, including the kind which frequently complicates mumps and the one which, rarely, occurs with cold sores. But there is another form in which the infection plays a role different from that of actually infecting the brain. For example, the encephalitis which sometimes complicates measles, German measles and chicken pox, and that which follows the injections to prevent rabies, is probably not caused by the viruses of these diseases, but is the result of a process related to an allergic reaction, a hypersensitivity.

There are other forms of encephalitis which are not due to infection, but to direct damage by a toxic agent, as for example, lead encephalitis which occurs as part of lead poisoning.

There is also the type that follows repeated brain concussion. A blow to the head as in a prize fight may result in a concussion or many small hemorrhages in the brain. These small bleedings often are absorbed, leaving no ill effect. But if they are repeated many times, small scars may form, leaving the characteristic picture of the "punch-drunk" person.

Polio is not primarily a disease of the brain, but in some cases the polio virus does affect the brain. It is then known as the encephalitic form of polio.

Symptoms: Usually encephalitis causes fever, dizziness, crossing of the eyes, double vision, headache, stiff neck, vomiting, drowsiness even to the degree of coma, and often marked irritability and convulsions.

Treatment: Since it is not easy to determine what causes an isolated case of encephalitis, it is well to treat them all alike until an accurate diagnosis is made. It is most important to differentiate between encephalitis and polio or some forms of bacterial meningitis which can be treated with antibiotics.

Treatment is general. The patient is kept in as good condition as possible while he overcomes the disease. Antibiotics are not effective, neither are the sulfa drugs. Effective serums are not available. In the type of disease which complicates measles, anti-allergic drugs, including cortisone, have been tried, but the results have been questionable. Gamma globulin in large amounts has been tried with negative results.

Encephalitis calls for urgent medical attention, and in the more severe forms, hospitalization.

Prevention: Vaccines or other preventive immunizations are not generally available.

Isolation and Quarantine: The patient is isolated for the duration of the disease. Members of the household are usually not quarantined, but local health department regulations pertaining to this type of disease must be used as a guide to the problems of isolation, quarantine and school attendance.

QUESTIONS & ANSWERS

Q. *How can you tell which virus causes the encephalitis?*

A. In some instances the pattern of the disease strongly suggests what type it is. In others the virus can be found in the spinal fluid or the blood or the throat of the patient, and identified. In some instances it is possible to determine which virus caused the disease only by testing the immunity the patient develops as he recovers.

Q. *Is the immunity to one virus different from the immunity to others?*

A. Yes, in most cases the immunity is usually specific. That is, if you become immune to one virus, you become immune to that one alone and not to others. There is some relationship between the viruses which cause the Russian, Australian and Japanese B forms of encephalitis. The immunity which results from any one of these infections is carried over to some extent to the others.

Q. *Is encephalitis different from meningitis?*

A. Usually encephalitis is limited to the brain tissue itself, while meningitis involves the membranes covering the brain, but there may be no absolute boundary to the spread of the infection. For example, tuberculosis can produce both meningitis and encephalitis. So can the mumps virus and other viruses.

Q. *How can encephalitis be distinguished from meningitis?*

A. An examination of the spinal fluid is the surest way of telling the difference, though sometimes the symptoms are
so characteristic that this is not necessary.

Q. *How common is encephalitis complicating measles,
mumps and chicken pox?*

A. It occurs in about one out of five hundred to two thousand
measles cases, and in at least 10 per cent of mumps cases.
Accurate figures for the number of times it complicates
chicken pox are not available, but in any case it is very
rare with chicken pox. It is practically zero after the
measles vaccine.

Q. *Is encephalitis spread directly from person to person?*

A. No. Most forms are transmitted through insects like mosquitoes. One form is known to be spread by eating food
contaminated by mouse excreta. When this occurs, infected mice are found in great numbers in the area. The
exact manner of spread is not known for every type. Those
which occur only as a complication of diseases like measles
or chicken pox or as a result of injury or a toxic agent are
not contagious.

Q. *Should all cases of encephalitis be treated in hospitals?*

A. Yes, except those which are very mild. Most cases associated with mumps are like that. They pass off in a few
days or a week and can be cared for at home. If they are
more severe, the hospital is a better place for the necessary
care.

Q. *Are large doses of gamma globulin effective in the treatment of measles, mumps and polio encephalitis?*

A. No.

Q. *Would you give gamma globulin to a child who had
measles, mumps or polio encephalitis?*

A. No.

Q. *Is the convalesence long?*

A. It is usually rapid after mumps encephalitis, but slower
after the other types.

Q. *If a child gets well from encephalitis, does he recover
completely?*

A.   Many do, but some are left with personality changes, sight or hearing disturbances, or other disturbances associated with brain damage. The more effort one exerts in follow-up of these children the more problems one discovers.

Q.   *Are there any vaccines or protective serums or drugs for prevention or treatment of encephalitis?*

A.   The vaccines against polio, measles and yellow fever, and against some of the Adeno viruses prevent the infection and therefore also prevent the encephalitis. A mumps-virus vaccine is now available. A vaccine against German measles will probably be available soon, and there will undoubtedly be many other vaccines against viruses which produce encephalitis in man and in cattle and other animals. We have no drugs at present which are effective against the viruses which produce encephalitis, or drugs which cure the encephalitis itself.

Q.   *How else can the various forms of encephalitis be prevented?*

A.   By preventing the infection which causes the encephalitis, as indicated in the answer to the previous question. In addition, it is important to avoid exposure to mosquitoes and other disease-conveying arthropods (mosquitoes, ticks, mites), particularly in areas where it is known that the arthropods are live and may be carriers of the viruses. Elimination of these mosquitoes are, of course, matters of public health.

Q.   *May the child with encephalitis be kept at home?*

A.   Most encephalitis patients should be in hospitals where the proper care can be rendered promptly as the indications arise. It may become necessary to insert a tube which will clear the airway to the lungs. In some instances a tracheotomy (the insertion of a tube into the windpipe) may become necessary and if it does it is usually *very urgent*. A child with 105° to 106° temperature may require a cooling mattress, wet packs, etc. Except in the mild form of mumps encephalitis, the child should be moved to a hospital. Your doctor will undoubtedly tell you to do so in every instance in which it is indicated. Do not try to argue with such a request because your child "does not like hospitals," or "he is frightened by hospitals," or "he will not stay there unless his mother can be with him all the time." Incidentally, you may be able to stay with him in many hospitals.

Intestinal Diseases

34: Acute Gastroenteritis

Acute gastroenteritis is due to an irritation of the stomach and intestines. It can be caused by irritants of different types, but we shall discuss only those caused by infection, or by the toxins liberated by bacteria. We shall subsequently describe typhoid fever, dysentery of various types, and salmonella infections. There are still many types of infections probably caused by viruses.

Different bacteria and viruses have been incriminated in acute gastroenteritis.

The condition may occur in epidemic form or sporadically. The symptoms vary from sudden intense nausea and vomiting, and diarrhea resulting in rapid dehydration (loss of body fluid), to mere cramps or stomach ache, or a few loose stools.

Staphylococcus toxin is liberated by the staphylococcus germ. The toxin can cause illness even if the contaminated food is cooked. Within hours after eating, one becomes terribly sick with uncontrollable vomiting, followed by diarrhea. The disease is short-lived, but many are so sick as to require prompt treatment with intravenous fluid. Antibiotics are useless. Most who have this experience recover in a day or two. This can occur in children's camps and in large group outings, and at large parties.

Salmonella infections, usually acquired from eating creamed food, foods with mayonnaise, éclairs, cream puffs and contaminated smoked fish which stand overnight without refrigeration, may cause similar violent outbreaks within hours after eating.

The treatment is usually the same as for the staphylococcal toxin.

Various viruses may produce vomiting and diarrhea of intense degree. These may be accompanied by fever, chills, severe distress and rapid debilitation. This condition may last one to three days and requires essentially the same treatment as other forms of the condition. The diagnosis or causative agent is often undetected. Treatment must therefore be directed toward curing the symptoms.

The younger the child the more dangerous these conditions may be. An infant may become very ill in less than a day. This demands urgent medical attention. The older child should be kept in bed. If vomiting is the major problem, do not force fluids or food. He will only vomit more. Depending on the size of the child, a half ounce or an ounce of liquid, diluted fruit juice with equal amounts of water, or any of the carbonated sweetened drinks, e.g., ginger ale or one of the cola drinks or fruit-flavored drinks, may be given every half hour. If the child can retain five to six consecutive doses, he will be able to tolerate larger amounts. Thereafter, hard candy, lollipops, cereal cooked with water, with sugar and salt added, may be tolerated and be helpful. Dietetic drinks are not to be given for such conditions since the glucose contained in the soft drinks is very important. Do not offer a full diet. Get to it in a few days.

Diarrhea: When diarrhea is severe, the infant may require prompt hospital treatment. He may require fluid given by injection into the blood before he can tolerate fluids by mouth.

Viral gastroenteritis may run through a family. All may get it at about the same time, or one after another in the course of a few days. When this occurs it usually involves the local community, and sometimes it is more widespread.

QUESTIONS & ANSWERS

Q. *Is gastroenteritis always severe?*

A. No. It may be very mild, sometimes just a mild stomach ache, sometimes slight nausea alone, sometimes one or two loose stools or any combination of these in one day or only for a few hours.

Q. *How does one treat this type of upset?*

A. Rest and a bland diet.

Q. *May it be severe in one person and not severe in another member of the family, group, etc?*

A. Yes. Of twenty children who became sick at the same time, some had diarrhea, others just nausea, others vomited or had stomach ache and a few had fever.

Q. *Are drugs used for treatment of gastroenteritis?*

A. Paregoric may be given for cramps and/or diarrhea, and some of the common medicines which your doctor will advise may be soothing.

35: Appendicitis

Appendicitis is a condition which occurs universally and at all ages. It is usually due to a secondary type of infection.

It is an inflammation of the appendix, a long, narrow, tubular structure at the junction of the small intestine and the cecum, or large intestine. It is a rudimentary organ in the human. It becomes obstructed with fecal impactions, sometimes with pinworms and is secondarily infected with bacteria. Occasionally the infection spreads by way of the bloodstream, as in tonsillitis, measles and in other infections.

It begins with pain in the abdomen, usually around the navel and to its right, and after a while settles to the right of the midline and in the lower part of the abdomen. Infrequently the pain may be higher and infrequently in the back, almost always on the right side. Nausea may be present and vomiting may occur once or repeatedly. The abdomen may hurt more when the child coughs, yawns or straightens out his legs. The pain is sufficient to make him double up. Temperature may be low-grade, 100.5° to 101° or 102°F., but temperatures of 103° and 104° are not rare. Occasionally when appendicitis complicates a sore throat or measles, the temperature may be very high. The pain continues and becomes more localized to the right lower quadrant of the abdomen.

The blood count reveals increased white blood cells. The urine is usually clear, but may contain an excess of red blood cells or pus cells.

It is most important that the diagnosis be made promptly to avoid rupture of the appendix and peritonitis.

Appendicitis may be confused with an ordinary upset intestine or stomach ache and more often with viral gastroenteritis and various infections such as those with salmonella germs.

Occasionally pneumonia, rheumatic fever and other ailments can be confused with appendicitis because of the abdominal pain and its location. An inflamed or ruptured Meckel's diverticulum can simulate appendicitis.

Treatment is usually surgical removal of the appendix.

If the appendix has ruptured and an abscess has formed, the doctor may want to treat the child with bed rest and antibiotics. He may continue this for several weeks, then decide to remove the appendix. This must be the physician's decision.

QUESTIONS & ANSWERS

Q. *Can a child as young as two or three years have appendicitis?*

A. Yes, but rarely. I have seen rare cases soon after birth and several times at two to five years. Most cases occur after six to seven years.

Q. *Is appendicitis seasonal?*

A. It is not necessarily seasonal, but we do see more cases in the late spring.

Q. *Can appendicitis cause diarrhea?*

A. Yes, on occasion. If the appendix ruptures and peritonitis results, diarrhea is more likely to occur.

Q. *Should one treat acute appendicitis without surgery?*

A. It may be possible in some cases, but I believe it safer to have the appendix removed as soon as the diagnosis is made, except as already mentioned, if an abscess is present. In every instance where appendicitis is possible, it is urgent and important that the doctor help you to determine how to proceed.

36: Salmonella Infections

These gastrointestinal diseases are caused by a large group of bacteria, most of which affect animals—rats, dogs, pigeons, poultry and most farm animals. The bacteria are sometimes found in eggs. About fifty varieties have been isolated in human beings, but only a few of these fifty account for most of the salmonella infections observed in children. These are *Salmonella paratyphi B, Salmonella typhimurium* and *Salmonella cholera suis*. The rest are caused by other representatives of the group, of which there are many. Each may be responsible for an outbreak or an epidemic.

The diseases occur everywhere, more often in warm climates. Salmonellosis is especially common in children and occurs usually in outbreaks but is occasionally found as a single case in a home. More than half of all the children who get it are under two years old, except for typhoid fever which occurs in older children.

Infection with one of the organisms leads to immunity to it, but we do not know how long the immunity lasts. There is also some cross-immunity; that is, if you are infected by one type, you develop some immunity to closely related members of the group. But this cross-immunity is not usually as strong as the immunity to the bacterium which actually caused the disease.

Manner of Spread: The infection is usually acquired through food contaminated by the droppings of animals, or through human convalescent carriers. Improperly prepared and poorly refrigerated foods, particularly eggs and milk, smoked fish and meats and roast fowl, pastry made with whipped cream, custards, salads containing infected egg and cream, are often the sources of epidemics. Explosive outbreaks of vomiting and diarrhea resulting from eating these foods, which originally contained the bacteria and which have not been cooked or refrigerated enough to control them, are reported frequently. Susceptibility seems to be closely tied to the amount of the infecting organism in the food, so outbreaks most often occur on occasions where large amounts of infected food are allowed to become warm, thus encouraging the rapid multiplication of the bacteria. Salmonella may produce three different types of disease.

Severe Gastrointestinal Type: There is an explosive outbreak of abdominal cramps, vomiting and diarrhea which comes rapidly six hours to three days after eating heavily infected foods. The interval is usually within twelve hours. A child so affected may become desperately ill with high fever and prostration due to vomiting and diarrhea. This type may last only a day or two, but sometimes it continues for seven to ten days with mucus and blood in the stools. This form of salmonella infection resembles the infection caused by botulism, staphylococcus toxin and dysentery and is distinguished from them mainly by finding the salmonella in the stool of the sick child.

Mild Gastrointestinal Type: The second type is one which produces a milder form of illness: diarrhea which is not very severe, but continues over a period of weeks or even months. From time to time, I have observed children who had little or no fever, looked and acted fairly well, though slightly below par, and continued to have three to five stools a day instead of their usual one or two. The stools were loose and contained mucus and, rarely, blood. Dietary treatment is not effective for this. Either the child recovers spontaneously or, after the cause of the disease is found, he is cured by an appropriate antibiotic. Questioning the family, I often have found that at about the time the child's illness started, other members of the household also had had a "stomach upset." This type may start in about three days.

Typhoid Type: A third type of salmonellosis resembles typhoid fever. The incubation period is longer, three to ten days. This one may also start with nausea and vomiting, but sometimes there is only fever, headache and malaise. In infants, fever and abdominal distention may be all the child shows, and these may last three to five days or as long as two or three weeks. With the paratyphoid infections (which are usually caused by *Salmonella paratyphi B*), rose spots on the trunk similar to those found in typhoid fever may appear.

Complications: Occasionally in infants the abdominal signs resemble those of acute appendicitis. Other parts of the body are sometimes affected. These are apt to be the joints, bones, and less frequently the lungs, kidneys and meninges, and occasionally the heart.

Treatment: A child ill with any of the salmonella infections should be kept in bed. If he has the acute gastrointestinal form, he needs hospital care because he will require fluid injections into the bloodstream to prevent dehydration and collapse. If he has the typhoid-fever-like disease, hospital care is probably more efficient and the disease is less likely to spread to other members of the family.

His diet should be bland, with plenty of fluids and no roughage. If he can eat, he should be given milk, meat, fish, poultry, purée of vegetables and fruits, cereals, white bread and so forth. The treatment can only be symptomatic until the bacterium causing the infection is found. Then the most suitable antibiotic will be prescribed and it should be continued until the child's temperature is normal and also after that until specimens of three consecutive daily stools are found to be free of the bacteria.

Prevention: Salmonella infection is prevented by observing the usual rules of cleanliness. It is very important to wash your own and your child's hands before handling food, before eating and after toilet. Food should be protected from contamination by rat droppings. All food should be properly refrigerated, especially foods containing eggs, cream and custard, and cold meats and smoked fish. There should be sanitary control of food handlers, delicatessen shops and restaurants; cases of infection should be reported to the health department.

Injections of vaccine against paratyphoid A and B are usually given along with typhoid vaccine and they may also protect against some of the other salmonella organisms. Children going to summer camps, and children and adults traveling abroad who expect to visit rural areas, or even large cities in some parts of the world, should have these injections. Vaccine against other specific members of the salmonella group is not recommended.

Isolation and Quarantine: An infected child is isolated only during the illness, but his stools are examined repeatedly until three consecutive specimens are free of salmonella. People exposed to the infection are not quarantined, but their stools are examined for the infection. If any of them is found to be a carrier, he is treated until he is free of the infection. While some people do carry salmonella infection without showing symptoms, chronic carriers are less common than typhoid carriers, except in the case of paratyphoid carriers. Household contacts of paratyphoid patients and carriers should be immunized.

Hygiene: The patient's laundry and excreta should be handled with caution and disinfected to avoid spreading the infection to the rest of the household. After the patient is well, the room may be cleaned with soap and water to make it safe for others.

QUESTIONS & ANSWERS

Q. *Can common household pets—dogs, cats, birds—transmit salmonella infection to my children?*

A. Yes, if they are infected. This is not very likely, however, with pets kept at home and fed prepared foods. It is more likely with stray dogs and cats which feed on garbage or whatever they can find in the way of food.

Q. *Can a person infect a dog or a cat?*

A. It is possible, if hygiene is poor.

Q. *Is treatment the same for dogs as for children?*

A. Yes, essentially.

Q. *Is handling of uncooked fowl a common source of infection?*

A. No.

Q. *Can you tell whether a fowl is infected?*

A. If it is abscessed because of paratyphoid there will be some white spots on the liver, but you cannot tell otherwise.

Q. *Are eggs a source of infection?*

A. Yes, commonly—particularly cracked and soiled eggs and some products made from them. A large outbreak in many hospitals in New York, New Jersey and Pennsylvania was due to Salmonella Darby found in such eggs.

Q. *Can you have the disease more than once?*

A. Yes, but the bacteria causing it would probably be different each time.

Q. *Why does the severity of the disease vary so widely— some cases so acute and some so mild?*

A. The gastrointestinal types are local infections of the intestines. When the infection is a heavy one and vomiting and diarrhea begin within twelve hours, it is usually because there are a great many infecting organisms. They liberate a toxin which acts quickly. There are fewer in the type that takes three days or more to begin. In the typhoid type the germ gets into the bloodstream and produces a more general disease which takes three to ten days to start.

Q. *Are there any especially good antibiotics for this group of diseases?*

A. There are several. Your doctor will select the one which is most effective against the germ causing your child's infection.

Q. *Is it necessary to treat all types of salmonella infection with antibiotics—those which only last two or three days as well as the typhoid type?*

A. It is preferable, but we cannot always discover quickly which bacterium is responsible for the disease, and until we can, we can only treat the symptoms because the antibiotic must be a specific one to be effective. Most people recover without antibiotics.

Q. *My child has the low-grade type of illness with no fever. Must she be kept in bed until she is entirely well?*

A. Not if you and she can be careful about hygiene so that the infection will not be spread.

Q. *How soon after recovery may my boy go to school?*

A. As soon as he is released from isolation, if he feels well enough.

Q. *Why is vaccination against salmonellosis not recommended?*

A. You would need frequent injections of vaccine against many different strains of the salmonella and numerous boosters to maintain a high level of immunity to all the different bacteria, so they would be impractical. Vaccination is routinely recommended against paratyphoid A and B, for people who live in or are about to travel in areas where paratyphoid is prevalent. This is usually given with typhoid immunization.

Q. *Are carriers isolated?*

A. No, but they are not allowed to work as food handlers and they should not take jobs involving small children.

Q. *Do children ever become carriers?*

A. They may, but this does not happen very often.

Q. *If one of my children gets ill, may his sister go to school?*

A. Yes, but her stool will be examined by the board of health.

Q. *Is she a danger to other children?*

A. Not unless her stool reveals the presence of salmonella.

Q. *May she go to the circus or the movies or beaches?*

A. Yes, as long as she is not ill with the infection.

37: Dysentery

The term *dysentery* means inflammation of the colon, which is part of the large intestine. There are several forms of dysentery, but the two I am discussing here are amoebic and bacillary.

AMOEBIC DYSENTERY AND AMOEBIC COLITIS

This disease is widespread all over the world. It occurs in about 10 per cent of the North American population and more frequently in the tropics. While it does occur in the northern part of the United States, it is much more of a problem in the southern states and even more so in the tropics and the Orient, especially where human excreta are used as fertilizer and the water supply is not properly treated. The acute disease is rarely seen in large cities where the water supply is free of contamination.

People of all ages are susceptible. The disease is produced by a protozoan, *Endamoeba histolytica,* a single-cell form of animal life.

Contagion: Amoebic dysentery is communicable, and it can be spread as long as the patient harbors the organism in his intestines. It is usually spread through contaminated food, especially food which is served cold and moist, and occasionally perhaps by contamination of water, or through flies, or by direct contact with infected excreta.

Incubation Period: The incubation period can be as short as three days in severe infections and as long as several months in some of the low-grade infections. Uusually, however, it is between three and four weeks.

Symptoms: The disease occurs in several forms. Acute amoebic dysentery is a severe, acute infection with fever, bloody diarrhea, abdominal pain and general discomfort. The chronic form consists of recurrent attacks of diarrhea or relatively mild inflammation of the colon. There is still a third form, called amoebic colitis, without dysentery, which produces general abdominal discomfort, occasional diarrhea alternating with constipation, and symptoms which frequently suggest chronic appendicitis. A fourth type is the carrier state in which the person does not feel ill, but harbors the amoeba in his intestinal tract or his liver.

Treatment: An acutely ill child must stay in bed. He is given enough fluid to make up his loss of it through diarrhea and enough nourishment to sustain him. Drugs are given to stop the pain in the abdomen and the discomfort from straining, and antibiotics and other drugs are given to combat the amoebae. There are many effective drugs for this, but none of them is universally effective.

Complications: The most usual complication is infection of the liver, occasionally with abscess formation. Usually, treatment with drugs is effective for this, but sometimes there must be an operation to drain the abscess.

Prevention: Preventive measures against amoebic dysentery consist primarily of the hygienic control of the disease. Human feces must be disposed of by sanitary methods; the public water supply must be protected against fecal contamination. Water obtained from doubtful sources should be boiled or chlorinated. There must be supervision of the general cleanliness, personal health, and the sanitary practices of people preparing food in public places. This is especially important in the case of foods eaten raw in countries where human excreta are used as fertilizer. Education in personal cleanliness and washing hands with soap and water before eating and after defecation are very important. Fly control and protection of food by screening and proper use of insecticides are of some help. Instructing convalescents and chronic carriers in personal hygiene is extremely important. There is no vaccine for immunization.

Isolation and Quarantine: The patient who is acutely ill with amoebic dysentery is isolated until he is free of symptoms and his stools become free of the amoebae. If, after the diarrhea has stopped, the temperature is normal and the patient feels well, he still has amoebae in his intestines, he may be free to go about. He may not work as a food handler, however, until he is free of the amoebae, and, of course, he must be careful about personal hygiene.

Carriers are not isolated, and people exposed to the infection are not quarantined.

Hygiene: While the patient is ill, his stool is treated with antiseptic. His dishes, clothes, and bedding must be boiled. Measures must be taken to eliminate flies from his room.

After the illness is over, the room should be cleaned with soap and water to make it safe for a healthy person.

BACILLARY DYSENTERY
(SHIGELLOSIS)

Bacillary dysentery is also called shigellosis because the bacterium which causes it was first discovered by a Japanese scientist named Shiga. Like amoebic dysentery, it is a worldwide disease and is more frequent in the tropics and in the Orient than in this country. But it is quite prevalent in the United States, particularly in warm climates, in the summer months in the temperate zones and in areas where hygienic measures are still primitive.

The disease is caused by one of several types of dysentery bacteria, which are named for the people who first discovered them. All ages are susceptible, but it is more common and more severe in children than in adults. Adults are more likely than children to have developed some immunity as a result of previous contact with the germs. This may explain why people traveling in countries where dysentery is common quickly catch it whereas the natives, who eat the same food, drink the same water and are surrounded by even more infected flies, remain well.

The disease occurs both in epidemics and sporadically. It is not so common where the water supply is made safe, sewage disposal is sanitary, milk is pasteurized and bottled, and infant hygiene is good.

Contagion: The disease is communicable during the entire acute phase and until cultures of the stools show that they are free of bacteria. This usually takes a few weeks unless specific treatment is given, in which case the period is considerably shortened. Occasionally, an individual remains a carrier. This disease is spread through contaminated milk or food. The contaminating bacteria are usually discharged by sick patients or by carriers who handle food. It is also spread by flies which light on infected stools and then on food and water.

Incubation Period: The incubation period is usually two to four days, but occasionally it is as short as one day or as long as seven.

Symptoms: The disease usually starts acutely with diarrhea, fever, abdominal cramps, straining and rectal pain on defecation. The stools contain blood, mucus and pus. It may be so mild as to be indistinguishable from a slight stomach or intestinal upset, or it may be so devastating that within a few hours, a child who has been perfectly healthy is prostrate and requires urgent medical attention. His body may be so dried out because of the water he loses in his stools that he is very seriously ill.

Treatment: Many of the antibiotics and sulfa drugs are effective in the treatment of bacillary dysentery and more are steadily becoming available. Your doctor will know which are the most effective, so do not try home remedies. While the treatment is almost identical with the treatment for amoebic dysentery, the antibiotics and sulfa drugs used are different ones. The doctor must decide which drug is best, what dosage to give and how long to give it.

Isolation and Quarantine: The patient is usually isolated until the acute phase is over and three successive stools are found to be free of the dysentery bacteria. If all measures taken to rid the patient of the bacteria fail and he remains a carrier, he may be discharged by the department of health after instruction in personal hygiene to show him how not to spread the disease.

People who are in an area highly infected with bacillary dysentery are not quarantined, nor is quarantine enforced on members of a family in which one person is sick. But all members must submit stool specimens to the health department for examination to be sure that they are not carriers.

Prevention: There is no effective vaccine for immunizing against bacillary dysentery. The only preventive measures are good hygiene, both personal and public. Carriers are prohibited from becoming food handlers in public places. In places where dysentery is very prevalent, breast feeding is a safeguard against infecting infants with contaminated food.

Hygiene: Hygienic measures to be taken both during the illness and after it are the same as for amoebic dysentery.

QUESTIONS & ANSWERS

Q.   *If you have bacillary dysentery once, is it possible to get it again?*

A.   Yes. You may be reinfected with the same type of bacteria that caused it in the first place or with any one of the many other types.

Q.   *Do you become immune to amoebic dysentery?*

A.   No.

Q.   *Are there any skin tests for the detection of either amoebic or bacillary dysentery?*

A.   There are no skin tests, but there are laboratory tests which indicate whether the child has the infection or has recently had it.

Q.   *Can these tests be done in any laboratory?*

A. Probably, but some laboratories are better equipped for them than others. The city, county or state health departments are usually well equipped.

Q. *Is prevention of dysentery largely a question of hygiene?*

A. Yes.

Q. *Can I take care of my child at home if she has bacillary dysentery?*

A. Yes, if you are instructed in how to do it and are able to carry out the directions.

Q. *Is it preferable to hospitalize a child with dysentery?*

A. Under some circumstances it is. If the child is very ill, especially if he is too sick to take fluids by mouth and must have them injected into a vein, a hospital is certainly preferable. Also it is much wiser if your home has no separate room with separate toilet facilities. If you cannot give all of your time to taking care of him, he would be better off in a hospital, because caring for a child ill with dysentery can be a full-time job.

Q. *Can I carry the germ to the other members of my family?*

A. You certainly can, if you are not meticulous about the disposal of excreta and about your personal hygiene.

Q. *Can I take care of my older child who is ill and at the same time care for my six-months-old baby?*

A. I do not think that is safe, but it can be done.

Q. *Is it safe to look after the sick child and cook for the rest of the family?*

A. No. Send the sick child to a hospital if there is no one but you to cook for your family. It can be done if you are careful, however.

Q. *Can you be vaccinated against either amoebic or bacillary dysentery?*

A. Not against amoebic dysentery, and while you can be vaccinated against bacillary dysentery, the results are too poor to make it worthwhile.

Q. *Are there any antiserums for treating either type of dysentery?*

A. Not for amoebic dysentery. There are some for some
    forms of bacillary dysentery and the results are reported
    to be good, but they are not used very much now because
    we have so many antibiotics which are more effective than
    the serum.

Q. *Is gamma globulin effective against any form of dysen-
    tery?*

A. I do not believe it has been tried enough to answer that
    question, but I doubt that it would be useful.

Q. *How soon after recovering from dysentery may my child
    go to school or the movies or the beach?*

A. Once he is fully recovered and has been released from
    isolation by the health department, he is free to do any-
    thing he is strong enough to do.

Q. *Must I be careful about diet for my child after he has had
    dysentery?*

A. Not after he is completely recovered.

Q. *My son recovered from dysentery several weeks ago, but
    he still gets diarrhea quite frequently. Is that to be ex-
    pected?*

A. Yes, for several weeks, or even months. The intestines go
    through a period of healing even after the amoeba or bac-
    teria have been eliminated, and during this time they are
    more easily irritated than they would be normally. You
    should make sure that he does not have the infection and
    that his intestine is not ulcerated.

38: Typhoid Fever

Typhoid fever is another infection which is prevalent all over the world, especially in areas where good hygiene is the exception and where primitive sanitary conditions prevail. It used to be a very common disease in the United States. Forty years ago when I was a hospital intern, typhoid patients—children as well as adults—were always present in the wards. Today it is one of the rarer types of infections we see in American hospitals. From a real scourge, it has become a relatively infrequent disease in this country except in the areas where poor hygiene still prevails, especially as it applies to proper sewage disposal.

Typhoid fever may occur in any season, but it is more common in the warmer months. It attacks anyone from newborn babies to old people, but it is not so frequent in children under five. It is caused by the typhoid bacillus. More than one attack is rare. Immunity seems to be of long duration.

Means of Infection: The disease is often spread by carriers. About 2 to 5 per cent of people who have had typhoid fever remain carriers; that is, they harbor the germ in their intestines or gall bladder while feeling perfectly well. They excrete the typhoid bacillus in their stool, and by soiling their hands they contaminate food which is eaten by someone else who then becomes infected. One of the most common causes of outbreaks of typhoid is the careless carrier who becomes a food handler. About ten years ago a localized epidemic of over twenty cases occurred in Coney Island, New York, in a children's camp where a carrier contaminated the food. Typhoid Mary was notorious because of the numerous outbreaks she caused by working in one place after another where she contaminated food. Flies lighting on infected excreta of carriers may also spread the infection by contaminating the food we eat.

Another common source of infection is infected shellfish which are taken from polluted waters and eaten raw. Typhoid may also be caused by drinking unboiled water from streams or wells which are contaminated by the excreta of carriers. Occasionally a large epidemic is caused by contamination of water or milk. In a large city in Germany in 1926 there were over two thousand cases as a result of contaminated water. In a Canadian city in 1927 there were over four thousand cases caused by contaminated milk.

Incubation Period: The incubation period of typhoid fever is seven to fourteen days.

Symptoms: The typhoid bacteria enter the body by way of the mouth with food, but cause no ill effects until they reach the intestines. After the incubation period the patient may feel ill at ease, he may have fever, headache, abdominal discomfort, cramps and distention. Some have mild diarrhea, or the opposite, mild constipation. In adults the course of the disease is characteristic and quite regular. The fever lasts about twenty-one days. The first week the temperature increases daily, the second week it remains quite high, and the third week it drops progressively, so that by the end of the twenty-one days the temperature becomes normal. In infants and children typhoid may be quite different. It may last only seven days, or fourteen, or twenty-one. It is usually milder; the child is not quite so knocked out. But in some cases infants and children may have it just as severely as adults do.

Relapse of the entire illness may occur several days or a week after the first attack seems to be finished. The relapse is often milder and shorter than the first attack, lasting seven or fourteen days instead of twenty-one. There are sometimes two, three or more relapses before the disease is finished.

Diagnosis: Typhoid fever is accompanied by a rash which appears late in the first week or during the second one. The rash consists of pink, round, flat spots, sometimes very few, usually seen on the abdomen. But in some patients the rash covers the entire body and looks very much like a pale measles rash. These spots are known as rose spots. The spleen, one of the organs below the ribs on the left side of the abdomen, becomes enlarged at the end of the first week. It is possible to make the diagnosis of typhoid wholly by the combination of these symptoms and a relatively low white blood cell count, a relatively low pulse, a high persistent fever, a doughy feeling of the abdomen, and by finding the typhoid bacillus either in the urine, stool or blood of the patient.

Treatment: The child is kept in bed. He is much too sick to want to, or to be allowed to, be active. His diet should be low in roughage and vegetables, otherwise it should be as usual. When the child's temperature is high, extra fluids are helpful. Your doctor will probably advise you to keep his temperature down with small doses of drugs and with sponge baths. You should not give him large doses of aspirin as they may cause a sharp drop in temperature with exhaustion.

Some antibiotics are quite effective in typhoid fever, but they must be given in large doses and for about two weeks, or they do not seem to prevent relapse. Chloromycetin is the drug of choice, but be sure to inquire whether newer drugs are better. The doctor must decide on the amount to give and how long to give it for each patient separately. No one should try to diagnose or treat typhoid fever without medical advice.

Unless there are adequate facilities for taking care of a patient with typhoid fever at home, he should be removed to a hospital. It is much safer and easier for the family and the community at large.

Hygiene: The urine and the stool must be disposed of carefully. You put enough water in the bedpan containing the excreta to cover them, and add a tablespoonful of a strong antiseptic like Lysol or CN. You let this stand for at least an hour before disposing of it in the toilet. Bedclothes, pajamas, towels, and so forth should be boiled before being sent to a public laundry, but they may be laundered at home if boiling water is used. Eating utensils should be either boiled or kept apart for the patient, in which case the usual washing is enough. A person taking care of a patient with typhoid fever should wear a gown in the patient's room and take the gown off and wash his hands carefully with soap before leaving the room.

Convalescence: Typhoid fever is a serious and debilitating disease. The child who has just recovered from it is quite weak and not in condition to resume all his usual activities. After he has been released by the local department of health, he may be allowed to leave the sickroom. Before going back to school, however, he should exercise an increasing amount each day, or as much as he seems to be able to take without getting tired. When he appears to be capable of the effort involved in going to school, he may go. This takes seven, ten or fourteen days— even longer in some cases.

Complications: The complications of typhoid fever in childhood are infrequent except for relapse of the disease, bronchitis and temporary changes in the mental picture. Typhoid fever may cause a child to be delirious, overactive almost to the point of being manic, and occasionally drowsy to the point of stupor. Hemorrhage from and perforation of the intestines are rarely seen in children.

Prevention: You can be vaccinated against typhoid fever. The vaccine produces immunity which protects you in most instances, though occasionally a person is exposed to such a large amount of contaminated material that the immunity is not enough to protect him. Vaccination against typhoid consists of three injections given about one week apart. The immunity which results reaches its height about six weeks after the first injection. Therefore, if your child is going to camp, it is important for him to be injected early enough so that the immunity is at its height by the time he arrives at camp. If the injections are given during the last few days before he leaves for camp, the peak is attained just about two weeks before he is ready to come home. After immunization with three injections of vaccine, a single booster given each year will keep the child's immunity at a safe level. If more than two years lapse after the immunization, the three injections should be repeated. Some doctors think it is safer to give the three injections every third year and one booster in each of the intervening years.

Prevention of typhoid is largely a question of hygiene. Isolation of the patient and careful supervision of contacts and carriers are most important. Eliminating flies from kitchens, dining rooms and sickrooms is essential. If a child is taught such simple precautions as washing his hands before eating, if he will not drink water of doubtful purity such as water from streams, brooks and old wells, if he will not eat shellfish from questionable sources, he is not likely to get typhoid. When you travel in countries where typhoid is prevalent, these precautions are even more important.

Isolation and Quarantine: Typhoid fever patients are isolated until the temperature has been normal for ten days, and after that until three stools taken on consecutive days are free of germs which cause the disease. People who have been exposed to typhoid are immunized and watched for possible illness, but are not quarantined. Nevertheless, the board of health does not allow exposed persons to work as food handlers until their stools are found to be free of the typhoid bacilli.

QUESTIONS & ANSWERS

Q. *Is it possible to get typhoid fever more than once?*

A. Second attacks are very rare.

Q. *Do flies carry typhoid?*

A. Yes. They may feed on infected excreta, then contaminate food. They should be eliminated from the kitchen and dining room.

Q. *Does one always find typhoid germs in the stool of a person who has the disease?*

A. Usually, but not always. They may be found in the blood and not in the stool, but if several stools from the patient are examined, the chance of finding the typhoid bacilli is considerably increased.

Q. *Can a child who has had typhoid go about his business as soon as his temperature is normal?*

A. No. The doctor reports the disease to the department of health. The health department usually investigates the condition of the patient's home and tries to discover the source of the infection. They try as quickly as possible to correct the conditions which allowed the disease to spread. Health department regulations indicate that the child must have three negative stool cultures two days apart after he has had at least seven to ten days of normal temperature before he is released. In any event, a child who is recovering from typhoid fever is usually quite weak for some time after his temperature becomes normal. His convalescence should be prolonged for two to four weeks, or longer if necessary. There is also the possibility of a relapse within a period of seven days after the temperature becomes normal. One or two relapses are not rare, even when the child has been treated with antibiotics. Of course, this would preclude return to normal activity right away.

Q. *Does typhoid affect other parts of the body besides the intestinal tract?*

A. Yes, it is a general infection. The bacteria may be found in the blood of the patient and may settle anywhere in the body. Typhoid may involve the bones; it can produce pneumonia and meningitis. But all of these complications are relatively uncommon. The one condition that is universally present in typhoid fever is the involvement of the intestinal tract.

Q. *My child goes to a private summer camp. The director of the camp says he has city water and does not have typhoid injections himself, nor do his children. Should my child be injected?*

A. Yes, no matter how well the camp is managed. Children go on hikes, sometimes overnight, and they may drink contaminated water. There may be an unrecognized typhoid carrier who handles food. Food brought into the camp might be contaminated with typhoid germs.

Q. *Is the vaccine used for typhoid immunization the same everywhere?*

A. The strength of the vaccine is standardized in this country, but all vaccines are not identical. Nevertheless, all those produced by the state departments of health and licensed pharmaceutical firms are good. Typhoid vaccine

is put up alone, but more often it is mixed with paratyphoid A and B vaccine.

Q. *Is there a skin test for typhoid fever?*

A. No.

Q. *Can you prevent typhoid with gamma globulin?*

A. No.

Q. *Suppose a child with typhoid fever continues to have positive stool cultures for several weeks after the disease is
over—may he go to school?*

A. No. The health department will make every effort to rid
the child of the carrier state, and will only let him free
when the infection is completely gone. If, after many
attempts at treatment, he remains a carrier, the health
department may free him from isolation. In the case of
an adult, he is only freed with the provision that he will
not become a food handler. Families of carriers should be
immunized.

Q. *Suppose a person continues to be a carrier indefinitely.
What can be done with him?*

A. About the only thing to do is to abide by the public
health regulation that forbids his taking a food-handling
job. Sometimes a carrier harbors the typhoid germ in the
gall bladder and removing it may cure him.

Q. *If my child has typhoid fever, am I quarantined at home?*

A. No. Usually the health department will examine the stools
of all persons living with the patient. If they are free of
typhoid infection, they may go where they please.

Q. *If one of my children has typhoid, may the other one go
to school?*

A. Yes, if the well child has a negative stool culture.

Diseases of the Mouth & Eyes

39: Diseases of the Mouth

The mouth is frequently involved in general infections. For example, in measles there are Koplik spots on the membrane lining the mouth and the palate and in the throat. In scarlet fever, the throat is very inflamed, the tonsils are red and the tongue, too, is red, with peeling of the upper layers of cells giving it the appearance of a strawberry. In diphtheria, the membrane usually seen in the throat sometimes involves the mouth also. Chicken pox sometimes causes blisters in the throat, in the mouth and on the lips. So does the virus which causes cold sores.

All sorts of infections may involve the mouth locally, those caused by bacteria, by fungi and by viruses. In Greek, *stoma* means mouth and the term *stomatitis* is often used for an inflammation of the mouth, but it is really too broad a term since an infection may cause an inflammation only of the gums, called gingivitis, or inflammation only of the tongue, which is called glossitis.

COLD SORE (HERPETIC STOMATITIS)

Many infections of the mouth are caused by the virus responsible for cold sores, the herpes simplex virus. It usually causes small blisters on the lips, but it may also cause uncomfortable sores on the tongue which make it difficult for the child to eat or drink. The infection often occurs with no fever, but there may be a little, lasting for a day or two. A more severe form of this disease is accompanied by fever ranging from 101° to

104° or 105°. It may last for four to six days, causing the child a great deal of discomfort and restlessness, and making him unable to eat, drink or even to sleep. The treatment is simple mouth hygiene, rinsing with warm water, salt solution, bicarbonate of soda solution or any of the simple mouth antiseptics. There are no specific drugs for this infection. If antibiotics are given, they do not alter the course of the disease except to prevent secondary infection. Sometimes the child may get a great deal of relief when the ulcers in the mouth are touched with a solution of silver nitrate.

Occasionally the lymph glands below the chin and jaws become swollen and tender. If this occurs, it usually is a sign of a secondary infection and antibiotics may be helpful.

Cold sores which are confined to the lips do not usually cause fever. Antibiotic ointments are helpful for preventing impetigo which often follows them, but they do nothing for the cold sores themselves.

THRUSH (MONILIASIS)

Thrush is a very common fungus infection of the mouth, especially in infants during the first few weeks of life.

Thrush of the newborn is usually acquired from the vaginal infection (moniliasis) of the mother. Thereafter it may be spread by contaminated nipples or fingers of the attendant.

Thrush also infects infants who are malnourished and children of all ages who are debilitated, and particularly those who are being treated with large doses of cortisone and antibiotics, and anti-tumor or anti-leukemia drugs.

When a baby has thrush, there are small white patches, like curds of milk, on the tongue, the sides of the mouth and on the gums. These little white patches sometimes become numerous enough to run together and give the appearance of a white membrane. The tongue looks completely coated and thick. If the membrane is scraped off, there are often little bleeding areas where the fungus has been removed. When thrush is limited to the mouth, it is annoying but not serious, but once in a while it extends into the throat, and even into the larynx, and then it can be a cause of great concern.

The doctor will treat thrush by applying with a cotton swab a 1 per cent solution of gentian violet or a 1 per cent solution of borax and glycerine to the parts involved. This usually clears up the disease in a few days. Currently, mycostatin seems to be the drug of choice for swabbing the areas of the mouth involved. The prevention of thrush is simple hygiene—being sure that everything you put into the baby's mouth is clean.

TRENCH MOUTH (VINCENT'S ANGINA, ULCERATIVE STOMATITIS)

In children, the infection commonly known as trench mouth is an infection due to the Vincent's organism, which is actually two organisms, a spirochete and a bacillus. *The organisms are commonly found together in the mouth around the teeth, and therefore there is some doubt as to whether or not Vincent's angina is truly a separate disease.* It is probably a secondary invader.

Vincent's infection is not found in infants before the eruption of their teeth, or in adults who have lost all their teeth. The illness usually occurs with only local symptoms in the mouth, but occasionally begins with malaise and some headache and a general feeling of being sick, with temperature of 101° to 102° or higher. The gums become swollen and inflamed and they hurt. Ulcers develop not only on the gums, but on the lips and tongue. The ulcerations become gray after a while and look as if they were covered by membrane, which disappears leaving raw surfaces. Usually, there is a characteristic odor which can be identified by people who are well acquainted with the disease. The glands under the jaw may be swollen and painful.

When the disease is limited to the gums, it lasts two to four days and gradually clears up by itself. When it involves the lips and tongue and the inside of the mouth, it is more extensive and lasts longer. Occasionally Vincent's angina spreads to the tonsils and they become swollen, dirty-gray and ulcerated. Pieces of tonsil are eaten away by the infection, leaving them irregular and scarred.

The treatment varies with the child's symptoms. If he has fever, he should be in bed; otherwise he may be up and about. Washing his mouth out with antiseptic solutions is soothing, and the doctor may prescribe antibiotics. He may not go to school until the infection is cured, but he is not isolated at home. He should have his own glass, towel, etc., to keep other members of the family from catching the infection.

HERPANGINA

Herpangina is an infection caused by a member of the Coxsackie group of viruses. Other members of this group cause epidemic pleurodynia (Devil's grippe) and aseptic meningitis (a condition sometimes confused with polio and other forms of meningitis). The virus attacks children, causing sore throat and high fever, up to 105°, which lasts one to four days and then disappears without treatment. When the doctor examines the child, he finds small blisters on the throat near the tonsils. These break, become coated, ulcerate and gradually heal.

It is contagious, with an incubation period said to be two to four days, so children who have it should be isolated, but those exposed to it need not be quarantined. Although immunity does occur after infection, we do not know how long it lasts.

There is no special treatment for herpangina other than reducing fever and relieving pain.

QUESTIONS & ANSWERS

Q. *Should I wash out my new baby's mouth?*

A. I would not put anything into the baby's mouth except water, food and the nipple, and a pacifier when needed —and, of course, whatever the doctor orders. Do not put your finger into his mouth and under no condition use cotton or gauze to swab the inside of the mouth.

Q. *Do pacifiers cause mouth infections?*

A. It can happen, but it rarely does.

Q. *Does thumb sucking ever introduce infection into the mouth?*

A. Hardly ever.

Q. *How can I tell whether my child's tongue is just coated or whether he has thrush?*

A. In some instances you may not be able to. If the tongue is coated, it is usually fairly uniform and not heavily whitened, nor is it coated in patches as in thrush. Usually thrush is not confined to the tongue and you can see the patches on the gums and the sides of the mouth. Furthermore, the ordinary coated tongue causes no symptoms. The child is able to eat and drink comfortably and he is not sick and unhappy. With thrush, the opposite may be true. If there is any doubt in your mind, you ought to have a doctor look at it.

Q. *Is infection of the mouth ever caused by poor teeth?*

A. Yes. The gums can certainly be inflamed because of infected or destroyed teeth. Occasionally you can see a reddened swelling of the gum at the level of the root of a tooth. It is called a gum boil and actually is an abscess of the bone. Vincent's angina often begins near a diseased tooth.

Q. *What should I do about a gum abscess?*

A. I believe you should show it to your dentist because it may take some special kind of attention to save the tooth if it is desirable to do so.

Q. *Do cold sores ever occur anywhere besides the lips?*

A. Yes, on any part of the body (the eyes, ears, mouth, throat, genitalia), and in the very young infant they sometimes occur as a generalized eruption all over the body. They are particularly likely to infect the skin of a child who has weeping eczema. They can even cause encephalitis, or infection of the brain.

Q. *I have heard that vaccinaton against smallpox stops repeated cold sores. Is that true?*

A. It was considered helpful by a few doctors, but this is not a widespread opinion. I would discourage this practice.

Q. *Are cold sores catching?*

A. Yes, they may be.

Q. *Does one become immune to the herpes virus?*

A. One builds antibodies to it, but may not become immune. Some people have repeated bouts of cold sores, as the virus lived in the body for years, possibly indefinitely.

Q. *What can I feed my child when his mouth is sore? He says that many foods hurt him.*

A. Give him milk and smooth milk products like junket, custard and ice cream, and foods that are not tart or acid. Drinking through a straw is sometimes less annoying.

Q. *If he can take food, may he have any kind he wants?*

A. Yes.

Q. *Orange juice, too?*

A. Yes, if he doesn't object to it because it is uncomfortable.

Q. *I have heard that fungus infections are increasing since antibiotics have been used so widely. Is that true?*

A. Yes, and they may also be more severe than they used to be. Monilia (a species of fungus) more often cause infection in the nose, throat, lungs and intestines than they did before antibiotics. Because of this, a new antibiotic has been developed which controls fungus infections. This is sometimes combined with an antibacterial antibiotic. The antibacterial antibiotic controls the disease and the anti-fungus antibiotic prevents fungus infections which are apt to occur after a course of antibiotics.

Q. *What are some of the other conditions of the mouth?*

A. Recurrent canker sores, or Aphthous Stomatitis, similar sores secondary to the use of antibiotics, to drugs used for leukemia, irritations due to chewing of cheeks and lips, etc. If the condition is due to drugs, change or stop using them.

40: Infections of the Eye

The conjunctiva is the mucous membrane which covers the outside of the eyeball and folds back to line the insides of the eyelids. The most common infectious eye diseases are infections of the conjunctivae and the eyelids. It is these we are primarily concerned with in the first part of this chapter.

GONORRHEAL CONJUNCTIVITIS

It is a rule in most hospitals in the United States and elsewhere that a solution or jelly of silver nitrate be instilled into the eyes of every newborn infant to counteract possible infection acquired as the infant passes through the birth canal of the mother. This rule was established because gonorrheal conjunctivitis was a very frequent disease. It became rare, but now it has again become a problem. When it does occur, it is in the first few days after birth. The eyes are red, the lids are so swollen that they may be closed, and thick white pus pours out between them. There is usually no fever. The infection responds very quickly to treatment with sulfonamide and penicillin. Since penicillin has come into use, one sees less gonorrheal conjunctivitis in maternity hospitals, even though more mothers have gonorrhea. Nevertheless, preventive measures are generally recommended. In some hospitals penicillin, instead of silver nitrate, is given as a preventive. A solution or ointment of penicillin is placed in the eyes or penicillin is injected into the baby shortly after birth.

Silver Nitrate Irritation: Inflammation caused by the use of penicillin is rare, but silver nitrate is sometimes irritating. The eyes seem inflamed and puslike material pours out of them for a day or two, sometimes longer, but almost always they improve without treatment or by simple washing with salt water.

VIRUS CONJUNCTIVITIS (INCLUSION BLENORRHEA)

Another eye condition of the newborn is called inclusion blenorrhea. It is an infection caused by a virus which has recently been identified. The newborn baby's eyes look very much as they do in the gonorrheal infection except that inclusion blenorrhea occurs about seven days after birth whereas the gonorrheal infection occurs early, as does silver nitrate irritation. There are no gonococci in the pus. It is quite contagious and may spread rapidly through a nursery, affecting several infants. It usually corrects itself, but it sometimes becomes a chronic eye irritation which persists for months.

PINKEYE (ACUTE CONJUNCTIVITIS)

Acute conjunctivitis can occur at any age. It is usually caused by the streptococcus, the staphylococcus and the pneumococcus, and we now know that the influenza bacillus causes the epidemic type called pinkeye. Treatment of acute conjunctivitis is similar to the treatment of the other eye infections I have mentioned; usually antiseptic drops or ointment are instilled into the eyes. Antibiotic ointments are commonly used. They should be put into both eyes even when only one appears to be involved because the infection is almost sure to spread to the other eye and sometimes this can be prevented, or at least the infection can be kept to a minimum. There is usually no need for antibiotics given by injection or taken by mouth. If, in the course of conjunctivitis, the eyelids or the skin around the eyes become inflamed as if they are involved in the infection, antibiotics are given internally. Local applications of warm water are soothing and helpful.

In the instances cited so far, there is rarely any disturbance of vision except the temporary effect of the inflammation. The infection is either rapidly corrected with antibiotics or it takes care of itself. In the case of the virus infection, inclusion blenorrhea, the antibiotics are useful only to fight bacteria which might complicate the original infection. They do not destroy the virus.

Prevention: To prevent eye infections in newborn babies, it is important that they be given penicillin or silver nitrate. In some institutions they changed to using just salt-water rinse of the eye right after birth to avoid secondary infections, and it seems to have been quite successful. But the law says that silver nitrate must be used unless permission is granted by the board of health to use penicillin or some other substitute. This is currently more stringently enforced because gonorrhea has become more common, particularly in young women and in adolescent girls.

In the first few months after the baby is born, the mother often tries to wash his eyes out with water or a boric acid solution. This is not necessary. In washing the face, if there is an accumulation of secretion in the corners of the baby's eyes, it can easily be washed out with water. Beyond doing that, it is best to leave the eyes alone. In the older child, prevention of conjunctivitis is a matter of cleanliness. A child who has conjunctivitis should have his own towel and washcloth and they should not be used by others. Tissues used to wipe away the discharges should be carefully discarded.

ALLERGIC CONJUNCTIVITIS

In older children it is often necessary to distinguish between infections and allergies involving the eyes. For example, children who have hay fever may develop redness and irritation of the eyes, itching and some discomfort. This is not to be confused with an infection, and it will not respond to treatment with antibiotics or other ointments used for the treatment of conjunctivitis, but it may respond to other medication, such as antihistaminic ointments or drops.

STY (HORDEOLUM)

The *hordeolum*, or sty, is an inflammation at the edge of a lid, usually involving the follicle of an eyelash. Sties frequently come in series. The child may have one and be almost finished with the first one when another starts. Sometimes they repeat themselves over quite a long period of time. If they are uncomfortable and cause extensive swelling and inflammation, hot compresses are very comforting. A sty which becomes very large may have to be opened. If your child has sties very frequently, you should take him to your doctor since he needs expert treatment of a general type. The doctor will probably treat him in the same way as he would for boils, because the bacteria which cause sties are similar to those which cause boils, and repeated sties are the same, in a sense, as boils.

CHALAZION (MEIBOMIAN CYST)

The sty is often confused with chalazion. A chalazion is an inflammation of a gland inside the eyelid resulting from obstruction of the duct. These glands are called meibomian glands and they secrete a fluid which lubricates the eyes. This fluid is what makes it possible for you to move your eyelids over your eyes without any noticeable friction. When the duct of the gland is clogged, the secretion fills up the gland, causing it to swell. It may become infected secondarily, causing a great deal of swelling, redness and discomfort. Here, too, hot compresses are very comforting. In the event that the chalazion is very large and uncomfortable and fails to clear up in a few weeks, the doctor may want to open it and drain it. The large majority of chalazions take care of themselves. They may empty, fill up again and repeat this cycle several times and yet cause no other disturbance than a slight temporary disfigurement. They are never dangerous except when they become infected. When the chalazion occurs at the margin of the eyelid, you should be very careful not to handle it even though it is very annoying, because when a chalazion in this position becomes infected, it may heal with scarring and cause irregularity of the eyelid. If it does become infected, the doctor may feel that something specific should be done.

TRACHOMA (CONJUNCTIVITIS GRANULOSA)

Trachoma is a virus infection of the conjunctiva and cornea. The cornea is the tough membrane which covers the colored part of the eye. Behind the center of the cornea, you can see the opening (pupil) through which light gets into the back of the eye. Trachoma causes inflammation of both the conjunctiva and the cornea. If the disease is treated early with sulfa drugs it responds favorably. Otherwise, it is a chronic disease which may last for years, causing disfigurement and scarring of the conjunctivae and the cornea and, in many instances, resulting in partial or complete loss of vision. Trachoma is present in the United States even though it is not generally known in our larger communities that the disease exists here. But in other parts of the world—in Egypt, the Near East and the Far East —trachoma is a major health problem and is one of the leading causes of blindness. It is contagious and is spread by contact with the secretions of the eyes and noses of infected people and with their tears. Previously difficult to cure, trachoma is now a curable disease.

OTHER CAUSES OF EYE INFLAMMATION

Other organisms may be responsible for eye infections, for example, the tubercle bacillus, the syphilis spirochete, the bacteria which cause tularemia, and occasionally fungi. While these are relatively infrequent, they can be serious when they do occur.

The eye is often involved in other diseases, especially measles. Occasionally chicken pox and shingles lesions appear on the eyes, as do cold sores. Some colds and the grippe are accompanied by conjunctivitis and excessive tearing and light-sensitivity. Syphilis produces the so-called interstitial keratitis, inflammation and scarring of the cornea which sometimes interfere with vision if they occur in front of the pupil. This disease occurs between the ages of five and fifteen and is one of the late developments of congenital syphilis. It has become a relatively uncommon disease since we have had penicillin.

QUESTIONS & ANSWERS

Q. *If a child is born at home, should anything be done about his eyes at birth?*

A. Yes. The doctor should give him the same treatment he would in a hospital.

Q. *Did you say that the eyes of infants and small children should not be cleaned?*

A. Yes. They should be left alone, except as the eyelids are normally washed along with the rest of the face. The eye is equipped to keep itself clean without any outside assistance.

Q. *How do I put drops of medicine into my baby's eyes?*

A. Separate the eyelids with the thumb and first finger of one hand and drop the drops into the eye right out of the dropper with the other. If the baby wiggles, rest the hand holding the dropper on the forehead and the bridge of the nose. This will give your hand support as you squeeze the bulb and when the baby moves, your hand will move too so that you cannot hurt his eye with the dropper.

Q. *Is there never fever with a sty?*

A. There may be, especially if the inflammation gets into the soft tissues around the eye, as well as the lid itself. Any fever means that the infection is more severe and needs more urgent attention.

Q. *Is there ever fever with a chalazion?*

A. Not unless it is secondarily infected, in which case the eye is swollen, red and painful.

Q. *Is pinkeye contagious?*

A. If the pus from the infection gets into the eyes of another child, he may catch it. This may happen when children use common washcloths and towels.

Q. *Can you tell pinkeye from other forms of conjunctivitis?*

A. Not without a laboratory test to find which bacteria are responsible for the infection. Technically, pinkeye is the acute conjunctivitis caused by the influenza bacillus.

Q. *What is phlyctenular conjunctivitis?*

A. It is a raised inflammation on the part of the conjunctiva that covers the eye, usually at the edge of the cornea. It looks rather like a pimple or a blister. It produces light-sensitivity, tearing and some discomfort. It used to be associated almost exclusively with early tuberculosis, but we know now that it also occurs with eye allergies.

Q. *Is it all right to use yellow oxide of mercury for pinkeye?*

A. It may be very good for conjunctivitis, though the mercury is irritating to some children.

Q. *You say that trachoma is a virus infection and that sulfa drugs stop the infection. Didn't you say that sulfa drugs do no good for virus infections?*

A. They are not effective in *most* virus infections. The exceptions are a few of the larger viruses, such as the ones which cause psittacosis and trachoma. These two viruses belong to the same group. Antibiotics are also effective against them.

Q. *Are bloodshot eyes always infected?*

A. No. Infection causes them to be bloodshot, but so does ordinary irritation, which is not the same thing. Allergy and injury cause bloodshot eyes, too.

Skin Conditions

41: *Fungus Infections*

There are so many different skin diseases that we could not possibly cover them all in a book of this kind, but there are some we see so frequently that they warrant at least a short discussion. Some are caused by viruses, some by bacteria and some by infestation, but the most widespread group is caused by fungi.

A fungus is a low form of plant life. There are thousands of them, only some of which produce disease in man. For purposes of identification these diseases are divided into two groups, the deep mycoses which involve the deeper layers of the skin or the whole body, and the superficial mycoses, or *tineas*, which involve only the superficial structures of the skin. They are further classified by the kind of lesion they produce, by the location of the lesions or by the name of the infecting fungus.

The deep mycoses cause conditions such as sporotrichosis, blastomycosis and actinomycosis which are relatively rare in the United States but are quite serious when they do occur. The superficial mycoses cause the more common fungus infections such as athlete's foot, scalp ringworm, body ringworm and thrush. One of the newer causes of fungus infections is the use of antibiotics. After antibiotics have been given to cure bacterial infections, we often see fungus infections of the mouth, pharynx, bronchial tubes, intestines and vagina because the antibiotics have eliminated the bacteria which kept the fungus under control.

ATHLETE'S FOOT (TINEA PEDIS, DERMATOPHYTOSIS)

This is called, after its location, tinea pedis or, after its causative agent, dermatophytosis. It is very common in both children and adults. In a children's school I found that 50 per cent of the children were infected before they were ten years old. Among soldiers and college students the percentage is much higher.

Athlete's foot appears between the toes where the skin is warm and moist. It causes swelling, redness and tiny blisters which may ooze and cause the skin to peel. It itches intensely and the child usually scratches and rubs the toes, thus causing further damage to the skin. It is a stubborn disease, lasting weeks, months or even years in some cases. It improves in the winter and becomes worse in the summer. There seems to be no lasting immunity, for it can be contracted over and over again in public showers and school and club gymnasiums.

There are numerous ointments to treat it with and they cause rapid improvement, but the cure is not easy. Secondary bacterial infection may have to be eliminated before the fungus can be. If you suspect that your child has athlete's foot, let your doctor recommend treatment. To be effective, any treatment must be carried out very diligently. The best treatment will fail unless it is continued for as long as the doctor advises. Socks and shoes become contaminated by the fungus when a child has athlete's foot, so the socks should be boiled after each wearing and the shoes should be disinfected and changed daily. If one member of a family has athlete's foot, he should wear slippers in the bathroom and step on to a mat different from the one used by the rest of the family. In gymnasiums and shower rooms and swimming pools children should rinse their feet in the special solution provided for elimination of the fungi. Because these solutions rapidly become diluted with water they should be changed often to be effective.

THRUSH

This is also called moniliasis after the infecting agent, *monilia albicans.* It is discussed under mouth diseases elsewhere in this book. It is a common complication following the use of antibiotics, and I have seen it appear three days after antibiotic therapy, often in the vagina in female children.

RINGWORM OF THE SCALP
(TINEA CAPITIS, FAVUS)

This is called, after its location, *tinea capitis* and, after its appearance, *favus* (Latin for honeycomb). It is more of a problem in middle Europe and elsewhere outside of the United States than it is here, but it does occur here. It is spread from person to person through contaminated combs and brushes. It causes round, yellowish, raised areas of inflammation with tiny blisters. As the center of the lesion heals, the outer edges resemble a ring. Wherever the patches are, the hair breaks off close to the scalp.

Favus is difficult to cure. The ointment which is generally ordered must be in contact with the infected scalp. Doctors usually recommend that the hair be removed by X-ray so that it will not grow back during the treatment. The reason for this is that while shaving it off is also helpful, it must be done repeatedly until the scalp is cured, and X-ray removal lasts much longer. The ointment should be applied twice a day. When you apply it, wash the crusts first with soap and water. The child should wear a cap night and day which should be boiled frequently and destroyed when it is no longer needed. This is necessary not only because scalp ringworm is very contagious, but because it itches and children may infect their fingernails by scratching the infected scalp. Fungus infection of the fingernail is very difficult to cure.

BODY RINGWORM (TINEA CORPORIS)

Tinea corporis is an infection of the nonhairy skin. It may affect any part of the body. It is usually acquired by contact with infected persons or infected dogs and cats. The treatment for it is applying ointments or lotions three or four times a day until it is cured, usually within seven to ten days.

RINGWORM OF THE CROTCH (TINEA CRURIS)

Tinea cruris is slightly different from body ringworm in that the lesions are arc-shaped instead of being a full circle, but the treatment is the same.

QUESTIONS & ANSWERS

Q. *Are there many different fungi?*

A. Yes, thousands of them. Some are found all over the world, and others are found only in certain areas.

Q. *Do they all produce disease in man?*

A. No. Some of them do, but most of them do not.

Q. *What other fungus diseases are there besides the ones you have discussed?*

A. Coccidioidomycosis or "valley fever" is a fungus disease which resembles tuberculosis. It is caused by a fungus which grows in the soil and is found on grass. It is found in the San Joachin Valley in California, in Mexico and in the Chaco region of Argentina and Uruguay. Histoplasmosis, another fungus infection, also resembles tuberculosis—so much so in fact that sometimes skin tests must be made to distinguish it from tuberculosis and from coccidioidomycosis. The fungus grows in the soil of the southern and midwestern United States and is particularly common in the central part of the Mississippi basin.

Q. *Are histoplasmosis and coccidioidomycosis spread from one child to another?*

A. No, not usually. The infection is transmitted by air-borne dust which contains the fungi.

Q. *Is skin ringworm serious?*

A. No, but annoying and difficult to cure.

Q. *How do fungus infections complicate diseases being treated with antibiotics?*

A. If bacteria are eliminated by antibiotics, the fungi have less competition and they seem to attack the tongue, mouth, throat, bronchial tubes and intestines. Babies get diaper rashes caused by overgrowth of fungi, and female children may get severe itching of the vagina.

Q. *Are these fungus complications serious?*

A. Usually they are merely annoying, but they may be serious.

Q. *May my child go to school with a fungus infection?*

A. He may if it is not on an exposed surface. For instance, he may go if he had athlete's foot or ringworm of the crotch, but he may not if he had scalp ringworm or lesions on his hands.

Q. *Aren't molds fungi?*

A. Yes.

Q. *Aren't molds troublesome, in that many people are allergic to them?*

A. Yes. Mold extracts are commonly used along with dust and pollen extracts in the treatment of vasomotor rhinitis.

Q. *Are antibiotics effective against fungi?*

A. Yes. Mycostatin is effective against monilia infection, such as thrush. Griseofulvin is now the drug of choice for ringworm of the scalp and against dermatophytosis, or athlete's foot. The treatment is long and tedious but often necessary.

42: Impetigo
(Impetigo Contagiosa)

Impetigo is an infection of the skin caused by germs similar to those which cause boils—the staphylococcus or the streptococcus. It occurs in anyone, from birth to old age, in all months of the year. It is most common in summer when children are scantily clad and more of their skin is exposed to injury and insect bites. Immunity to impetigo does not last, and a child can have repeated attacks within a short time, or a single attack may continue for weeks if it is not treated.

It is impetigo when your child has, on any part of his body, a yellowish crusted sore which remains and spreads to the skin around it and to other parts of the body unless it is adequately treated. Wherever people live night and day in the same clothes, where hygiene is primitive, especially where soap is scarce and where scabies (the itch) is widespread, impetigo is a common complication. It results from scratching the scabies-infested skin. I have seen several large hospital wards full of adults with impetigo which was superimposed on scabies.

Contagion: Impetigo is very contagious as long as there are any unhealed sores. The germs usually get into broken skin, especially skin that is scraped, for instance, by falling on gravel. Children may get it through contact with infected playmates or siblings when the germ is transmitted by discharges from the sores. They sometimes get it by using towels, washcloths, hairbrushes and other toilet articles which have been recently used by a child with impetigo. They occasionally get it by scratching and infecting insect bites.

Incubation Period: Impetigo usually appears within five days, sometimes as little as two days, of infection with the discharges.

Symptoms: Once the germs get into the skin, they produce little blisters which later break and ooze a yellowish fluid. These sores then become crusted. The crusts are pale yellow and are not firmly attached to the skin. When they are lifted, the yellowish material under them is pus. When a crust becomes dark and dry, it is usually a sign that the impetigo is healing at that particular spot. The skin under the crust looks pale for some time after the infection heals and the crust falls off, but eventually the normal skin color returns to the pale spots.

Impetigo is most often found on the hands, around the mouth, on the cheeks, and along the knees and shins, but it can infect any part of the skin, including the scalp. Impetigo is usually painless and does not cause fever unless the lymph glands in the area near the sore become swollen—then there may be some. The lymph glands in the groin may swell if the sore is on the thigh. If it is on the arm, the glands in the armpit may swell. If the sore is on the neck or scalp, the glands of the neck may be swollen. These glands are often painful and tender.

Treatment: Impetigo can be cured quickly with any of several different drugs, provided the treatment is continued without interruption until the skin is clear. The drugs are usually in the form of ointments to put on the sores. If the sores on the arm or leg are numerous, bandaging may be helpful for keeping the ointment on and avoiding further spread of the infection. The disease must be treated faithfully or it will spread. Occasionally, impetigo is quite resistant to treatment. This probably means that the bacteria which caused the infection have become resistant to the drug being used. In that case, your doctor will want to change to another form of treatment. If impetigo infects the scalp, it is sometimes necessary to cut the child's hair very short so that the medicines can get to the sores. If they cannot, the treatment will be unsuccessful.

Complications: Impetigo is not a harmless disease. If it is caused by one of the streptococcus germs and is not cured quickly, children may develop complications like erysipelas and kidney disease. In the New York area and in places with similar climates, about 2 or 3 per cent of the cases of acute nephritis (kidney inflammation) in children follow impetigo. The rest follow tonsillitis or scarlet fever. In some of the southern parts of the United States, impetigo may account for 25 per cent of the cases of nephritis, and in other parts of the world 75 per cent of the cases are caused by impetigo rather than tonsillitis or scarlet fever.

Prevention: The only preventive for impetigo is cleanliness. Teach your children to keep their hands and fingernails clean, and not to use other people's towels and washcloths. Skin sores, scratches, breaks in the skin and any condition which makes the skin itch so that the child scratches it should be treated promptly. Then the chance of the child's getting impetigo is very remote.

Isolation and Quarantine: Because impetigo is so easily spread, a child who has it is not allowed to go to school until it is healed. Impetigo sometimes occurs in nurseries for the newborn. It is a most unpleasant disease in the newborn and is sometimes quite troublesome. The infant who is infected has to be removed from the nursery and isolated and treated diligently to avoid spreading the infection to the other infants.

Hygiene: If a child has impetigo, his bedding and clothes ought to be changed daily and boiled or sterilized in some other way before they are used again. His towels and washcloths should be kept in a place where they will not be used by his brothers and sisters, and they should also be changed daily and sterilized. The toilet seat should be washed with soap after each time he uses it, especially if his thighs or buttocks are infected.

QUESTIONS & ANSWERS

Q.   *Do you develop any immunity to impetigo?*

A.   Probably not. A child may have it more than once, even within a short time. Each attack may be caused by a different germ.

Q. *How can you tell an ordinary infected sore on the skin from impetigo?*

A. It may be very difficult to tell the difference, except that in impetigo usually little blisters form at first, and if you inspect a sore carefully and see the blisters around the sore or in the center of it, it is more likely to be impetigo.

Q. *Is impetigo like a cold sore?*

A. In some ways. They both start with little blisters. When the cold sore becomes infected, it usually is impetigo. For that reason impetigo is common around the mouth and nostrils.

Q. *Does impetigo also infect the inside of the mouth?*

A. Rarely.

Q. *Does impetigo leave scars when it heals?*

A. In some cases impetigo injures some of the deeper layers of the skin and then it may leave some scarring. Usually it leaves only the pale area which is typical. This is particularly true in Negro children in whom the contrast between the dark skin and the pale spots of the healed impetigo is greater. Ultimately, pigment appears in the healed skin—after which it looks normal.

Q. *After my child has a runny nose for many days, he develops sores around his nose and upper lip. Is that impetigo or boils?*

A. Usually it is impetigo and has to be treated vigorously. Occasionally the skin gets red and swollen and a boil forms.

Q. *Can I treat impetigo myself or do I need a doctor?*

A. I think you need a doctor to make the diagnosis the first time you see it to advise you how to treat it, and later to tell you when it is cured.

Q. *Is there any way to avoid kidney complications with impetigo?*

A. Yes, by treating the impetigo immediately upon noticing it, and continuing the treatment until it is completely healed. This reduces the chances of complications a great deal. If a culture of the pus reveals the cause to be a streptococcus, penicillin treatment should be given promptly and for a ten-day period.

Q. *Is there any vaccine against impetigo?*

A. One can be made, but it is not generally recommended.

Q. *How soon may I send my child back to school after impetigo?*

A. A child usually is accepted at school once the sores have healed. If there is any doubt in the mind of the person who receives him at school, you will be asked to get a doctor's certificate saying that the child is well and that it is safe for him to be with other children.

Q. *What do I do about my child's clothes and bedclothes when he has impetigo?*

A. The bedding should be changed daily and so should the clothes. They should then be boiled before being used again. If the child has many impetiginous sores on the arms or legs to which you apply ointment, they ought to be bandaged to keep the ointment in place and limit the spread of the disease.

43: Diseases Caused by Staphylococci

Ritters Disease, pemphigus and Scalded Skin Syndrome are diseases that can occur in early infancy and childhood.

RITTERS DISEASE

This is a skin condition of the infant which causes severe illness. The skin is red over the entire body, including the face, and looks raw. It is usually caused by a staphylococcus and requires intensive treatment.

PEMPHIGUS

Pemphigus is a very severe, usually generalized disease. The body is studded with blisters containing pus and is often confused with impetigo. It is usually caused by staphylococci and requires urgent treatment. Pemphigus can occur in both children and adults—older people especially. Fortunately it occurs rarely, whereas impetigo is very common. (Almost every child who runs about barefoot has stubbed his toes, scuffed his knees and had impetigo, or he has developed it on top of "cold sores" around his mouth.)

SCALDED SKIN SYNDROME

This, too, is caused by staphylococci, usually of a particular strain or group. The child's skin looks as if scalded by hot water. The superficial skin layer peels off by itself or from friction with bedding or from rubbing or just handling. It is a very serious illness and, like the other generalized diseases, is caused by the staphylococcus. It, too, requires immediate and active treatment.

44: Boils (Furuncles) and Carbuncles

Boils are the result of an infection by the same germs that cause impetigo. But while impetigo is an infection of the superficial skin layers, a boil is an infection at the root of a hair. Sties are little boils resulting from an infection at the root of an eyelash. Boils have a tendency to spread to parts of the skin near the original infection as well as to quite distant parts. A cluster of boils which communicates is known as a carbuncle.

Incubation Period: The incubation period is very short, sometimes less than twelve hours.

Symptoms: Boils are painful. They start as a small red swelling of a hair follicle (the depression which contains the root of the hair). The swelling becomes larger, redder and more tender. It radiates a considerable distance from its center, which is the most prominent part. As the boil ripens, a white spot appears in the center of the swelling. If this white spot is broken or cut, a surprisingly large amount of pus is released. The boil may have a thick core of pus, and when this is removed it leaves quite a hole. This heals quickly. A carbuncle is often seen on the back of the neck. It is extremely painful, and pain is increased by moving the neck in any direction.

Boils, like other skin infections, may cause painful swelling of the nearby lymph glands, and they often cause fever.

Treatment: A single boil is usually treated by applying hot compresses to make the infection come to a head more quickly.

This is done by wetting a pad of cotton or a folded washcloth with hot water and holding it on the boil. The pad is reheated after it cools. This process is continued for fifteen to thirty minutes out of every two or three hours. When the child goes to bed, a wet dressing may be applied for the night. It will reduce the swelling and the soreness of the skin around the infection.

If a child has a chill while he has boils (which suggests the presence of a blood infection), it is urgent that he receive expert treatment. You should call your doctor without delay. The doctor should also be called if the child complains of severe pain in any of the bones or joints, with or without fever. Expert treatment is necessary, too, if he develops boils on different parts of the body at the same time, or if a boil causes fever or swelling of the lymph nodes near it. Antibiotics should be introduced promptly, and one should be chosen which destroys the staphylococcus since it is the cause in most cases involving infants and children.

Carbuncles should be treated very actively with local applications and antibiotics taken internally. If the pain is too severe to tolerate, surgical incision may be necessary. After the carbuncle is opened, the patient is quickly relieved of most of the pain and healing progresses more rapidly.

Prevention: A child may have boils or sties or both repeatedly over a period of weeks or months, even years in some cases. They often occur in more than one member of the family at once. When this happens or when the boils occur in rotation in one member of the family after another, it is important that the whole family be treated for seven to ten days with antibiotics at the same time, even those who have no boils at the moment. Otherwise, one person might be cured only to be reinfected by another.

Vaccines made from the germs causing the boils may be helpful. Many doctors prefer this vaccine treatment, either by itself or along with antibiotics. A sample of the pus obtained from a boil is sent to a laboratory where it is cultured. The bacteria are killed by heat and suspended in sterile or salt water. The child is given several injections of this suspension of dead bacteria. This stimulates his body to produce antibodies against the germs causing the boils, thus helping to prevent further boils from developing.

Everyone in the family must be very careful about cleanliness, and soaps or detergents (some of which have greater antiseptic properties than soap) are useful for this. It is important for a person who has boils repeatedly to be examined thoroughly to be certain that his general health is good, since boils are more likely to trouble sick or weakened people.

QUESTIONS & ANSWERS

Q. *Are boils the same type of infection as impetigo?*

A. No, not quite. Impetigo attacks the superficial layers of the skin. A boil usually starts as an infection of a hair follicle or a gland in the skin and works its way upward, spreading in all directions. Sometimes boils can be multiple, that is, there are several small boils in one group. When they produce a more extensive area of infection, it is called a carbuncle.

Q. *Do boils have to be operated on?*

A. Not necessarily, but sometimes it is easier to cure them by opening them when the boil has worked its way to the surface. If antibiotics are used early enough, a boil may be cured before it has formed pus.

Q. *Is that equally true of a carbuncle?*

A. It is possible to cure carbuncles without having to operate if treatment is vigorous, and is started early and continued as long as necessary. But sometimes it is wiser to open them early, as soon as liquid pus is formed. A good deal of time is saved and the patient is spared a great deal of discomfort.

Q. *When my son gets a sty, he almost always gets another one after a while. Sometimes they keep on coming for months. What can I do about it?*

A. Sties are the same as small boils in other parts of the body. As in boils, the infection of the follicle of one eyelash is likely to spread to others close by so that when one sty seems healed, others start up. In order to get rid of them and prevent their recurring so frequently, it is necessary to treat the first one vigorously. This is usually done with an antibiotic eye ointment. If a sty appears on another part of the eyelid, antibiotics taken internally should be added to local treatment.

Q. *What do you do when a child has boils repeatedly?*

A. It is possible to make a vaccine of the germ that is causing the boils and give him injections of it. We believe that this vaccine may be helpful, but treatment with antibiotics is preferable.

Q. *Are antibiotics and vaccines given at the same time?*

A. It is not a matter of choosing one or the other. They have different purposes. The drugs cure the disease when it is present. The vaccine is thought to make the child more resistant to it.

45: Warts and Mollusca

WARTS (VERRUCAE)

Warts are presumed to be caused by viruses. They are definitely not caused by handling toads. There are several varieties: the common wart, raised and rough-topped, which is usually found on children's hands; juvenile smooth and flat warts; thin threadlike warts; and plantar warts which appear on the soles of the feet. Only the plantar warts cause discomfort; the others are entirely a cosmetic problem unless they happen to be located at a point where they are constantly irritated, which may lead to bleeding or infection.

The art of curing warts probably has more practitioners than any other branch of medicine. All of the methods are said to work, and very likely they do—because most warts disappear eventually without any treatment. Professor Bruno Bloch, a famous Swiss dermatologist, believed that warts could be wished away, and he did cure many of his patients by simple suggestion. He had collected many tales of how warts were cured, as did Mark Twain, who described the many cures for warts. All of the cures had one thing in common: that they held promise that the warts would quickly disappear after the treatment, no matter how extraordinary the treatment was. So Dr. Bloch tested out his theory on his own patients and cured over 80 per cent of them by suggestion. Many of us have followed his lead and have had success with a fairly high percentage of our patients.

Warts which become irritated and plantar warts, which are usually painful, require removal through other techniques—injection of novocaine, cauterization, surgery or X-ray treatment. Plantar warts are often seen in several pupils of a school or among several children attending the same gymnasium.

Since I began treating warts by injection of novocaine and/or suggestion, I have not had to resort to cauterization, X-ray treatment or surgery for years. The simpler treatment seems to have been quite successful.

MOLLUSCUM CONTAGIOSUM

This is a virus infection of the skin which causes waxy, semi-globular elevations of pinhead to match-head size. They itch. They become larger and whiter as they age. The centers of the elevations cave in as the lesions dry. These pulpy nodules (*molluscus* means soft in Latin) spread about the skin, but at first they are usually limited to one area, such as the face, neck, back, chest or arms. They are not very contagious.

They cause no symptoms and are easily destroyed, but do not try to treat them yourself. Your child will not like it or like you for doing it. The doctor is likely to do a better job and to get rid of them more quickly. He will pinch off the mollusca with forceps and squeeze out the white globular mass he finds under them. Unless the mass is expressed, the mollusca may grow back. After this is done, the center is touched with tincture of iodine or silver nitrate.

QUESTIONS & ANSWERS

WARTS

Q. *Do warts occur in several members of a family because they spread the infection from one to another?*

A. We do not know exactly how the infection is spread. Warts usually are found in children, but they may occur at any age—particularly plantar warts.

Q. *Do antibiotics cure warts?*

A. No.

Q. *How can you prevent warts?*

A. We do not know except in the case of plantar warts. In this case they are transmitted from one person to another in places such as swimming pools and gymnasiums, and preventing them requires wearing slippers when swimmers are out of the water or rinsing the feet with antiseptics.

Q. *Why are plantar warts painful and the other kinds not?*

A. Because ordinary warts grow on the surface and have room to expand outward. Plantar warts grow on the pressure points of the feet, and pressure makes them grow inward. They form a hard conelike mass which extends into the sole of the foot more or less like a corn.

Q. *Do warts ever disappear without treatment?*

A. Most of them do.

Q. *Have you, yourself, tried treatment by suggestion successfully?*

A. Yes, and it has worked in four out of five children. All that seems to be necessary is to convince the child that the treatment will be successful. The treatment itself can consist of anything from rubbing oil on it twice a day to turning three somersaults every night before he goes to bed. If he really believes it, it will usually do the trick.

Q. *Do warts disappear more quickly with treatment by suggestion than they would ordinarily?*

A. They seem to, in general, and often they disappear within the exact time the doctor says the treatment will require.

Q. *Is the novocaine treatment suggestion?*

A. Possibly.

MOLLUSCA

Q. *Do mollusca look like any other infections?*

A. Yes, flat warts.

Q. *Is there any urgency in treating them?*

A. No, except that the longer the child has them, the more they will spread.

Q. *Can mollusca be cured with antibiotics?*

A. There have been some reports of success with antibiotics, but they have not been confirmed regularly.

Q. *Should other members of the family do anything to avoid catching mollusca?*

A. No. Nothing needs to be done unless they develop the lesions.

Q. *May a child with mollusca go to school?*

A. Yes. They are not very contagious. But if he rolls on a mat in the gymnasium he will contaminate it, so that others using the same mat may become infected.

46: Scabies and Lousiness

SCABIES (ITCH)

Scabies is caused by infection with the itch mite (*Sarcoptes scabiei*). This is a very common disease, annoying because of the intense itching, but serious only when scratching causes secondary infection of the skin.

Children get the itch from other children who are infested, from clothes or bed linen contaminated by another person or by a cat or a dog. It can also be acquired through direct contact with a cat or a dog, and cats and dogs may acquire it from humans. One of my patients developed a widespread skin eruption shortly after his family got a new cat. The cat was thought to have the mange, but turned out to be infested with the itch mite.

The female mite burrows into the outer layers of the skin where it lays its eggs. With a magnifying glass you can see where the mite entered at one end, black fecal dots in the burrow and the head of the mite at the blind end. Children often have scabies on the palms, soles, between the fingers and toes and on the body. It rarely appears on the face except in nursing infants whose mothers have scabies on the breast. Unless it is treated, scabies can go on for a long time—months—spreading over the skin until a large part of the body is involved.

Scabies used to be treated with sulfur ointment or balsam of Peru successfully, but these have been largely replaced by ointments containing DDT and other newer drugs. Before you apply the ointment, the child should be bathed. A shower is preferable to a tub bath. The drug is applied twice at twelve-hour intervals, and this is followed by another bath. The child's clothes should be cleaned or set aside. If they are set aside, the mites usually die in a day or two, but a thorough cleaning is more likely to destroy the mites and their eggs. If other members of the family are infested, they should all be treated at once to avoid reinfestation.

Prevention of scabies depends on cleanliness. When you sleep away from home, be sure that the linen is fresh. Children should be taught not to throw their clothes on beds. Cats and dogs which seem to have the mange may actually have scabies. Keep them off beds.

LOUSINESS (PEDICULOSIS)

Being infested by lice is common and universal. It is unpleasant, but not serious except in countries where body lice transmit diseases such as typhus fever and relapsing fever. At times typhus attains epidemic proportions involving thousands of people. It is especially likely to occur during war and famine. The body louse thrives where there is a shortage of soap, laundering and changes of clothing. While it is relatively harmless ordinarily, under these specified conditioned the body louse can become a great menace.

The head louse (*Pediculus capitis*), the body louse (*Pediculus corporis*) and the crab louse (*Pediculus pubis*) are the three species of lice which infest humans. Their movements, their bites and the irritation which results from becoming sensitive to their excreta produce severe itching so that the child scratches, especially at night. Lice lay eggs which hatch in about a week and become mature lice in about two weeks. The head louse lays its eggs, which are called nits, on the scalp or hair and the larvae attach themselves to the hair. The body louse lays its eggs in the seams of the clothing. The crab louse lays its eggs on the hair around the genitals. Head and body lice commonly infest children, while crab lice are more likely to affect adults.

DDT preparations and other chemical agents rapidly destroy the lice. Two applications, twelve hours apart, usually get rid of them. Epidemics of typhus have been stopped through disinfection of clothes, introducing cleanliness and body hygiene, such as bathing and using soap and water liberally, and by vaccination against the rickettsia transmitted by the lice which cause typhus.

QUESTIONS & ANSWERS

SCABIES

Q. *What kind of infection is likely to occur when a child scratches his skin because of scabies?*

A. Usually impetigo and occasionally erysipelas.

Q. *Is scabies a summer disease?*

A. No. It is more likely to occur in seasons when outer garments are worn because the mites get under the clothes.

Q. *Is scabies easily diagnosed?*

A. Yes.

Q. *Is it always easily cured?*

A. Usually it is cured by the first course of treatment, but sometimes two or more are needed. When it is not rapidly cured, it probably means that the child is being reinfested.

Q. *Do infested cats and dogs itch and scratch?*

A. Yes, and they make sores on the skin.

Q. *Is a child with scabies allowed to go to school?*

A. Usually not, if it is detected. It often escapes notice.

Q. *Is scabies prevalent in child-care institutions?*

A. Yes, it is always more common among children who live in groups.

LOUSINESS

Q. *When DDT is used for lousiness, is it dangerous to children?*

A. It would be if it were used excessively and repeatedly in products which have a high concentration of DDT. But it is rarely toxic in the doses used for one or two applications of the usual DDT products.

Q. *Can head lice be killed without DDT?*

A. Yes, by cutting the hair very short and using shampoo.

Q. *Does the common head louse carry disease?*

A. It may, but only when the louse itself is infected. This happens only when a disease like typhus is prevalent.

Q. *Then head lice are not dangerous here in the United States?*

A. No, they are not.

Q. *What about body lice and "crabs"? Do they carry disease?*

A. No, not unless they are infected or if open skin caused by scratching becomes infected.

Venereal Diseases

47: Syphilis (Lues)

Syphilis is a venereal disease caused by a spirochete, *Spirochaeta pallidum*. It is a widespread, very destructive disease. The name *lues* means, in Latin, pestilence. In many countries 3 to 10 per cent of the population used to have syphilis until the discovery of antibiotics which made it possible to prevent or cure syphilis in a high percentage of children. Today fewer adults have it, but the real decrease in the number of cases is in congenital syphilis in children.

A child who has syphilis harbors the disease throughout his life, unless he is treated. He never develops enough immunity to cure himself. If he is cured by penicillin or some other drug, he does not have enough immunity to keep from being reinfected.

CONGENITAL SYPHILIS

Syphilis in young children is mainly a congenital disease, one that is acquired before birth. The fetus is usually infected in the early months of the mother's pregnancy because the mother either had syphilis when she became pregnant or developed it during her pregnancy. If the mother contracts the disease later in the pregnancy and is not treated, the child will usually be syphilitic, too. A fetus affected by the disease in the first nine weeks of pregnancy undergoes changes in basic cell development so that if it survives at all, it may be defective in that some part of the body remains completely undeveloped. If it is affected later, the basic structure has already been laid down, but although the infant's body continues to develop in all its parts, some parts may develop defectively.

If the mother receives treatment before the fifth month of pregnancy, and if the infant survives, it will be free of syphilis. But if the fetus has been infected in the first two or three months of pregnancy, it may be damaged when born or it may be aborted. Children born with syphilis are also more likely to be premature, or small full-term infants.

In the newborn infant infected with syphilis, signs and symptoms of the disease may be present at birth or soon afterward. Sometimes the infant appears quite normal at first and develops evidence of infection some time later, at four to six weeks. The infected infant may have changes in the skull, the nose and the skin. The liver and spleen may be large and the kidneys smaller than normal and functioning poorly. The brain may be small, and in almost 100 per cent of syphilitic children the bones are involved.

LUES TARDA

In many instances, syphilis acquired before birth makes itself known much later, at six or eight years. Then it may be noticed, for instance, that the child does not hear well. There may be disturbances of the cornea of the eyes, the bone structure of the bridge of the nose may be caved in (saddle nose) and the permanent teeth may be peg-shaped or serrated (saw tooth).

ACQUIRED SYPHILIS

Rarely, small children are infected after birth. This usually happens when they are kissed by a person who has the disease. Acquired syphilis in children is very similar to acquired syphilis in adults. It occurs in three sharply defined stages. In the first stage, after an incubation period of about two to four weeks, a sore (chancre) develops on the child's lip where he has been kissed. A hard round edge develops around the sore. After a few weeks of this primary sore, the infection spreads throughout the body and produces a rash which is salmon pink and widespread. This is the second stage. A third stage of the disease shows up months later with syphilitic abscesses in the liver, spleen, bones, or in any other part of the body, including the brain. When syphilis invades the brain it is known as general paresis. When it affects the spinal cord it is known as *tabes dorsalis.*

Manner of Spread: When syphilis is not congenital, it is spread mainly through sexual intercourse and by kissing. Occasionally it is transmitted accidentally by transfusions of infected blood.

Wassermann Test: The Wassermann test and many others such as the Kahn or Kolmer tests indicate that there is a syphilitic infection when they are positive. Occasionally a positive Wassermann test occurs even when there is no syphilis. This false reaction takes place during infectious mononucleosis, infectious hepatitis, malaria and other conditions because of changes in the blood that occur during these diseases. These changes are not permanent, however, and after the disease is over, the Wassermann test will be negative again.

In the newborn baby who does not have syphilis, a positive Wassermann may mean only that the mother has had syphilis and been only recently cured. She may show a positive Wassermann for six months to a year after treatment, and in rare instances, indefinitely. She transfers the antibodies to the infant before it is born through their common bloodstream, and since these antibodies give only a temporary immunity, the infant's Wassermann test will become less and less positive as he becomes older until at about three months of age it will be negative. The degree of positivity is indicated by +, ++, +++, ++++, + being a mild reaction and ++++ a maximum reaction.

Treatment: Even in these presumably enlightened days, syphilis is a word which to many people has evil social connotations. Certainly this cannot apply to the child who acquires the disease through no fault of his own. It is an infection like many others—only more destructive because it is not self-limiting. It is nothing to be ashamed of. It can be eliminated with modern drugs, and it must be wiped out so that the child can develop into a normal, healthy adult.

Syphilis is a reportable disease. Any city, state or federal department of health is anxious to know of anyone who has syphilis and will gladly treat the patient without cost if he cannot afford private care. Penicillin and many other antibiotics are very effective. Arsenic, bismuth and mercury drugs are still used, but infrequently; these metallic drugs are not as effective as the antibiotics. Treatment should be continued until the patient is discharged by the doctor. Occasionally more than one course of treatment is necessary to accomplish a cure, but the disease can be made noncommunicable in a very short time. For instance, open sores, when untreated, are a source of infection because they are teeming with spirochetes, but twenty-four hours after treatment is started the organisms can no longer be found in the sores.

Prevention: The prevention of syphilis in children depends almost entirely on the prevention and cure of syphilis in adults. Penicillin taken before or soon after intercourse is usually successful in avoiding the disease. If the disease has already developed, treatment should be started immediately, not only for the sake of the person who has it, but to avoid communicating it to others.

Isolation and Quarantine: Syphilis patients are not isolated unless they have open sores. If they do, they are isolated for twenty-four hours after treatment is started. Persons with communicable syphilis should not be allowed to work in personal service jobs, particularly those which involve intimate contact with children. People who have been exposed to syphilis are not quarantined, but families of those who are found to have syphilis should be examined.

QUESTIONS & ANSWERS

Q. *Will a child get syphilis if his father has it before he is born?*

A. Probably, but not from the father. He will get it only because the mother will be infected.

Q. *If the mother acquires syphilis when she is six or seven months pregnant, will the baby have it?*

A. Probably—almost surely.

Q. *How will a mother know she has syphilis so that she can be treated?*

A. If she has not discovered it before she becomes pregnant, it will be discovered later. It has become customary for doctors to examine the blood of all women during pregnancy. Also, her blood will surely be examined at the hospital when she arrives to give birth to the baby.

Q. *If the mother is treated during pregnancy, is the baby likely to be normal and healthy?*

A. Yes, if she is treated at the beginning, soon after becoming pregnant. If she is treated later in pregnancy the infant will be free of syphilis, but it may have been damaged before treatment was begun.

Q. *Is all syphilis curable?*

A. Just about all, though occasionally a case is found to be resistant to treatment. There are cases, of course, where the disease has caused serious damage before it is cured, and the damage may be permanent even though the infection has been eliminated. This is particularly true of syphilis of the brain.

Q. *Are all syphilitic children necessarily damaged?*

A. No. Once cured, most of them are perfectly normal except for what has been damaged beyond repair, such as the bridge of the nose and the shape of the teeth, or brain damage.

Q. *If an infant's Wassermann test remains positive after he is three months old, does it mean he has syphilis?*

A. Yes, in most cases.

Q. *Do children ever have a Wassermann that stays positive indefinitely after the infection is cured?*

A. Yes, but it is rare.

Q. *How soon after penicillin treatment does the Wassermann become negative?*

A. Within six months in most children, up to a year in some.

Q. *Once the Wassermann becomes negative, can it become positive again?*

A. Yes, if the child is reinfected. This is quite rare in children, though they can become infected again as adults.

Q. *How can I enroll my child in a board of health clinic for treatment?*

A. Your doctor will refer you to the clinic, or you may go there directly. If you do not know where to go, call your department of health.

Q. *May a child with syphilis attend school?*

A. Yes, unless he has open sores.

Q. *May he play with other children?*

A. Yes.

Q. *Will he infect other children?*

A. Not unless there are open sores.

Q. *When a child has congenital syphilis which is not treated, and she grows up and marries, will she pass it on to her children?*

A. This occurs rarely, if at all. If the mother has been infected recently, the infant is almost sure to have syphilis, but the older an infection is, the less active it becomes, and a less active infection is much less likely to be transmitted to the infant. In the case of a mother who was herself infected before birth, the infection is very inactive.

Q. *Is the blood test the only way to detect syphilis?*

A. No, the doctor usually suspects it when he examines the child.

Q. *Is there a vaccine to prevent syphilis?*

A. No.

Q. *What can be done to avoid syphilis?*

A. To avoid it in your child, avoid getting it yourself, and if you do get it, have it treated.

Q. *Is syphilis on the increase?*

A. Yes, particularly in teen-agers. It requires urgent attention. Homosexuals spread it many times more than others.

Never make the mistake of delaying treatment because of shame.

Q. *How can we prevent our teen-age children from getting it?*

A. Give them early sex education. Teach them about prophylactic treatment if they should indulge in intercourse or sex play with homosexuals. Above all, try to maintain good relations with them so that they will want to live by your example and with your guidance, and be always ready to be helpful should they acquire the disease.

48: Gonorrhea

Gonorrhea is a venereal infection caused by an organism called the gonococcus. The forms of gonorrhea most common among children are gonorrheal conjunctivitis and gonorrheal vaginitis in the female child. Previously a very common infection in infants and young children, gonorrhea has become relatively rare because it is quickly eradicated by penicillin. At one time gonorrheal infection of the eyes of the newborn was the leading cause of blindness in children. Now it is less common but it is unfortunately on the increase. In the United States, for instance, a pregnant woman who has gonorrhea is cured before her baby is born if she has any medical supervision at all. And if the birth of the baby is attended by a doctor or a nurse, the baby has silver nitrate or an antibiotic instilled into his eyes as soon as he is born as a cure or preventive for gonorrheal infection.

Gonorrheal vaginitis used to be a very common and highly contagious infection in hospital wards. If a child was admitted for this disease, it was likely to spread in a short time to all female children and even boys, in whom the disease affects the urethra.

Vaginal discharges in female children are common, but most of them are not due to gonorrhea. If there is a profuse, pussy discharge that persists, it should be examined by a physician, and if gonorrhea is the cause, it should be treated. The child with gonorrheal conjunctivitis or vaginitis should be isolated only until the gonococcus has disappeared from the discharges, usually a matter of twenty-four hours after treatment is begun.

Adult gonorrhea is usually acquired through sexual intercourse, but in children the infection usually results from the use of common towels, sponges, washcloths and from actual contact. An adult with gonorrhea should be careful to avoid spreading it to children by boiling all objects that may come in contact with the discharges, including underclothes, and should never touch the infant without first thoroughly washing her hands with soap and water. The old idea that it can be spread through the indirect contact of using toilet seats is obsolete.

In the last few years gonorrhea has become much more common, particularly among teen-agers and young adults. What causes added concern is that many of the strains of the gonococcus have become resistant to treatment with several of the drugs which were very effective a few years back.

QUESTIONS & ANSWERS

Q. *Do older children get gonorrhea?*

A. Yes, but not of the eyes. They get vaginal or urethral and occasionally rectal gonorrhea.

Q. *How does this happen?*

A. Children become infected by towels or other infected objects handled by adults. Most often it happens during a bath when the child washes the genital area with a contaminated washcloth or touches the genital area with dirty hands. Of course, sex-play as a cause increases with age.

Q. *Is vaginal gonorrhea easily cured?*

A. Yes. Penicillin cures most cases in one day. Some cases require more intensive and longer treatment, and some recur after treatment and have to be re-treated.

Q. *Are other antibiotics besides penicillin effective?*

A. Yes, many of them are quite good.

Q. *Do children who catch gonorrhea have difficulties later?*

A. Sometimes, but this is less common now because the disease is usually cured rapidly. Usually gonorrhea must go untreated for quite a while to produce permanent damage.

Q. *Is gonorrhea disappearing?*

A. No, on the contrary, it has increased greatly in the past few years. Teen-agers are particularly involved. In addition, many of the gonorrheal germs, the gonococci, have become resistant to some drugs and antibiotics. Larger doses, longer treatment and other antibiotics have to be employed when drug resistance is discovered.

Q. *What can be done about this increase in gonococcal infection?*

A. This is very difficult to answer, but I shall repeat what I have already said. Teach your children about sex matters. As they approach adolescence, teach them about sex hygiene. Tell them what to do if they have been exposed to possible infection. Try to convince them that you want to be helpful, not critical. Make your family life as wholesome and as free of strife as possible.

Glossary

While all of the more technical words I have used in this book are explained at some point in the text, it would be very cumbersome and make very slow reading to explain each one every time it is used. Then too, there are a number of words which have different or more specific meanings in medical usage than in ordinary English. Some people who read this book will want further information about a given term, while others will be satisfied not to know any more than is necessary for understanding the text. For these reasons, I have prepared a rather extensive glossary. It is not required reading; you can get everything you need from the text of the book without ever referring to it. But if you are interested in knowing more about a word or a phrase or a process, or if you read medical articles in newspapers and magazines, I believe this glossary will be helpful to you.

When the definitions contain words which are italicized, you will find these words elsewhere in the glossary as cross-references.

abortive. An abortive case of a disease is one in which the disease is of shorter-than-usual duration, and does not develop fully, often having no obvious or identifiable *symptoms*. For example, a child may have an abortive attack of poliomyelitis which is passed off as an insignificant cold or intestinal upset.

abscess. A localized collection of *pus* in any part of the body.

A.C.T.H. A hormone or chemical substance which is produced by the pituitary gland and which stimulates the adrenal glands to secrete *cortisone* and other similar substances.

active immunity. The *immunity* acquired as a result of having a disease or by having injections of a *toxin, toxoid* or *vaccine* which stimulate the body to produce *antibodies* against a disease.

acute. Having a sudden *onset*, definite *symptoms* and a short course; not *chronic*.

adenoids. The adenoids are actually called the pharyngeal *tonsils* since they are composed of the same kind of *tissue*. The adenoid is not divided, but is in one piece, at the back of the throat behind the nose.

adolescence. The period of youth which starts at *puberty* and ends at maturity.

adrenalin. Epinephrine. A drug produced by the adrenal gland which constricts the blood vessels; often used to relax the *bronchial tubes* in *asthma,* and as a heart stimulant.

allergic rhinitis. *Inflammation* of the *mucous membrane* of the nose caused by *allergy* rather than *infection.*

allergy. Altered reactivity to a substance. Sensitivity to a specific substance which causes no reaction in those who are not sensitive. The allergic reaction of the body may manifest itself as *hives, asthma, hay fever, eczema,* etc., or as skin rashes, *serum* sickness, or drug-sensitivity.

amoeba coli. A colorless, jellylike, one-celled organism found in the stool of persons infected with it. It causes dysentery, *diarrhea* and liver disease.

anaphylactic shock. When a substance such as horse *serum* which stimulates the body to produce *antibodies* against it is injected, and at a later date reinjected, the reaction of the patient to the second injection is sometimes severe—even *shock* and collapse. The reaction is due to hypersensitivity to the horse serum. Experimentally, anaphylactic shock in animals can be produced by repeated injection of many substances, not only horse serum.

anesthetic. A drug which pro-

duces loss of sensibility. A topical anesthetic produces loss of sensibility at the site when applied locally to the skin. A local anesthetic can be a topical anesthetic or one which is injected and affects only the nerves in the injected area. A general anesthetic is one which works by affecting the brain. It can be inhaled like ether, nitrous oxide, etc., or injected into the blood like sodium pentothal.

animal host. An animal which normally harbors an *infectious agent* which, if transmitted to man, may produce disease. For example, the mosquito in malaria.

antibiotic. A chemical substance produced from *bacteria* or molds, or produced synthetically, having antibacterial properties which make it useful for treatment or prevention of bacterial *infection.* For example, penicillin, Aureomycin, Terramycin, streptomycin, etc. There are also antibiotics which affect the growth of *fungi* and *viruses.*

antibody. A protective substance in the blood which the body produces as a reaction to *infection* or to the injection of *toxin, toxoid* or *vaccine.* It serves to fight the *infectious agent.*

antihistamine. A substance capable of preventing or diminishing some of the effects of histamine, which, when liberated in the body, causes allergic *symptoms.* There are many antihistaminic drugs which are helpful against *hives, hay fever,* etc.

antiseptic. A substance which stops or inhibits the growth of *bacteria,* molds or *viruses* or kills them, and thus prevents putrefaction and fermentation.

antiserum. The fluid part of blood —human or other animal—which contains protective substances against a particular *infectious agent*. It is ordinarily injected to help fight an *infection*.

antistreptolysin titre. Antistreptolysin is an *antibody* formed in the blood against the *toxins* liberated by the hemolytic *streptococcus*. The blood test is often done in doubtful cases of rheumatic fever to find out whether the patient has recently had a hemolytic streptococcus *infection*. The antistreptolysin titre is the measure of the amount of antistreptolysin in the blood.

antitoxin. A substance, usually *serum* contained in blood, produced by the human or animal body when a specific *toxin* has been introduced into it, causing it to produce *antibodies* against that toxin. For instance, *serum* against diphtheria or tetanus toxins.

arthritis. *Inflammation* of one or more joints.

aseptic meningitis. A form of *meningitis* which is not caused by the usual *bacteria,* but which may be due to an *infection* with a *virus* or possibly some other agent, and which is usually not severe.

asphyxiation. Suffocation due to lack of oxygen in the body.

asthma. A condition characterized by spasms of the *bronchial tubes,* swelling of their linings and excessive secretion of *mucus.* These cause coughing, wheezing, breathing difficulty and a feeling of constriction in

the chest and are usually due to an *allergy.*

attenuated. Reduced virulence and toxicity of a vaccine or toxin.

bacillus. A rod-shaped *bacterium.* Bacillary, in disease, means caused by bacilli.

bacterial allergy. Sensitivity to *bacteria* which produces *allergic symptoms* on top of the symptoms of the bacterial *infection.*

bacterium. Any one of a large group of single-celled vegetable *microorganisms,* relatively few of which produce disease in man. They are classified as *cocci, bacilli, spirilli, spirochetes* and vibrios.

bile. A bitter, greenish-yellow fluid *secreted* by the liver and poured into the gall bladder, then into the intestines to aid in digestion and absorption of fats and calcium salts.

blood cells. See *white blood cells* and *red blood cells.*

blood count. The process of finding out how many *red* and *white blood cells* are in a cubic millimeter of blood. It is used in the *diagnosis* of many diseases in which the number and character of red and white cells are altered.

blood pressure. The pressure exerted by the blood in the arteries, depending on the force of the heart beat, the elasticity of the walls of the arteries, the volume of blood, etc.

blood product. Any substance made from blood, such as plasma, immune *serum* or *gamma globulin.*

blood type. Human beings have four different types of blood, usually called O, A, B and AB.

If one type is mixed with a type "foreign" to it, as in a transfusion, the result is the destruction of the red blood cells. None of the *serums* will destroy type O cells, so this type is safe for transfusion in anyone. In type AB the serum does not destroy any cells, so a person with this type could receive a transfusion from anyone. But type A must receive A or O and B must receive B or O.

booster injection. An additional injection of *toxoid* or *vaccine* given some time after the initial ones to stimulate a higher level of *immunity* in a person whose immunity is weakening. The increase of immunity is called a *booster* or recall reaction, and the amount of material injected is called a booster or recall dose.

botulism. Food poisoning caused by a *bacterium* called *Clostridium botulinum,* found in improperly canned foods.

broad-spectrum antibiotics. *Antibiotics* which are effective against a large number of organisms. For instance, Aureomycin, Terramycin, Achromycin, Chloromycetin, Tetracyn. Penicillin, while it is effective against some disease-causing organisms, does not cover nearly as broad a field as those above.

bronchial tubes. The two principal branches of the *trachea.*

bronchiectasis. A condition in which the *bronchial tubes* are distended into little pockets. It is usually caused by *chronic inflammation.*

calamine lotion. A soothing lotion used to relieve itching. It is often combined with *antihistamines* or with 1–2% phenol.

camphor. A drug which is a mild irritant and *antiseptic.* It is used internally to relieve colic, and as a stimulant for the heart and lungs.

carbohydrate. An organic substance containing carbon, hydrogen and oxygen. Sugars, dextrins, starches and celluloses are carbohydrates.

carrier. A person or animal who carries the *germ* of a disease without showing *symptoms* of it. In some diseases the *infected person* acts as a carrier during the *incubation period* of the disease, e.g., scarlet fever, typhoid, dysentery.

caseous. Resembling cheese. Caseation is the process of *cell* destruction which turns *tissue* into a soft, cheeselike substance, as in tuberculous *infection.*

catarrhal vaccine. *Vaccine* made from organisms found in the nose and throat which may act as a preventive against the *complications* of colds.

causative agent. A *bacterium, virus, protozoan* or any other substance or object which causes a disease.

cell. A unit of body structure or mass of protoplasm containing a nucleus.

cellulitis. Any *inflammation* of the body cells. Specifically, inflammation of the *tissues* just under the skin, usually caused by *pus*-forming *germs* like the *streptococcus* and the *staphylococcus.*

centigrade. Having 100 divisions or degrees. Specifically a scale of measurement used on thermometers in all countries except

England and the United States. To find the *Fahrenheit* equivalent in degrees, multiply centigrade degrees by 9/5 and add 32.

central nervous system. The brain and *spinal cord.*

cervical adenitis. *Inflammation* of the *lymph* glands in the neck.

chlorinate. To add chlorine to water. Chlorine becomes a powerful germicide in the presence of moisture and is used to decontaminate or prevent *contamination* of drinking and swimming water.

choriomeningitis. A *virus* disease, usually benign, involving *inflammation* of the covering *membrane* of the brain. It is transmitted by the house mouse to man, probably by *contamination* of food.

chronic. Lasting a long time, as opposed to *acute.*

clinical. Pertaining to the *symptoms* and course of a disease as the doctor sees them, without laboratory tests, etc.

coccidioidomycosis. A disease similar to tuberculosis, which involves the lungs, caused by inhaling spores of a *fungus,* commonly found in the San Joachim Valley of California.

coccus. A spherical *bacterium.*

colic. Abdominal pain or cramps coming in spells or paroxysms due to *spasms* of the muscle of the intestines.

collagen. A substance existing in some tissues of the body, especially bone-cartilage and in the connective tissue (tissue which binds together skin to underlying structure). Cement substance of the body.

coma. Unconsciousness from which the patient cannot be aroused. The patient in this condition is said to be comatose.

communicable. An *infection* is communicable when the *causative agent* can be transmitted from one person or animal to another. The period of communicability is the time during which the causative agent may be transmitted directly or indirectly.

complication. An accidental condition or a second disease which occurs during the course of, or as a result of, a primary disease.

compress. A folded cloth or a pad of soft material, wet or dry, cold or hot, applied to a part of the body for the relief of *inflammation* or the prevention of *hemorrhage.*

congenital. Existing at birth, but not inherited.

conjunctivitis. *Inflammation* of the conjunctiva, which is the tissue that lines the eyelids and covers the eyeball.

contact. A person who has been exposed to a *communicable* disease.

contagion. The process by which a disease is transmitted, either by direct contact or contact with an intermediate object. The medium of transmission of disease.

contamination. The presence of an *infectious agent* in a wound, on an eating utensil, on clothes, in water, milk, other foods, etc.

convalescence. 1. The recovery of health after a disease. 2. The time spent in recovering.

convalescent serum. *Serum* made from the blood of a patient who is *convalescing* from an *infectious* disease. It may be injected as a preventive or a cure for that disease in other persons.

convulsion. A sudden involuntary contraction of muscles all over the body which is often the result of infection, injury or degeneration of the brain. In *infants* and small children it may accompany the *onset* of high fever and is the equivalent of a chill in an adult. It may occur with or without loss of consciousness.

cortisone. A substance excreted by the adrenal gland, in greater amounts when it is stimulated by some sudden disturbance. It has a powerful effect on many functions of the body.

cresol. A powerful *antiseptic* and germicide obtained from coal tar.

cross-immunity. The *immunity* to a subgroup of a *bacterium* or *virus* which is acquired by having been infected with the bacterium or virus itself. The immunity to the subgroup will be less than the immunity to the original *infectious agent*.

croup. A condition of the *larynx* in which there is a harsh crowing cough and difficult breathing. It is caused by swelling, *inflammation* or *spasm* of the larynx.

culture. 1. Growth of *microorganisms* on artificial mediums. A culture of *bacteria* is made when it is impossible to identify them under a microscope because there are too few of them. The material from an infected part which contains the bacteria is grown so that the bacteria multiply and form colonies of millions. They are then more easily identified. 2. The act of growing the microorganisms. 3. The microorganisms thus grown.

dehydration. The removal of water, as from a body.

delirium. A state of mental excitement and confusion in which the senses are clouded. Usually there are hallucinations.

Devil's grippe. An epidemic disease with fever and pain in the chest, upper abdomen and midback which was so called because it "felt like the Devil's grip" on the chest. The present-day name is epidemic pleurodynia.

diagnosis. 1. The act of determining the nature of a disease. 2. The decision reached.

diaphragm. A partition between the chest and the abdomen which is muscular around the edges and similar to tendon tissue at the center. It is the chief muscle of respiration.

diarrhea. Excessive rate of excretion of intestinal contents manifested by more frequent and more fluid *stools* than normal. A common *symptom* of many *gastrointestinal* diseases.

Dick test. A *skin test* which determines whether or not a person is *immune* to scarlet fever.

diphtheritic membrane. See *membrane*.

discharge. 1. To evacuate or secrete or emit. 2. The product which is emitted.

disinfection. The destruction of the agent or *germs* which produce disease.

distention. A state of being stretched, as when the abdominal muscles are relaxed and gas within the intestines causes them to balloon out.

droplet infection. *Infection* transmitted by droplets of moisture from the nose and throat of a patient. The droplets contain the *bacteria* or *viruses* responsible for the disease and are propelled into the air by breathing, sneezing, coughing or speaking.

duct. A tube or channel, especially one which carries the *secretions* of a gland.

eczema. An allergic skin condition in which the skin is rough, reddened, swollen and finely blistered in patches. The blisters are so small that they are almost invisible. They ooze *serum* which dries and crusts. A dry form of eczema appears scaly.

electrocardiogram. A pictorial record of tracings of the electric current traversing the heart muscle. It makes it possible for the doctor to tell whether any part of the heart tissue is damaged, and if so, which part it is. The record is made by attaching electrodes to the body surfaces.

electroencephalogram. A chart recording the electric activity of the brain, obtained by attaching electrodes to the scalp.

electron microscope. A microscope which will enlarge detail 50 to 100 times more than an ordinary optical microscope. It is based on the fact that electrons carry waves much smaller than light waves. The images are studied on a fluorescent screen or recorded photographically.

enanthum. An *eruption* on the *mucous membrane.* For instance, the lining of the mouth, nose, throat, intestines, vagina, etc.

encephalitis. *Inflammation* of the brain.

endemic. Peculiar to a certain geographical area. Used when a disease occurs frequently in an area and is localized there.

enzymes. Substances formed by living cells which produce chemical ferment. They are in the digestive juices and many of the *tissues* of the body.

epidemic. Widespread in a certain region. Used to describe a disease affecting an unusually large number in one area at one time.

epidemic spinal meningitis. A type of *inflammation* of the covering of the brain which is caused by the *meningococcus.* It is the most common kind of *meningitis* which occurs in *epidemics.*

epilepsy. A disorder of the *central nervous system* in which there are transient periods of unconsciousness, sometimes with *convulsive* movements.

eruption. 1. Skin *lesions*, especially of diseases with rashes. 2. The appearance of a tooth through the gum.

erysipelas. An acute *infectious streptococcus* disease of the skin characterized by a spreading *inflammation* of both the skin and the *tissues* beneath it. It is treated very effectively with the *sulfonamides.* It used to be called "St. Anthony's Fire" because of the vivid redness of the patches.

exanthum. An *eruption* on the skin.

excreta. Waste material cast out of an organism. Specifically, bowel excretions and urine.

exposure. Contact with a person with a *contagious* disease, or with an intermediate object *contaminated* with the *germs* of it.

Fahrenheit. A scale of measurement of degrees which divides the distance between the freezing point of water, 32°, and the boiling point, 212°, into 180°. To find the *centigrade* equivalent, subtract 32 from Fahrenheit degrees and multiply the result by 5/9.

febrile. Pertaining to fever, or having fever as a characteristic.

feces. The product of evacuation of the bowels, or defecation.

fibrin. A fibrous material which forms a network surrounding blood corpuscles in the clotting of shed blood.

follicular tonsillitis. An *inflammation* of the *tonsils* in which dirty white spots or a *membrane* forms on them. It is often difficult to distinguish from diphtheria.

fungus. A low form of plant life, some of which cause disease in man.

gamma globulin. 1. One of the proteins of human blood. 2. A preparation made from human blood *serum* which contains *antibodies* to many *infectious* diseases. It is generally used to give *passive immunity* after *exposure* to a disease or when exposure is probable. The immunity it gives lasts only two to five weeks.

gastrointestinal. Pertaining to the stomach and intestines.

genitalia. The male and female organs of reproduction.

germ. Any *microorganism*, especially those *bacteria* which produce disease.

glucose. A colorless or yellowish, thick syrupy liquid. Also a granular powder. A *carbohydrate*, a sugar which has a sweet taste

and no odor. It is often used for nourishment and given intravenously to patients who are unable to take food by mouth.

gown. An outer garment used to cover the clothing of persons entering a sickroom to prevent carrying in of germs from the outside and carrying out of germs from the patient.

hay fever. An allergic condition, a reaction to *pollen*, involving the nose, eyes and *sinuses*, in which there is sneezing, running nose, intense itching of the eyes and inside of the nose, and often headache.

heart murmur. An abnormal sound accompanying the heart sounds and heard over the heart. There are various names for heart murmurs, according to which part of the heart they originate in, and at which part of the heart's cycle they are heard.

hemorrhage. An escape of blood from the blood vessels, through either intact or broken walls.

herpes. An *inflammation* of the skin or *mucous membranes* characterized by groups of blisters on an inflamed base. Herpes zoster is a name for shingles, and herpes simplex for cold sore.

histoplasmosis. A disease caused by a *fungus*, more frequent in some of the southern states in the United States, causing changes in the lungs similar to those caused by tuberculosis.

hives (urticaria). An allergic skin condition in which there appear intensely itchy red blotches with white raised centers, either in a few places or distributed widely over the body. They appear and disappear in crops.

Hodgkin's disease. A fatal disease of the *lymph* glands of unknown origin. The patient has painless swollen glands, anemia, fever, itching and weight loss.

homologous. Corresponding in structure, or being of the same type or series. We speak of homologous *serum* when we inject human blood serum into other humans, dog serum into dogs, etc.

hormones. Chemical substances which are produced in some of the organs and most of the glands of the body, which are carried by the blood to other areas where they have a regulatory effect. Sex hormones are the ones which are produced in the male (testicles) and female (ovaries) reproductive systems. *Adrenalin* and *cortisone* are produced by the adrenal glands; thyroid extract or thyroxin by the thyroid gland.

hygiene. The science that deals with the rules of health and the methods of observing them.

hyperimmune. The state of possessing an excess of *antibodies* to an *infectious agent.* For example, if a person is already *immune* to whooping cough and is given an injection of whooping cough *vaccine,* his body produces far more antibodies than are necessary for his protection. His blood *serum* is then hyperimmune serum.

immunity. The ability to withstand *infection* because of the presence in the body of *antibodies* to the *infectious agent.* It may be temporary, long-lasting or lifelong. (See *active immunity* and *passive immunity.*)

inapparent infection. One in which the *infected person* shows no evidence of being ill. A large proportion of the population is *immune* to many infectious diseases because of this type of infection. Also called latent and subclinical infection.

incubation period. The time between the first *infection* with an agent-causing disease and the *onset* of the first *symptoms.*

infant. A baby under one year old.

infected person. One who harbors an *infectious germ,* whether he is sick or is a *carrier.*

infection. 1. The entrance into the body of *bacteria, viruses* or other agents which produce disease. 2. The transmission of disease from one subject to another. 3. An infectious disease.

infectious. A disease is said to be infectious when it can be transmitted from one person or animal to another.

infectious agent. A *bacterium, virus, protozoan* or other organism which is capable of being transmitted from one person or animal to another.

infestation. The presence of animal parasites (fleas, lice, worms, ticks) on or in the human or animal body.

inflammation. Swelling, redness, tenderness and heat of *tissue* resulting from *infection.*

influenza bacillus. Certain strains of these *bacteria* cause *conjunctivitis* and influenzal *meningitis.* They also cause respiratory diseases.

influenza virus. The *virus* which causes influenza.

inherited. Derived from an ancestor.

inoculation. The introduction of a disease agent into the body, either by contact with the *germ* or by injection of live germs.

invasion period. The period during which the *infectious agent* is dispersed through the body, which usually corresponds to the *onset* of the *symptoms* of a disease, the period which follows the *incubation period* and before the height of the disease.

ipecac. A drug which, when given in the proper dosage (one teaspoon for an infant), will induce vomiting in fifteen to thirty minutes. When given in about one-tenth of this amount every four to six hours, it helps to increase expectoration. For these purposes it is usually made in the form of syrup.

isolation. The separation from others of either a patient with a *contagious* disease or a *carrier,* to prevent the spread of the disease.

jaundice. A yellowness of the skin, *mucous membranes,* and the *secretions* of the body, caused by an increase of *bile* pigments in the bloodstream. This can be caused by an obstruction of the flow of blood from the liver to the intestine, or by an excessive destruction of *red blood cells* and thus liberation of the blood pigments.

joint fixation. Making a joint rigid so that it can no longer be bent.

laryngitis. *Inflammation* of the *larynx* or voice box.

larynx. The organ of the voice which is situated between the base of the tongue and the windpipe and contains the *vocal cords.*

latent infection. See *inapparent infection.*

lesion. Any localized structural change in the body due to injury or disease—such as a cut, a burn, a chicken pox blister or a cold sore.

leucocyte. A *white blood cell* (corpuscle) with more than one nucleus.

leukemia. A fatal disease of the blood-forming organs characterized by uncontrolled multiplication of immature *white blood cells,* and rarely of the *red blood cells.*

lymph. An almost colorless fluid which bathes most of the *tissues* of the body. It travels through the lymph vessels into the bloodstream. *Bacteria* in the lymph must pass through the lymph nodes (glands) which are packed with *white blood cells* called *lymphocytes* and are placed strategically along the lymph vessels. The lymphocytes and the leucocytes attempt to destroy the bacteria.

lymphatic. 1. Pertaining to *lymph.* 2. A vessel conveying lymph.

lymphocyte. One of the *white blood cells,* containing a single nucleus.

malaise. A feeling of indefinite general discomfort, uneasiness and illness, often preliminary to an attack of a disease.

mask. A gauze, muslin or paper shield to cover the nose and mouth. It is used to avoid *droplet infection.*

mastoiditis. *Inflammation* of the cells of the mastoid bone behind the ear.

medication. 1. Treatment with

medicines. 2. The medicines used in treatment.

membrane. A thin layer of *tissue* covering or connecting parts, or separating or lining cavities. A *diphtheritic* membrane is a congealed mass which forms on the surface of the *tonsils* and pharynx, *mucous membrane* or skin, consisting of *serum, fibrin,* destroyed cells, diphtheria germs and *white blood cells.*

meninges. The *membranes* covering the brain and the *spinal cord.*

meningitis. *Inflammation* of the covering *membranes* of the brain, the *meninges.*

meningococcus. A *coccus* which causes epidemic cerebrospinal *meningitis.*

meningoencephalitis. *Inflammation* of the brain and the *membrane* surrounding it.

microorganism. A microscopic organism, either animal or plant, especially *bacteria, protozoa* and *viruses,* some of which are capable of producing disease in man.

miliary. 1. Of the size of a millet seed. 2. Characterized by the formation of many *lesions* of millet-seed size distributed widely throughout one or more organs.

motor nerve cells. The nerve *cells* which control the movement of muscles. Unlike most other body cells, nerve cells cannot regenerate themselves. Dead ones are not replaced, but damaged ones can recover—how much depends on the extent of the damage.

mucous membrane. The thin layer of *tissue* which lines the canals and cavities of the body (mouth, nose, vagina, urethra, etc.) which communicate with the air. Its glands *secrete* fluid to keep it moist.

mucus. The thick liquid *secreted* by the mucous glands in the *mucous membrane.*

muscle transplant. The surgical removal of one end of a muscle from its normal location and insertion of it in an adjacent part of the body to take the place of a paralyzed muscle.

mycosis. An *infection* caused by a *fungus* of the whole body, or either a deep or superficial infection of the skin.

nephritis. *Inflammation* of the kidney.

newborn. An infant from birth to two weeks old.

occupational therapy. A form of treatment in which the patient is instructed in, and given a chance to pursue, work and hobbies for sedative and psychological reasons, and possibly as an aid or a means for a handicapped person to gain a livelihood.

onset of a disease. The beginning of *signs* and *symptoms* of the disease.

osteomyelitis. *Inflammation* of the bone marrow.

otitis media. *Inflammation* of the middle ear, the space just inside the eardrum containing the little bones which conduct sound waves to the inner ear.

outbreak. A small *epidemic.*

ovaries. The female reproductive glands in which the ova (eggs) and the *hormones* that regulate female secondary sex characteristics develop.

pancreas. A gland in the abdomen which *secrets* a fluid into the intestines that digests *proteins,* fats and *carbohydrates*. It also secretes insulin, a *hormone* which regulates the body's ability to utilize sugar.

pandemic. Epidemic of large proportions, over a wide geographical area, sometimes worldwide.

passive immunity. The *immunity* which is produced by the injection of *antitoxin, antiserum, gamma globulin,* etc. Its effect is immediate but temporary, about two to five weeks. Also the immunity transmitted from the mother to a *newborn* infant.

peritoneum. The *membrane* lining the inside of the abdominal cavity and surrounding the organs within it. This cavity is also called the peritoneal cavity, and *inflammation* of all or part of the peritoneum is known as peritonitis.

physiotherapy. Treatment of disease with physical agents, such as heat, water, light, electricity, massage, etc. Also called physical medicine.

pigment. A coloring matter or substance.

placenta. The organ which develops on the wall of the uterus during the third month of gestation to which the unborn baby is attached by means of the *umbilical cord,* and through which the baby receives nourishment and oxygen from the mother's blood and casts off waste materials from his own.

pneumococcus. A species of *bacterium* which causes pneumonia, especially the lobar type, but also causes other *infectious* diseases such as *meningitis,* middle ear infection, *arthritis, conjunctivitis,* etc.

pneumonia. *Inflammation* of the lungs.

pollen. The fertilizing element produced by flowering plants— usually a powdery substance which is found on the anthers and which is carried from one blossom to another by insects or wind.

polyps. Growths, found especially on *mucous membrane.* Nasal polyps project from the mucous membranes of the nose. Polyps are also found in the intestinal tract.

polyvalent vaccine. A *vaccine* made from two or more strains of the same species or of different *bacteria* or *viruses,* so that *immunity* against more than one type of *infection* can be stimulated simultaneously.

primary infection. First *infection* with an *organism,* as in primary tuberculosis.

prognosis. A forecast of the probable outcome of a disease.

prophylaxis. The prevention of disease, by hygienic measures, by drugs, *serums,* etc.

prostrate. In a state of exhaustion.

protein. One of three basic food elements; one of a group of nitrogenous substances, found in various forms in animals and plants, which furnish the body with nitrogenous compounds necessary for growth and maintenance; for example, eggs, gelatin, meat.

protozoan. A division of single-celled organisms of the animal kingdom. The lowest form of animal life.

psittacosis. Parrot fever. A disease which is transmitted by birds and which in man causes pneumonia, and in birds—parrots, parakeets, etc.—*inflammation* of the intestines.

psoriasis. A chronic skin disease which is characterized by inflamed red patches covered by silvery-white, overlapping scales.

puberty. The period at which the reproductive organs become capable of performing their adult function. In boys it is indicated by the voice change and the discharge of semen, in girls by the beginning of menstruation.

pulse. Each time the heart contracts to pump blood through the arteries, the arteries change in shape because of increased tension of their walls. This change can be felt with the fingers at any point where an artery is near the surface. The number of changes per minute is the pulse rate.

pus. A thick yellowish fluid produced by the body in its efforts to destroy *bacteria* causing *inflammation*. It is mainly composed of *leucocytes* and *serum*.

quarantine. The restriction of freedom of a person who has been exposed to a *contagious* disease, usually for the *incubation period* of the disease. Quarantine may be partial, e.g., exclusion from school or work, but not *isolation* at home. (See *surveillance* and *segregation*.)

rale. An abnormal sound in the lungs and air passages which the doctor can hear with a *stethoscope*. It is caused, usually, by air passing through abnormal moisture in the air passages.

recall injection. See *booster injection*.

red blood cells. *Cells* which are

produced by the bone marrow and which contain a coloring matter called hemoglobin. The function of the hemoglobin is to pick up oxygen from the lungs and carry it to the *tissues* by way of the arteries. In the tissues, the oxygen is exchanged for carbon dioxide, which is then carried back to the lungs by way of the veins and expelled from the body.

rehabilitation. Teaching a handicapped person to make the most of the faculties he has in order to live as normally as possible in society.

reinfection. *Infection* with an *organism* after the first infection with the same organism has been cured.

relapse. A return of the typical *symptoms* of a disease after a period free of them, but before *convalescence* has been entirely completed.

remission. 1. The abatement of the *symptoms* of a disease. 2. The period during which the symptoms are subsiding or during which the disease is quiescent.

resistance. The body mechanisms which repel or destroy an *infectious agent*, not only through *immunity* but by phagocytosis (ingestion of *bacteria* by *white blood cells*) and other ways which lead to a tendency to resist disease.

respiratory allergy. A sensitivity which gives rise to *symptoms* involving the respiratory system, as in *asthma*, *allergic rhinitis* (sneezing, swollen membranes in the nose and nasal drip).

Rh factor. A quality in *red blood*

cells which is similar to that found in the simians and named after rhesus monkeys. Rh positive blood has this factor and Rh negative blood lacks it. When Rh positive blood is injected into an Rh negative person *antibodies* against the Rh factor are formed. About 15 per cent of people are Rh negative and if given an injection or transfusion of Rh positive *serum* or blood, they produce antibodies to it so that further transfusions of Rh positive blood may cause serious, sometimes very dangerous, reactions. An Rh negative woman who marries an Rh positive man may have difficulties with her second and subsequent pregnancies.

salt solution. Any solution of salts, but the term commonly refers to a solution of sodium chloride and water which is favored for intravenous injection because it is isotonic or is in balance with the salts contained in the fluid part of blood.

scabies. A *contagious* skin disorder caused by an insect which burrows into the skin to lay eggs. This causes an irritation which is intensely itchy.

Schick test. A *skin test* which determines *immunity* or lack of immunity to diphtheria. A little diphtheria *toxin* is injected into the skin, and the resulting reaction indicates whether or not the person is immune.

scrotum. The pouch of skin which contains the *testicles* and their coverings.

secondary infection. An *infection* or disease implanted on another which already exists.

secretion. 1. The act of forming certain substances, such as milk, bile, etc., in the glands out of materials furnished by the blood, which are either eliminated by the body or used in carrying on special functions. 2. The substance secreted.

sedative. A drug which quiets activity.

sedimentation rate. The speed at which the *red blood cells* settle to the bottom of a glass tube filled with blood. The speed is increased in many diseases.

segregation. Separation of some from others. For instance, when several children in a camp are *exposed* to the same disease, they may be *quarantined* together, away from the rest of the camp during the *incubation period.*

serum. The fluid part of blood. (See *antiserum.*)

shock. Shock causes a derangement of many body functions, but basically it reduces the amount of blood returned to the heart through the veins and reduces the *blood pressure,* sometimes to the point of circulatory failure. There are many causes of shock.

signs. The outer manifestations of a disease, such as red eyes, rash, sores, blisters, etc.

silver nitrate. A chemical used locally as a germicide, especially on the *mucous membranes,* particularly as a preventive against gonorrheal *conjunctivitis* in *newborn* babies.

sinus. A hollow or cavity or pocket. The nasal sinuses are cavities lined with *mucous mem-*

brane which are connected with the nose.

skin tests. Tests made on the skin to determine *immunity* or lack of it, the presence of *infection,* and sensitivity to certain substances. Skin tests are made by injecting material into the skin, by applying material to a scratch on the skin or by keeping the material in contact with the skin for a day or two.

smear. A preparation of *secretions,* of blood or of bacteria, which is spread on a glass slide so that it can be examined with a microscope.

soft palate. The soft fleshy part at the back of the roof of the mouth from which the *uvula* projects downward.

spasm. A sudden muscular contraction.

spinal cord. The part of the *central nervous system* which is inside the canal formed by the vertebrae and extends from the base of the brain down the middle of the back to the first or second lumbar vertebra at the base of the spine.

spinal fluid (cerebrospinal fluid). The fluid which bathes the brain and the *spinal cord* inside the framework of the skull and the vertebrae.

spirillum. A spiral-shaped *bacterium.*

spirochete. A spiral-shaped *bacterium.*

spleen. One of the abdominal organs located below the *diaphragm* on the left side. Its function is not clearly understood, but it is thought to be concerned with the breaking down and disposal of worn-out

blood cells as well as production of new blood cells. It is the largest *lymphatic* organ of the body.

sporadic. Describes an isolated or occasional case of a disease, as opposed to an *epidemic.*

sputum. Spit. Material discharged from the surface of the air passages, the throat or the mouth which is expelled by spitting or swallowing.

stain. 1. To dye minute transparent structures in order to make them visible under a microscope. 2. The dye used in this process.

staphylococcus. A *coccus* which is responsible for many *pus*-producing *inflammations,* usually localized. Sometimes it produces more general diseases such as *pneumonia* and *meningitis,* and infection of the blood.

staphylococcus toxin (staphylotoxin). A *toxic* substance liberated by staphylococci.

sterile. 1. Not capable of reproducing. 2. Free from germs.

stethoscope. An instrument which aids in hearing sounds which arise from within the body. It consists of a bell- or cup-shaped end piece connected to two pieces of rubber tubing which conduct the sound to both ears of the listener.

stool. The product of evacuation of the bowels.

stool culture. A group of *microorganisms* from a *stool* grown in an artificial medium for purposes of identification.

streptococcus. A *bacterium* responsible for many *infections,* among them, scarlet fever, septic sore throat, childbed fever, *ery-*

sipelas, nephritis, bronchopneu-monia.

subclinical infection. See *inapparent infection.*

sulfa drugs. See *sulfonamides.*

sulfonamides. A group of compounds derived from sulfanila-mide, and used in the treatment of various bacterial *infections.* There are many different members of the group which is known popularly as the *sulfa drugs.*

surveillance. Close and frequent observation of an *exposed* person during the time he is likely to develop the disease, such as careful inspection at home by the parents or at school by the nurse, to detect early *signs* of the disease.

susceptible. The state of having neither natural nor acquired *immunity* to a disease or for other reasons being unable to resist an infection. The opposite of immune.

symptoms. The reactions of the body when the disease begins, such as cough, pain, nausea, *diarrhea,* vomiting, etc.

temporary immunization. See *passive immunity.*

testicles. The male reproductive glands which produce spermatozoa after sexual maturity.

tissue. An aggregate of similar cells and cell products which form a specific kind of structural material in an animal or plant, e.g., muscle tissue, bone, nerve tissue, blood, etc.

tonsils. Two structures, about the size of strawberries, consisting of *lymph* glands and lymph vessels, which are located on either side of the entrance to the throat. One of their functions is to filter out the *infectious germs* before they gain entrance to the throat.

tonsillectomy. Removal of the *tonsils* by surgery.

toxic. 1. Pertaining to the appearance or condition of a person who is poisoned with a *toxin* and who is very ill. 2. The nature of the effect of some poisons or *infectious agents.*

toxin. A poisonous substance produced by *bacteria* or other *infectious agents,* e.g., the *toxins* produced by diphtheria or tetanus *bacilli.*

toxoid. A *toxin* which has been treated with chemicals or heat to reduce its injurious aspects and retain its ability to stimulate the production of *antibodies,* e.g., diphtheria and tetanus *toxoids.*

toxoplasmosis. A disease caused by the parasitic *protozoan,* toxo-plasma. In infants it usually involves *inflammation* of the brain and *spinal cord.*

trachea. The windpipe, which extends from the lower part of the *larynx* (the voice box) to its division into the two *bronchial tubes.*

tracheotomy. The operation of cutting an opening in the windpipe *(trachea).* Usually a tube is inserted into the *larynx* (voice box) to insure the passage of air into the lungs when the *tissues* of the larynx and adjacent parts are swollen.

transmission. The passing on of a *contagious* disease directly or indirectly.

tuberculin. A material made from the tubercle *bacillus* which is able to produce *inflammation* of the skin in a person who has had tuberculosis or *inoculations* against it. It is used in the *skin test* for tuberculosis.

tuberculin test. A *skin test* which indicates, when positive, the presence of active or healed tuberculosis or, when negative, no tuberculosis and, rarely, healed *infection*.

tumor. A localized overgrowth of new *tissue* which serves no useful purpose.

ulcer. An open sore with an inflamed base on the surface of the body or on the wall of a natural cavity.

umbilical cord. A long tube attached to the *placenta* (afterbirth) at one end and the navel of the baby at the other. Within it are the arteries and vein which connect the bloodstream of the mother with that of the unborn child.

upper respiratory diseases. Those diseases which involve the nose, throat, *larynx, tonsils, adenoids, sinuses* and windpipe.

uvula. The conical projection which hangs from the free edge of the *soft palate* at the back of the mouth.

vaccination. 1. *Inoculation* with cowpox (vaccinia) *virus* to protect against smallpox. 2. Inoculation with any organism to produce *immunity* to an *infectious* disease.

vaccine. A material made from dead, weakened or in some cases live *bacteria* or *viruses* which, when injected into the body, stimulates the production of *antibodies* and produces *immunity*. (See *active immunity*.)

vaginal tract. The female genital organ, a canal from the opening of the uterus to the outside of the body through which the infant travels during the birth process.

vector. An animal which transmits disease by acting as a host for the *causative agent*, e.g., the mosquito in malaria, the louse in typhus fever.

virulence. Power to produce disease; infectiousness.

virus. A very small living substance, either plant or animal, which grows only on living *tissue*. Viruses are so small that they cannot be seen with the naked eye or the ordinary microscope, but they can be seen with the *electron microscope*. They are small enough to pass through porcelain filters. They cause many diseases in man, e.g., measles, mumps, chicken pox, smallpox, polio, etc., as well as in plants and animals.

vocal cords. Two folds of *mucous membrane* placed across the *larynx* which vibrate and produce sound when air passes across them. When tension or lack of it or swelling force them nearer together or farther apart, the pitch of the voice changes.

white blood cells. One of the colorless cells of the blood, called *leucocytes*, which are concerned with destroying disease-producing *microorganisms*.

white blood count. The determination of the number and kind of *white blood cells* in a cubic millimeter of blood. In certain diseases the white blood cells are greatly decreased and in others they are increased. Knowing the number and kind of white cells in the blood is a valuable aid to *diagnosis*.

zinc stearate. A dusting powder used in various skin diseases, particularly diaper rash, because it has a moisture-repelling quality which keeps urine off the skin of the diaper area.

Index

About the Author

DR. SAMUEL KARELITZ is one of the country's leading pediatricians. He took his Bachelor of Philosophy degree at Yale in 1920, and his M.D. at Yale Medical School in 1923. He was a resident at Mt. Sinai Hospital in New York in 1925–26; subsequently he did postgraduate study in Berlin and Vienna.

Dr. Karelitz served on the staff at Mt. Sinai Hospital from 1927 to 1955, where he was attending pediatrician and for some time was acting chief of the Department of Pediatrics. For eighteen years he was also associated with the well-known Willard Parker Hospital for Communicable Diseases, and he was appointed chief of pediatrics at the new Long Island Jewish Hospital. At present Dr. Karelitz is pediatrician-in-chief of the Long Island Jewish Hospital—Queens Hospital Center Affiliation and consulting pediatrician to the Mt. Sinai Hospital of New York and the Flushing Hospital in Flushing, New York.

Through the years, he has served on the Committee on Control of Infectious Diseases of the American Academy of Pediatrics. He has been associated with Columbia University College of Physicians and Surgeons, and has been a consultant to the New York City and New York State health departments. He is now clinical professor of pediatrics at the Downstate branch of the New York State Medical School.

Dr. Karelitz is still active in the evaluation of new antibiotics and vaccines, and has written some ninety articles on communicable diseases for journals in this country and abroad.

	Fever	Rash	Chill	Cough	Changed Voice	Sore Throat	Nasal Drip	Swollen Glands	Headache	Muscle Ache
CAT SCRATCH FEVER p. 265	✓							✓		
COMMON COLD AND GRIPPE p. 275	✓		✓	✓	✓	✓	✓	✓	✓	✓
INFLUENZA p. 283	✓		✓	✓	✓	✓	✓	✓	✓	✓
CROUP p. 294	✓			✓	✓	✓				
CERVICAL ADENITIS p. 302	✓		✓			✓		✓		
BRONCHITIS p. 309	✓				✓					
SINUSITIS p. 316	✓		✓	✓	✓	✓	✓	✓	✓	✓
TONSILLITIS p. 324	✓		✓		✓		●	✓	✓	●
PNEUMONIA p. 332	✓		✓	✓					✓	
POLIO p. 353	✓		●		●				✓	✓
BACTERIAL MENINGITIS p. 379	✓	●	✓		✓				✓	✓
ENCEPHALITIS p. 387	✓				✓				✓	
TYPHOID p. 413	✓	●	✓						✓	✓
DYSENTERY p. 406	✓		✓							
SALMONELLA INFECTIONS p. 400	✓		✓							
STAPHYLOCOCCAL INFECTIONS p. 449	✓	✓	✓	●	●			✓		
FUNGUS INFECTION p. 439		✓								
SYPHILIS p. 465		●						✓		

● = Could accompany other symptoms but not necessarily

Swelling	Malaise	Fatigue	Weakness	Diarrhea	Vomiting	Cramps	Nausea	Jaundice	Itching	Convulsion	Paralysis		Other
	√								√				Dry Scabs.
	√	√	√								●		Throat membrane.
	√												Possibly no rash.
	√	√	√	●	√		√	√	√				May have no jaundice.
	√	√	√					●					Throat membrane.
	√	√	√										Peeling skin.
	√												
	√									●			
	√												Pain along nerve. Dries with scabs.
	√	√											Dry Scabs. Toxic.
	√		√										
	√	√											
	√												
√	√	√	√										
	√	√	√										Pain in back. Pain behind eyes.
	√	√						●					Scab on site of bite.
	√	√	√	●	●								

Continued on back endpaper